Full View of Yangtze River Pharmaceuticals Group（Taizhou,Jiangsu,China）

扬子江药业集团全景（中国·江苏·泰州）

Newly Compiled
Practical English-Chinese Library
of Traditional Chinese Medicine
（英汉对照）新编实用中医文库

General Compiler-in-Chief Zuo Yanfu
主编 左言富

Translators-in-Chief
Zhu Zhongbao Huang Yuezhong Tao Jinwen Li Zhaoguo
编译 朱忠宝 黄月中 陶锦文 李照国（执行）

Compiled by Nanjing University of
Traditional Chinese Medicine
Translated by Shanghai University
of Traditional Chinese Medicine

南 京 中 医 药 大 学 主 编
上 海 中 医 药 大 学 主 译

OPHTHALMOLOGY OF TRADITIONAL CHINESE MEDICINE

中 医 眼 科 学

Examiner-in-Chief	Lu Mianmian
Compiler-in-Chief	Ding Shuhua
Vice-Compiler-in-Chief	Ni Yun
Translators-in-Chief	Zhang Dengfeng
	Yang Mingshan
Vice-Translators-in-Chief	Lou Jianhua
	Zhu Yuqin

主　审　陆绵绵
主　编　丁淑华
副主编　倪　云
主　译　张登峰
　　　　杨明山
副主译　楼建华
　　　　朱玉琴

PUBLISHING HOUSE OF SHANGHAI UNIVERSITY
OF TRADITIONAL CHINESE MEDICINE
上海中医药大学出版社

Publishing House of Shanghai University of Traditional Chinese Medicine

530 Lingling Road，Shanghai，200032，China

Ophthalmology of Traditional Chinese Medicine

Compiler-in-Chief Ding Shuhua Translators-in-Chief Zhang Dengfeng Yang Mingshan
(A Newly Compiled Practical English-Chinese Library of Traditional Chinese Medicine
General Compiler-in-Chief Zuo Yanfu)

ISBN 7 - 81010 - 655 - 4/R · 621　paperback
ISBN 7 - 81010 - 682 - 1/R · 647　hardback
Printed in Shanghai Xinhua printing works

图书在版编目(CIP)数据

中医眼科学/丁淑华主编；张登峰，杨明山主译．—上海：上海中医药大学出版社，2002
（英汉对照新编实用中医文库/左言富总主编）
ISBN 7 - 81010 - 655 - 4

Ⅰ.中…　Ⅱ.①丁…②张…③杨…　Ⅲ.中医五官科学：眼科学—英、汉　Ⅳ.R276.7

中国版木图书馆 CIP 数据核字(2002)第 058680 号

中医眼科学　　主编 丁淑华　　主译 张登峰 杨明山

上海中医药大学出版社出版发行　　　　　（零陵路 530 号　邮政编码 200032）
新华书店上海发行所经销　　　　　　　　上海新华印刷厂印刷
开本　787mm×1092mm　1/18　印张 12.666　字数 303 千字　印数 1—2 000 册
版次 2002 年 11 月第 1 版　　　　　　　印次 2002 年 11 月第 1 次印刷

ISBN 7 - 81010 - 655 - 4/R · 621　　　　　　定价 28.90 元

《（英汉对照）新编实用中医文库》编纂委员会

Translation Committee of the Library

Advisors Shao Xundao Ou Ming

Translators-in-Chief Zhu Zhongbao Huang Yuezhong Tao Jinwen

Executive Translator-in-Chief Li Zhaoguo

Vice-Translators-in-Chief (Listed in the order of the number of strokes in the Chinese names)

Xun Jianying Li Yong'an Zhang Qingrong Zhang Dengfeng Yang Hongying
Huang Guoqi Xie Jinhua

Translators (Listed in the order of the number of strokes in the Chinese names)

Yu Xin	Wang Ruihui	Tian Kaiyu	Shen Guang
Lan Fengli	Cheng Peili	Zhu Wenxiao	Zhu Yuqin
Zhu Jinjiang	Zhu Guixiang	Le Yimin	Liu Shengpeng
Li Jingyun	Yang Ying	Yang Mingshan	He Yingchun
Zhang Jie	Zhang Haixia	Zhang Wei	Chen Renying
Zhou Yongming	Zhou Suzhen	Qu Yusheng	Zhao Junqing
Jing Zhen	Hu Kewu	Xu Qilong	Xu Yao
Guo Xiaomin	Huang Xixuan	Cao Lijuan	Kang Qin
Dong Jing	Qin Baichang	Zeng Haiping	Lou Jianhua
Lai Yuezhen	Bao Bai	Pei Huihua	Xue Junmei
Dai Wenjun	Wei Min		

Office of the Translation Committee

Director Yang Mingshan

Secretaries Xu Lindi Chen Li

《（英汉对照）新编实用中医文库》编译委员会

顾　　问　邵循道　欧　明

总　编　译　朱忠宝　黄月中　陶锦文

执行总编译　李照国

副 总 编 译 （按姓氏笔画为序）

寻建英　李永安　张庆荣　张登峰　杨洪英　黄国琪　谢金华

编　译　者 （按姓氏笔画为序）

于　新　王瑞辉　田开宇　申　光　兰凤利　成培莉　朱文晓
朱玉琴　朱金江　朱桂香　乐毅敏　刘升鹏　李经蕴　杨　莹
杨明山　何迎春　张　杰　张海峡　张　维　陈仁英　周永明
周素贞　屈榆生　赵俊卿　荆　蓁　胡克武　徐启龙　徐　瑶
郭小民　黄熙璇　曹丽娟　康　勤　董　晶　覃百长　曾海苹
楼建华　赖月珍　鲍　白　裴慧华　薛俊梅　戴文军　魏　敏

编译委员会办公室

主　任　杨明山

秘　书　徐林娣　陈　力

Approval Committee of the Library

Foreword Ⅰ

As we are walking into the 21st century, "health for all" is still an important task for the World Health Organization (WHO) to accomplish in the new century. The realization of "health for all" requires mutual cooperation and concerted efforts of various medical sciences, including traditional medicine. WHO has increasingly emphasized the development of traditional medicine and has made fruitful efforts to promote its development. Currently the spectrum of diseases is changing and an increasing number of diseases are difficult to cure. The side effects of chemical drugs have become more and more evident. Furthermore, both the governments and peoples in all countries are faced with the problem of high cost of medical treatment. Traditional Chinese medicine (TCM), the complete system of traditional medicine in the world with unique theory and excellent clinical curative effects, basically meets the need to solve such problems. Therefore, bringing TCM into full play in medical treatment and healthcare will certainly become one of the hot points in the world medical business in the 21st century.

Various aspects of work need to be done to promote the course of the internationalization of TCM, especially the compilation of works and textbooks suitable for international readers. The impending new century has witnessed the compilation of such a

序 一

人类即将迈入 21 世纪,"人人享有卫生保健"仍然是新世纪世界卫生工作面临的重要任务。实现"人人享有卫生保健"的宏伟目标,需要包括传统医药学在内的多种医学学科的相互协作与共同努力。世界卫生组织越来越重视传统医药学的发展,并为推动其发展做出了卓有成效的工作。目前,疾病谱正在发生变化,难治疾病不断增多,化学药品的毒副作用日益显现,日趋沉重的医疗费用困扰着各国政府和民众。中医药学是世界传统医学体系中最完整的传统医学,其独到的学科理论和突出的临床疗效,较符合当代社会和人们解决上述难题的需要。因此,科学有效地发挥中医药学的医疗保健作用,必将成为 21 世纪世界卫生工作的特点之一。

加快中医药走向世界的步伐,还有很多的工作要做,特别是适合国外读者学习的中医药著作、教材的编写是极其重要的方面。在新千年来临之际,由南京中医药大学

series of books known as *A Newly Compiled Practical English-Chinese Library of Traditional Chinese Medicine* published by the Publishing House of Shanghai University of TCM, compiled by Nanjing University of TCM and translated by Shanghai University of TCM. Professor Zuo Yanfu, the general compiler-in-chief of this Library, is a person who sets his mind on the international dissemination of TCM. He has compiled *General Survey on TCM Abroad*, a monograph on the development and state of TCM abroad. This Library is another important works written by the experts organized by him with the support of Nanjing University of TCM and Shanghai University of TCM. The compilation of this Library is done with consummate ingenuity and according to the development of TCM abroad. The compilers, based on the premise of preserving the genuineness and gist of TCM, have tried to make the contents concise, practical and easy to understand, making great efforts to introduce the abstruse ideas of TCM in a scientific and simple way as well as expounding the prevention and treatment of diseases which are commonly encountered abroad and can be effectively treated by TCM.

This Library encompasses a systematic summarization of the teaching experience accumulated in Nanjing University of TCM and Shanghai University of TCM that run the collaborating centers of traditional medicine and the international training centers on acupuncture and moxibustion set by WHO. I am sure that the publication of this Library will further promote the development of traditional Chinese med-

主编、上海中医药大学主译、上海中医药大学出版社出版的《(英汉对照)新编实用中医文库》的即将问世,正是新世纪中医药国际传播更快发展的预示。本套文库总主编左言富教授是中医药学国际传播事业的有心人,曾主编研究国外中医药发展状况的专著《国外中医药概览》。本套文库的编撰,是他在南京中医药大学和上海中医药大学支持下,组织许多著名专家共同完成的又一重要专著。本套文库的作者们深谙国外的中医药发展现状,编写颇具匠心,在注重真实,不失精华的前提下,突出内容的简明、实用,易于掌握,力求科学而又通俗地介绍中医药学的深奥内容,重点阐述国外常见而中医药颇具疗效的疾病的防治。

本套文库蕴含了南京中医药大学和上海中医药大学作为 WHO 传统医学合作中心、国际针灸培训中心多年留学生教学的实践经验和系统总结,更为全面、系统、准确地向世界传播中医药学。相信本书的出版将对中医更好地走向世界,让世界更好地了解中医产生更

icine abroad and enable the whole world to have a
better understanding of traditional Chinese medicine.

为积极的影响。

Professor Zhu Qingsheng

Vice-Minister of Health Ministry of the
People's Republic of China

Director of the State Administrative Bureau of
TCM

December 14, 2000 Beijing

朱庆生教授

中华人民共和国卫生部副部长

国家中医药管理局局长

2000 年 12 月 14 日于北京

Foreword II

Before the existence of the modern medicine, human beings depended solely on herbal medicines and other therapeutic methods to treat diseases and preserve health. Such a practice gave rise to the establishment of various kinds of traditional medicine with unique theory and practice, such as traditional Chinese medicine, Indian medicine and Arabian medicine, etc. Among these traditional systems of medicine, traditional Chinese medicine is a most extraordinary one based on which traditional Korean medicine and Japanese medicine have evolved.

Even in the 21st century, traditional medicine is still of great vitality. In spite of the fast development of modern medicine, traditional medicine is still disseminated far and wide. In many developing countries, most of the people in the rural areas still depend on traditional medicine and traditional medical practitioners to meet the need for primary healthcare. Even in the countries with advanced modern medicine, more and more people have begun to accept traditional medicine and other therapeutic methods, such as homeopathy, osteopathy and naturopathy, etc.

With the change of the economy, culture and living style in various regions as well as the aging in the world population, the disease spectrum has changed. And such a change has paved the way for the new application of traditional medicine. Besides,

序　二

在现代医学形成之前,人类一直依赖草药和其他一些疗法治病强身,从而发展出许多有理论、有实践的传统医学,例如中医学、印度医学、阿拉伯医学等。中医学是世界林林总总的传统医学中的一支奇葩,在它的基础上还衍生出朝鲜传统医学和日本汉方医学。在跨入21世纪的今天,古老的传统医学依然焕发着活力,非但没有因现代医学的发展而式微,其影响还有增无减,人们对传统医学的价值也有了更深刻的体会和认识。在许多贫穷国家,大多数农村人口仍然依赖传统医学疗法和传统医务工作者来满足他们对初级卫生保健的需求。在现代医学占主导地位的许多国家,传统医学及其他一些"另类疗法",诸如顺势疗法、整骨疗法、自然疗法等,也越来越被人们所接受。

伴随着世界各地经济、文化和生活的变革以及世界人口的老龄化,世界疾病谱也发生了变化。传统医学有了新的应用,而新疾病所引起的新需求以及现代医学的成

the new requirements initiated by the new diseases and the achievements and limitations of modern medicine have also created challenges for traditional medicine.

WHO sensed the importance of traditional medicine to human health early in the 1970s and have made great efforts to develop traditional medicine. At the 29th world health congress held in 1976, the item of traditional medicine was adopted in the working plan of WHO. In the following world health congresses, a series of resolutions were passed to demand the member countries to develop, utilize and study traditional medicine according to their specific conditions so as to reduce medical expenses for the realization of "health for all".

WHO has laid great stress on the scientific content, safe and effective application of traditional medicine. It has published and distributed a series of booklets on the scientific, safe and effective use of herbs and acupuncture and moxibustion. It has also made great contributions to the international standardization of traditional medical terms. The safe and effective application of traditional medicine has much to do with the skills of traditional medical practitioners. That is why WHO has made great efforts to train them. WHO has run 27 collaborating centers in the world which have made great contributions to the training of acupuncturists and traditional medical practitioners. Nanjing University of TCM and Shanghai University of TCM run the collaborating centers with WHO. In recent years it has, with the cooperation of WHO and other countries, trained about ten thousand international students from over

就与局限又向传统医学提出了挑战,推动它进一步发展。世界卫生组织早在20世纪70年代就意识到传统医学对人类健康的重要性,并为推动传统医学的发展做了努力。1976年举行的第二十九届世界卫生大会将传统医学项目纳入世界卫生组织的工作计划。其后的各届世界卫生大会又通过了一系列决议,要求各成员国根据本国的条件发展、使用和研究传统医学,以降低医疗费用,促进"人人享有初级卫生保健"这一目标的实现。

世界卫生组织历来重视传统医学的科学、安全和有效使用。它出版和发行了一系列有关科学、安全、有效使用草药和针灸的技术指南,并在专用术语的标准化方面做了许多工作。传统医学的使用是否做到安全和有效,是与使用传统疗法的医务工作者的水平密不可分的。因此,世界卫生组织也十分重视传统医学培训工作。它在全世界有27个传统医学合作中心,这些中心对培训合格的针灸师及使用传统疗法的其他医务工作者做出了积极的贡献。南京中医药大学、上海中医药大学是世界卫生组织传统医学合作中心之一,近年来与世界卫生组织和其他国家合作,培训了近万名来自90多个国

90 countries.

In order to further promote the dissemination of traditional Chinese medicine in the world, *A Newly Compiled Practical English-Chinese Library of Traditional Chinese Medicine*, compiled by Nanjing University of TCM with Professor Zuo Yanfu as the general compiler-in-chief and published by the Publishing House of Shanghai University of TCM, aims at systematic, accurate and concise expounding of traditional Chinese medical theory and introducing clinical therapeutic methods of traditional medicine according to modern medical nomenclature of diseases. Undoubtedly, this series of books will be the practical textbooks for the beginners with certain English level and the international enthusiasts with certain level of Chinese to study traditional Chinese medicine. Besides, this series of books can also serve as reference books for WHO to internationally standardize the nomenclature of acupuncture and moxibustion.

The scientific, safe and effective use of traditional medicine will certainly further promote the development of traditional medicine and traditional medicine will undoubtedly make more and more contributions to human health in the 21st century.

Zhang Xiaorui

WHO Coordination Officer

December, 2000

家和地区的留学生。

在南京中医药大学左言富教授主持下编纂的、由上海中医药大学出版社出版的《(英汉对照)新编实用中医文库》，旨在全面、系统、准确、简要地阐述中医基础理论，并结合西医病名介绍中医临床治疗方法。因此，这套文库可望成为具有一定英语水平的初学中医者和具有一定中文水平的外国中医爱好者学习基础中医学的系列教材。这套文库也可供世界卫生组织在编写国际针灸标准术语时参考。

传统医学的科学、安全、有效使用必将进一步推动传统医学的发展。传统医学一定会在 21 世纪为人类健康做出更大的贡献。

张小瑞

世界卫生组织传统医学协调官员

2000 年 12 月

Preface

前　言

The Publishing House of Shanghai University of TCM published *A Practical English-Chinese Library of Traditional Chinese Medicine* in 1990. The Library has been well-known in the world ever since and has made great contributions to the dissemination of traditional Chinese medicine in the world. In view of the fact that 10 years has passed since its publication and that there are certain errors in the explanation of traditional Chinese medicine in the Library, the Publishing House has invited Nanjing University of TCM and Shanghai University of TCM to organize experts to recompile and translate the Library.

Nanjing University of TCM and Shanghai University of TCM are well-known for their advantages in higher education of traditional Chinese medicine and compilation of traditional Chinese medical textbooks. The compilation of *A Newly Compiled Practical English-Chinese Library of Traditional Chinese Medicine* has absorbed the rich experience accumulated by Nanjing University of Traditional Chinese Medicine in training international students of traditional Chinese medicine. Compared with the previous Library, the Newly Compiled Library has made great improvements in many aspects, fully demonstrating the academic system of traditional Chinese medicine. The whole series of books has systematically introduced the basic theory and thera-

　　上海中医药大学出版社于 1990 年出版了一套《（英汉对照）实用中医文库》，发行 10 年来，在海内外产生了较大影响，对推动中医学走向世界起了积极作用。考虑到该套丛书发行已久，对中医学术体系的介绍还有一些欠妥之处，因此，上海中医药大学出版社特邀南京中医药大学主编、上海中医药大学主译，组织全国有关专家编译出版《（英汉对照）新编实用中医文库》。

　　《（英汉对照）新编实用中医文库》的编纂，充分发挥了南京中医药大学和上海中医药大学在高等中医药教育教学和教材编写方面的优势，吸收了作为 WHO 传统医学合作中心之一的两校，多年来从事中医药学国际培训和留学生学历教育的经验，对原《（英汉对照）实用中医文库》整体结构作了大幅度调整，以突出中医学术主体内容。全套丛书系统介绍了中医基础理论和中医辨证论治方法，讲解了中药学和方剂学的基本理论，详细介绍了 236 味中药、152 首常用方剂和 100 种常用中成药；详述

peutic methods based on syndrome differentiation, expounding traditional Chinese pharmacy and prescriptions; explaining 236 herbs, 152 prescriptions and 100 commonly-used patent drugs; elucidating 264 methods for differentiating syndromes and treating commonly-encountered and frequently-encountered diseases in internal medicine, surgery, gynecology, pediatrics, traumatology and orthopedics, ophthalmology and otorhinolaryngology; introducing the basic methods and theory of acupuncture and moxibustion, massage (tuina), life cultivation and rehabilitation, including 70 kinds of diseases suitable for acupuncture and moxibustion, 38 kinds of diseases for massage, examples of life cultivation and over 20 kinds of commonly encountered diseases treated by rehabilitation therapies in traditional Chinese medicine. For better understanding of traditional Chinese medicine, the books are neatly illustrated. There are 296 line graphs and 30 colored pictures in the Library with necessary indexes, making it more comprehensive, accurate and systematic in disseminating traditional Chinese medicine in the countries and regions where English is the official language.

This Library is characterized by following features:

1. Scientific　Based on the development of TCM in education and research in the past 10 years, efforts have been made in the compilation to highlight the gist of TCM through accurate theoretical exposition and clinical practice, aiming at introducing authentic theory and practice to the world.

2. Systematic　This Library contains 14 sepa-

264 种临床内、外、妇、儿、骨伤、眼、耳鼻喉各科常见病与多发病的中医辨证论治方法；系统论述针灸、推拿、中医养生康复的基本理论和基本技能，介绍针灸治疗病种 70 种、推拿治疗病种 38 种、各类养生实例及 20 余种常见病证的中医康复实例。为了更加直观地介绍中医药学术，全书选用线图 296 幅、彩图 30 幅，并附有必要的索引，从而更加全面、系统、准确地向使用英语的国家和地区传播中医学术，推进中医学走向世界，造福全人类。

本丛书主要具有以下特色：(1) 科学性：在充分吸收近 10 余年来中医教学和科学研究最新进展的基础上，坚持突出中医学术精华，理论阐述准确，临床切合实用，向世界各国介绍"原汁原味"的中医药学术；(2) 系统性：本套丛书包括《中医基础理论》、《中医诊断学》、《中药学》、《方剂学》、《中医内

rate fascicles, i.e. *Basic Theory of Traditional Chinese Medicine*, *Diagnostics of Traditional Chinese Medicine*, *Science of Chinese Materia Medica*, *Science of Prescriptions*, *Internal Medicine of Traditional Chinese Medicine*, *Surgery of Traditional Chinese Medicine*, *Gynecology of Traditional Chinese Medicine*, *Pediatrics of Traditional Chinese Medicine*, *Traumatology and Orthopedics of Traditional Chinese Medicine*, *Ophthalmology of Traditional Chinese Medicine*, *Otorhinolaryngology of Traditional Chinese Medicine*, *Chinese Acupuncture and Moxibustion*, *Chinese Tuina (Massage)*, *and Life Cultivation and Rehabilitation of Traditional Chinese Medicine*.

3. Practical Compared with the previous Library, the Newly Compiled Library has made great improvements and supplements, systematically introducing therapeutic methods for treating over 200 kinds of commonly and frequently encountered diseases, focusing on training basic clinical skills in acupuncture and moxibustion, tuina therapy, life cultivation and rehabilitation with clinical case reports.

4. Standard This Library is reasonable in structure, distinct in categorization, standard in terminology and accurate in translation with full consideration of habitual expressions used in countries and regions with English language as the mother tongue.

This series of books is not only practical for the beginners with certain competence of English to study TCM, but also can serve as authentic textbooks for international students in universities and colleges of TCM in China to study and practice TCM. For those from TCM field who are going to go

科学》、《中医外科学》、《中医妇科学》、《中医儿科学》、《中医骨伤科学》、《中医眼科学》、《中医耳鼻喉科学》、《中国针灸》、《中国推拿》、《中医养生康复学》14个分册,系统反映了中医各学科建设与发展的最新成果;(3)实用性:临床各科由原来的上下两册,根据学科的发展进行大幅度的调整和增补,比较详细地介绍了200多种各科常见病、多发病的中医治疗方法,重点突出了针灸、推拿、养生康复等临床基本技能训练,并附有部分临证实例;(4)规范性:全书结构合理,层次清晰,对中医各学科名词术语表述规范,对中医英语翻译执行了更为严格的标准化方案,同时又充分考虑到使用英语国家和地区人们的语言习惯和表达方式。

本丛书不仅能满足具有一定英语水平的初学中医者系统学习中医之用,而且也为中医院校外国留学生教育及国内外开展中医双语教学提供了目前最具权威的系列教材,同时也是中医出国人员进

abroad to do academic exchange, this series of books will provide them with unexpected convenience.

Professor Xiang Ping, President of Nanjing University of TCM, is the director of the Compilation Board. Professor Zuo Yanfu from Nanjing University of TCM, General Compiler-in-Chief, is in charge of the compilation. Zhang Wenkang, Minister of Health Ministry, is invited to be the honorary director of the Editorial Board. Li Zhenji, Vice-Director of the State Administrative Bureau of TCM, is invited to be the director of the Approval Committee. Chen Keji, academician of China Academy, is invited to be the General Advisor. International advisors invited are Mr. M. S. Khan, Chairman of Ireland Acupuncture and Moxibustion Fund; Miss Alessandra Gulí, Chairman of "Nanjing Association" in Rome, Italy; Doctor Secondo Scarsella, Chief Editor of YI DAO ZA ZHI; President Raymond K. Carroll from Australian Oriental Touching Therapy College; Ms. Shulan Tang, Academic Executive of ATCM in Britain; Mr. Glovanni Maciocia from Britain; Mr. David, Chairman of American Association of TCM; Mr. Tzu Kuo Shih, director of Chinese Medical Technique Center in Connecticut, America; Mr. Helmut Ziegler, director of TCM Center in Germany; and Mr. Isigami Hiroshi from Japan. Chen Ken, official of WHO responsible for the Western Pacific Region, has greatly encouraged the compilers in compiling this series of books. After the accomplishment of the compilation, Professor Zhu Qingsheng, Vice-Minister of Health Ministry and Director of the State Administrative Bureau of TCM, has set a high value on the books in his fore-

行中医药国际交流的重要工具书。

全书由南京中医药大学校长项平教授担任编委会主任、左言富教授任总主编,主持全书的编写。中华人民共和国卫生部张文康部长担任本丛书编委会名誉主任,国家中医药管理局李振吉副局长担任审定委员会主任,陈可冀院士欣然担任本丛书总顾问指导全书的编纂。爱尔兰针灸基金会主席萨利姆先生、意大利罗马"南京协会"主席亚历山大·古丽女士、意大利《医道》杂志主编卡塞拉·塞肯多博士、澳大利亚东方触觉疗法学院雷蒙特·凯·卡罗院长、英国中医药学会学术部长汤淑兰女士、英国马万里先生、美国中医师公会主席大卫先生、美国康州中华医疗技术中心主任施祖谷先生、德国中医中心主任赫尔木特先生、日本石上博先生担任本丛书特邀外籍顾问。世界卫生组织西太平洋地区官员陈恳先生对本丛书的编写给予了热情鼓励。全书完成后,卫生部副部长兼国家中医药管理局局长朱庆生教授给予了高度评价,并欣然为本书作序;WHO传统医学协调官员张小瑞对于本丛书的编写给予高度关注,百忙中也专为本书作序。我国驻外教育机构,特别是中国驻英国曼彻斯特领事张益群先生、中国驻美国休斯敦领事严美华

word for the Library. Zhang Xiaorui, an official
from WHO's Traditional Medicine Program, has
paid great attention to the compilation and written a
foreword for the Library. The officials from the educational organizations of China in other countries
have provided us with some useful materials in our
compilation. They are Mr. Zhang Yiqun, China
Consul to Manchester in Britain; Miss Yan Meihua,
Consul to Houston in America; Mr. Wang Jiping,
First Secretary in the Educational Department in the
Embassy of China to France; and Mr. Gu Shengy-
ing, the Second Secretary in the Educational Department in the Embassy of China to Germany. We are
grateful to them all.

The Compilers
December, 2000

女士、中国驻法国使馆教育处一秘
王季平先生、中国驻德国使馆教育
处二秘郭胜英先生在与我们工作
联系中,间接提供了不少有益资
料。在此一并致以衷心感谢!

编　者
2000 年 12 月

Note for compilation

The basic theory and diagnostic and treating experience of ocular diseases in the ophthalmology of TCM are systematically presented in this fascicle with the theory of TCM as its base and emphasize not only the features of TCM but also the characteristics of its ophthalmology as well.

The diagnosis and treatment of every ocular disease in the book is objectively and characteristically discussed in a standard style with importance attached to clinical practice. The fascicle consists of the two parts—general introduction and discussions of specific diseases.

Of the three chapters in the first part, chapter one briefly expounds various physiological and pathological relations between the eyes and viscera. The second chapter contains the ophthalmologic diagnostic methods and common syndrome-differentiating methods in ophthalmology, including the differentiation of external and internal oculopathy, of nebula and of common symptoms and signs. Ocular internal and external therapies and common oral drugs are discussed in the third chapter.

The second part of the book is grouped into five chapters to introduce the diagnoses and treatments of 23 kinds of common ocular diseases that occur in the eyelid, canthi, bulbar conjunctiva, cornea and pupil. The discussion of each disease is precise and appropriate in TCM, and the treating methods introduced are dependable and practical.

编写说明

本书以中医理论为基础,突出中医特色,抓住中医眼科特点,系统地介绍了中医眼科学的基础理论和对眼病的诊治经验。

本书体例规范,特色鲜明,注重临床实用,客观地介绍了每一种疾病的中医药诊疗方法。全书内容分总论、各论两部分。

总论分三章,第一章眼与脏腑的关系,简要阐述了眼与人体各脏腑之间在生理、病理等各方面的关系;第二章诊断概要,介绍了眼科诊法和眼科常用辨证方法,包括辨外障与内障、辨翳、辨常见病证;第三章治疗概要,介绍了中医治法,包括内治法、外治法以及眼科常用内服药物等。

各论分五章,介绍了胞睑疾病、两眦疾病、白睛疾病、黑睛疾病、瞳神疾病等 23 种常见眼病的诊疗,每病中医理论阐述精当,治疗方法可靠实用。

Professor Ding Shuhua was in charge of compiling the first three chapters of general introduction and the fifth chapter of specific discussion, and the other four chapters in specific discussions were compiled by Dr. Ni Yun.

编写分工：总论第一章、第二章、第三章和各论第五章由丁淑华编写，各论第一章、第二章、第三章和第四章由倪云编写。

CONTENTS

目　录

1 General Introduction

总 论

1.1 The Relationship between the Eyes and the Viscera

第一章 眼 与 脏腑的关系

The eyes depend on the nourishment from the visceral essence to see things and distinguish colors. It is said in *Lingshu* that "The visceral essence flows upwards into the eyes." That's why dysfunction of the viscera leads to eye disorders.

眼之能够明视万物,辨别颜色,是赖五脏六腑精气的滋养,如《灵枢·大惑论》谓"五脏六腑之精气皆上注于目而为之精"。而脏腑功能失调则可致眼病。

1.1.1 The Relationship between the Eyes and the Heart and Small Intestine

一、眼与心和小肠的关系

1.1.1.1 The heart governs the vessels that are all related to the eyes

(一)心主血脉,诸脉属目

In the Chapter of Generation of the Five Zang-organs in *Suwen*, it says："All blood is related to the eyes", "the heart is associated with the vessels", "all the vessels are related to the eyes". In the Chapter of Pulse Abstruseness in *Suwen*, it says："The vessels house blood." The heart governs vessels. The blood in the vessels is propelled by heart qi to circulate throughout the body and into the eyes. That is why the eyes are able to see.

《素问·五藏生成》曰"诸血者,皆属于目","心之合脉也","诸脉者,皆属于目";《素问·脉要精微论》谓"脉者,血之府"。因此,心主全身血脉,脉中血液受心气推动,循环全身,上输于目,目受血养,才维持视觉。

1.1.1.2 The heart houses spirit and the eyes are commanded by the heart

(二)心主藏神,目为心使

Though the spirit is governed by the heart, its outward manifestations are in the eyes. In the Chapter of Treasure of Eyes in *Shenshi Yaohan*, it says："The heart spirit displayed in the eyes is vision and the kidney water

因心为神之舍,精神虽统于心,而外用则在目,故目为心之使。《审视瑶函·目为至宝论》曰:"心神在目,发为神

enables the eyes to see everything."

1.1.1.3 The relationship between the eyes and the small intestine

In the Chapter of Linglan Midian in *Suwen*, it says: "The small intestine is the organ responsible for reception and transformation." The small intestine separates the lucid from the turbid when food and water are taken into the body. The lucid part is transported to the whole body by the spleen to nourish the eyes. Besides, the heart and the small intestine are internally and externally related to each other. The functional state of the small intestine not only relates to the heart, but also affects the eyes.

1.1.2 The Relationship between the Eyes and the Liver and Gallbladder

1.1.2.1 The liver opens into the eyes

In the Chapter of Jingui Zhenyanlun in *Suwen*, it says: "The east is related to the green color and corresponds to the liver which opens into the eyes. The essence of the eyes is stored in the liver." This means that the eyes are the orifices for the liver to communicate with the external environment. Only when the essential substance stored in the liver is transported to the eyes can the eyes be nourished and see things.

1.1.2.2 The storage of blood in the liver enables the eyes to see things

The eyes are the outward orifices of the liver because the eyes are nourished by the blood from the liver. That is why it is said, in the Chapter of Generation of the Five Zang-organs in *Suwen*, that "Storage of blood in the liver enables the eyes to see things."

1.1.2.3 The liver qi enters the eyes

The provision of blood and fluid to the eyes depends

光,肾水、神光深居瞳神之中,才能明视万物。"

（三）眼与小肠的关系

《素问·灵兰秘典论》曰:"小肠者,受盛之官,化物出焉。"水谷经小肠分清别浊,清者由脾转输全身,从而使目受到滋养。此外,心与小肠相表里,小肠功能是否正常,既关系到心,也影响到眼。

二、眼与肝和胆的关系

（一）肝开窍于目

《素问·金匮真言论》曰:"东方青色,入通于肝;开窍于目,藏精于肝。"指出了目为肝与外界联系的窍道。故肝所受藏的精微物质,能输送至眼,使眼受到滋养,从而维持其视觉功能。

（二）肝受血而能视

目为肝之窍,尤以肝血的濡养为重要,故《素问·五藏生成》曰:"肝受血而能视。"

（三）肝气通于目

供给眼部的血液、津液,

on the propelling power of qi. The normal activity of qi is related to the diffusing and dispersing function of the liver. That is why it is said in the Chapter of Measurement of Pulse in *Lingshu* that "The liver-qi enters the eyes and the normal function of the liver ensures normal vision of the eyes."

依赖气的推动,而人体气机是否调畅,又与肝的疏泄功能密切相关。故《灵枢·脉度》曰:"肝气通于目,肝和则目能辨五色矣。"

1.1.2.4 The liver meridian is connected with the eyes

The liver meridian is connected with the eyes as it is mentioned in the Chapter of Meridians and Vessels in *Lingshu*. Among the twelve meridians, only the liver meridian is directly connected with the eyes. The liver meridian serves to connect the liver and the eyes internally and externally, associates the eyes with the liver and transports qi and blood.

（四）肝脉连目系

《灵枢·经脉》认为:足厥阴肝脉"连目系"。十二经脉,唯有肝脉是本经直接上连目系的。肝脉在眼与肝之间起着沟通表里、联络眼与肝脏、为之运行气血的作用。

1.1.2.5 The relationship between the eyes and gallbladder

The surplus of liver qi enters the gallbladder and accumulates into essence known as bile, the secretion and excretion of which is influenced by the diffusing and dispersing function of the liver. Bile is very important to the eyes. In the Chapter of Normal Span of Life in *Lingshu*, it says "At the age of fifty liver-qi begins to decline, the liver lobes become thin, the bile is reduced and the eyes become dim." In *Zhengzhi Zhunshen*, it further suggests that bile condenses into essence to nourish the eyes.

（五）眼与胆的关系

肝之余气溢入于胆,聚而成精,乃为胆汁。胆汁的分泌和排泄,受肝的疏泄功能的影响。胆汁于眼,十分重要。如《灵枢·天年》曰:"五十岁,肝气始衰,肝叶始薄,胆汁始减,目始不明。"《证治准绳·杂病·七窍门》进一步提出了胆之精汁积成珠内神膏,膏涵养瞳神之说。

1.1.3 The Relationship between the Eyes and the Spleen and Stomach

三、眼与脾和胃的关系

1.1.3.1 The spleen transports essence upwards into the eyes

In the Chapter of Yuji Zhenzanglun in *Suwen*, it says:"Deficiency of the spleen leads to the obstruction of

（一）脾输精气,上贯于目

《素问·玉机真藏论》论脾之虚实曰:"其不及,则令人

the nine orifices", indicating that deficiency of the spleen can also cause the disorder of the eyes. In the Chapter of Manifestations of yin and yang in *Suwen*, it says: "The lucid yang is emitted from the upper orifices." Spleen-qi ascends to transport essential substances to the eyes, so that the eyes are nourished by the lucid yang and can see things.

1.1.3.2　The spleen commands blood and the blood nourishes the eyes

In the Section of Blood Syndrome in the Chapter of Miscellaneous Syndromes in *Jingyue's Book*, it says: "Since the spleen commands blood, deficiency of spleen-qi makes it difficult to control blood. Since the spleen produces blood, deficiency of spleen-qi makes it fail to govern blood and leads to extravasation of blood." Circulation of blood in the ocular collaterals depends on spleen-qi to command blood. If the spleen-qi is deficient, it will lead to ocular hemorrhage.

1.1.3.3　The spleen governs muscles and monitors the opening and closing of the eyelids

In the Chapter of Flaccidity in *Suwen*, it says: "The spleen controls the muscles in the whole body." Since the spleen is responsible for the transportation and transformation of water and food, the essense derived from which can nourish the muscles. With the nourishment provided by the spleen, the eyelids are able to open and close.

1.1.3.4　The relationship between the eyes and the stomach

The spleen and stomach are internally-externally paired and regarded as the acquired base of life.

In the Chapter of Transmission and Transformation of Asthenia and Sthenia in *Piwei Lun* (Discussion on the Spleen and Stomach), it says: "The nine orifices are dominated by the five zang-organs. With the nourishment of stomach-qi, the five zang-organs can function normally."

九窍不通。"即包含脾虚能致眼病。《素问·阴阳应象大论》谓"清阳出上窍"，脾气上升，才能将精微物质升运于目，目得清阳之气的温养则视物清明。

（二）脾主统血，血养目窍

《景岳全书·杂证谟·血证》又曰："盖脾统血，脾气虚则不能收摄；脾化血，脾气虚则不能运化，是皆血无所主，因而脱陷妄行。"血液行于眼络中不外溢，赖于脾气的统摄。若脾气虚衰，失去统摄的能力，可引起眼部的出血病症。

（三）脾主肌肉，睑能开合

《素问·痿论》曰："脾主身之肌肉。"脾主运化水谷之精，以生养肌肉。胞睑肌肉得养则开合自如。

（四）眼与胃的关系

胃脾互为表里，为"后天之本"。《脾胃论·脾胃虚实传变论》曰："九窍者，五脏主之，五脏皆得胃气乃能通利。"并指出："胃气一虚，耳、目、口、鼻俱为之病。"此外，《素问·阴阳应象大论》曰："清阳

It also points out that "If the stomach-qi becomes deficient, the ears, eyes, mouth and nose will all be in disorder." Besides, in the Chapter of the Manifestations of Yin and Yang in *Suwen*, it says: "The lucid yang flows into the upper orifices while the turbid yin goes into the lower orifices." Since the spleen is responsible for ascending the lucid and the stomach for descending the turbid, the normal functions of both organs will direct the turbid to be discharged from the lower orifices and not to attack the upper orifices.

1.1.4 The Relationship between the Eyes and the Lung and the Large Intestine

1.1.4.1 The lung controls qi and the normal function of qi ensures nomral vision

The lung is associated with all vessels and controls qi. Qi can promote blood circulation to nourish and warm the whole body. With the nomral function of lung-qi and smooth flow of qi and blood, the visceral essence flows into the eyes to enable the eyes to see things. If lung-qi is deficient, the eyes will lose sufficient nourishment and become dim.

1.1.4.2 The dispersing and descending functions of the lung smooth the ocular collaterals

The normal functions of the lung make the blood vessels smooth. With the warming and nourishment of the defensive qi and body fluids, the eyes will maintain normal in functions because turbid substances descend and will not affect the eyes.

1.1.4.3 The relationship between the eyes and the large intestine

The small intestine transfers turbid materials into the large intestine which transforms them into waste. Such a tranference and transformation depends on lung-qi to

出上窍,浊阴出下窍。"脾主升清,胃主降浊,二者升降正常,则清浊分明,浊阴从下窍出,不致上犯清窍。

四、眼与肺和大肠的关系

(一)肺为气主,气和目明

肺朝百脉,主一身之气,气能推动血行,气血并行于全身,目亦受其温煦濡养。又,肺气调和,气血流畅,五脏六腑精阳之气皆能输注入目,故目视精明。若肺气不足,以致目失所养,则昏暗不明。

(二)肺主宣降,眼络通畅

肺之宣降正常,则血脉通利,目得卫气和津液的温煦濡养,卫外有权,且浊物下降,不得上犯,目不易病。

(三)眼与大肠的关系

小肠浊物下注大肠,化为粪便,有赖肺气肃降,以推送其排出体外。若大肠积热,腑

depurate, descend and discharge waste from the body. If heat is accumulated in the large intestine, it will affect the functions of the lung, leading to disorders of the eyes due to stagnation of qi, blood and body fluids.

1.1.5 The Relationship between the Eyes and the Kidney and Bladder

1.1.5.1 Superabundance of kidney essence enables the eyes to see things

In the Chapter of Genuine Discussion in the Antique in *Suwen*, it says: "The kidney controls water and receives and stores essence from the five zang-organs and six fu-organs." That is why the eyes are in close relationship with the kidney essence.

1.1.5.2 The kidney produces cerebral marrow and the eyes are connected with the brain

In the Chapter of the Manifestations of Yin and Yang in *Suwen*, it says: "The kidney produces cerebral marrow." In the Chapter of Sea Discussion in *Lingshu*, it says: "The brain is the sea of marrow." In Elucidation on Major Problems in *Lingshu*, it says: "The ocular system pertains to the brain in the upper and comes out from the middle of the nape. The brain and marrow are different in name but both transformed from kidney essence. The ocular system is connected with the brain and is related to the function of the kidney to store essence and produce cerebral marrow. If the kidney essence and marrow are abundant, the eyes are sharp in vision. If the kidney essence and marrow are deficient, tinnitus, vertigo and dim eyesight will be caused.

1.1.5.3 The kidney controls body fluids and moistens the ocular balls

In the Chapter of Reverse Regulation in *Suwen*, it says: "The kidney is a water organ and controls fluid." In

气不通,影响肺之肃降,则可导致眼部因气、血、津液壅滞而发病。

五、眼与肾和膀胱的关系

(一)肾精充足,目视精明

眼之能视,有赖于充足的精气濡养。《素问·上古天真论》强调"肾者主水,受五脏六腑之精而藏之",故眼与肾精关系至为密切。

(二)肾生脑髓,目系属脑

《素问·阴阳应象大论》谓"肾生骨髓",《灵枢·海论》谓"脑为髓海",《灵枢·大惑论》又指出,目系"上属于脑,后出于项中"。脑和髓异名同类,都由肾精化生,而目之系连属于脑,也就与肾藏精生脑髓功能相关。故肾精充沛,髓海丰满,则目光敏锐,若肾精亏虚,髓海不足,则脑转耳鸣,目无所见。

(三)肾主津液,上润目珠

《素问·逆调论》曰:"肾者水脏,主津液。"《灵枢·五

the Chapter of Differentiation of Five Kinds of Retention and Fluid in *Lingshu*, it says: "Fluid from the five zang-organs and six fu-organs all comes into eyes." In the eyes, fluid transforms into tears to moisten the eyes and vital liquids to nourish the eyes.

1.1.5.4 The relationship between the eyes and the bladder

The qi transformation in bladder depends on the state of kidney qi. If kidney qi is insufficient or if damp-heat is accumulated, it will lead to dysfunction of the kidney in transforming qi, resulting in retention of fluid and invasion of fluid into the eyes. Besides, the bladder meridian controls the surface of the whole body and is subject to attack by exogenous pathogenic factors which causes eye disorders.

1.1.6 The Relationship between the Eyes and the Triple Energizer

The triple energizer is a solitary fu-organ and functions to transport primordial qi, food and water as well as to dredge water passage. The dysfunction of triple energizer will lead to disturbance in digestion, absorption, distribution and discharge of water and food, depriving the eyes of sufficient nourishment. Unsmoothness of the triple energizer will result in retention of fluid, upward invasion of pathogenic water into the eyes and occurrence of eye diseases.

The relationships between the eyes and the viscera are different and have their own characteristics. Physiologically they depend on each other and pathologically they affect each other.

癃津液别》曰:"五脏六腑之津液,尽上渗于目。"津液在目化为泪,则为目外润泽之水;化为神水,则为眼内充养之液。

(四)眼与膀胱的关系

膀胱的气化作用主要取决于肾气的盛衰。若肾气不足,或湿热蕴结,引起膀胱气化失常,水液潴留,可致水湿上泛于目。此外,膀胱属足太阳经,主一身之表,易遭外邪侵袭,亦常引起眼病。

六、眼与三焦的关系

三焦为孤府,主通行元气与运行水谷、疏通水道的功能。若三焦功能失常,致水谷精微之消化、吸收和输布、排泄紊乱或发生障碍,则目失濡养。若三焦水道不利,致水液潴留,水邪上犯于目,引起眼病。

眼与五脏六腑之间的关系各具特点,其密切程度不同,它们在生理上是相互协调,相互依存的;在病理上是相互影响,相互传变的。

1.2 Diagnostic Essentials

第二章 诊断概要

1.2.1 Diagnostic Methods in Ophthalmology

第一节 眼科诊法

1.2.1.1 Optometry

Optometry include the examination of distant vision and near vision. In the examination, the eyes must be examined separately. Usually the right eye is examined first and then the left one. The other eye is covered with an eye shield or one of the patient's own hands without compressing the eyeball.

1.2.1.1.1 Distant Vision Examination

The international universal vision-test chart or the logarithmic visual chart is often used in the examination. The patient or subject to be examined must be five meters away from the test-chart, or a reflecting mirror can be used if the distance is not far enough. Take the international standard test chart as an illustrating example. The 1.0 line of the test-chart and the subject's eyes must be at the same high level. The examiner then points to the chart letters line by line with an indicating bar and asks the patient to tell or gesticulate the opening side of the pointed letter in order to find out the utmost line of the letters that the patient can completely identify with no mistake. The marked figure on the line will be the visual acuity of the patient. The standard of normal vision is 1.0. If he or she can not identify the biggest letter (0.1

一、视力检查方法

视力检查方法包括远视力和近视力,检查时须两眼分别进行,一般先右后左,可用手掌或其他物遮盖另眼,盖时不可压迫眼球。

(一)远视力检查法

常用国际标准视力表或对数视力表。被检查者距视力表 5 m,如距离不足 5 m,可采用反光镜法。现以国际标准视力表为例加以说明,视力表的 1.0 行应与被检者眼同高,检查者用杆指着视力表上的字符,嘱被检查者说出或用手势表示该字符缺口方向,逐行检查,找出被检查者最多能将哪一行的字符完全正确认识,该行标志的数字即表示被检查者的视力。正常视力标准为 1.0。如果患者在 5 m 处连最大的字符(0.1 的一行)也

line) on the test chart, the patient is permitted to come near the chart step by step till he can identify the biggest letter. Then the distance between the patient and the chart is measured and his or her vision is calculated according to the following formula:

Vision = (distance between the patient and chart/ 5m) × 0.1

If the patient can identify the 0.1 visual target of the test-chart in a distance of 4 meters, for instance, his or her vision should be $4/5 \times 0.1 = 0.08$, and 0.06 vision should be in a distance of three meters, 0.04 in a distance of two meters, 0.02 in one meter.

If he or she can not identify the visual target in a distance of one meter, the patient is asked to move forwards a distance of some centimeters to identify fingers or the moving hand of the examiner, and the result is recorded. If he or she still cannot identify the fingers or the hand, the light perception of the patient is examined in a dark room. If he or she can tell the on and off of the light with the sick eye, the distance of the light sense or ocular sensation of light is recorded. If he or she cannot identify the light in the dark room, he or she can be diagnosed as the absence of light perception.

1.2.1.1.2　Near Vision Examination

In this examination, the standard reading chart or the logarithmic visual chart is used, and the examination should be done in the natural sunlight or lamplight. With the vision-test chart placed 30 cm far away from the patient, both eyes must be examined respectively from the biggest visual target 0.1 downwards in order. If the visual targets above 1.0 can be identified, the near vision of the eye is normal. If the 1.0 visual target cannot be identified in 30 cm distance, the vision-test chart is moved forward or backwards the patient till the patient can identify the

不能认出,则嘱患者逐步向视力表走近,直到认出为止,测量其与视力表的距离,然后按照下列公式计算:

视力 = (被检查者与视力表之距离/5 m) × 0.1

如检查者在 4 m 处才能辨别 0.1 视标,则该眼视力为 $4/5 \times 0.1 = 0.08$,3 m 为 0.06,2 m 为 0.04,1 m 为 0.02。

如被检查者已前至距视力表 1 m,仍未能辨别视标时,则嘱其辨别距离眼前若干厘米的指数或手动,并加以记录。若被检者连手动都不能辨别,则应进入暗室,测其光感。患眼如能辨别灯光明灭,亦应记录距离,写出几米光感或眼前光感。如在暗室内完全不能辨认灯光,则该眼视力为无光感。

(二)近视力检查法

近视力检查法用标准近视力表或对数近视力表。检查须在充足自然光线或灯光下进行,把近视力表置于眼前 30 cm 处,分别检查两眼,由最大视标 0.1 开始,顺序向下。凡能辨认出 1.0 以上视标字向者,该眼近视力正常。如不能在 30 cm 处分辨出 1.0,则将视力表向眼前或后移动,直至

smallest visual target, and the result is recorded, such as 1.0/20 cm, or 0.5/30 cm. The normal reading is 1.0/30 cm.

1.2.1.2　Visual Field Examination

The visual field is the portion of space which the fixed eye can see. Compared with the central vision, it is the extent of the peripheral field of vision. The central visual field is termed as the 30°extent around the fixed visual point. The field beyond that extent is called the peripheral visual field. When the eye field is less than 10°extent, according to the WHO's standard, the case can still be determined as a kind of visual field defect even if the vision is normal.

Visual field defect can be caused by many internal ocular disorders, so visual field examination plays an important part in the diagnosis of different diseases of fundus, especially the pathogenic changes concerning the central nervous system.

1.2.1.2.1　Contrast Examination

With no need of any facilities, this is a simple and convenient method. During the examination the doctor and the patient are sitting face to face in a distance of 0.5 meter and at the same height of eyesight. If, for instance, the right eye of the patient is to be examined, the left eye of the patient and the right one of the doctor are covered to have the patient's right eye fixed on the doctor's left eye. The doctor then places his fingers in the space between himself and the patient and moves his fingers from the outside to the center in every direction. If the patient can see the doctor's fingers in any direction at the same time as the doctor see them, his visual field can be determined as normal. The visual field of the other eye

能辨出最小视标字向的距离为止,然后分别记录,如1.0/20 cm,或0.5/30 cm等,正常为1.0/30 cm。

二、视野检查方法

视野是当眼球向正前方固视不动时所见的空间范围。与中央视力相对而言,它是周围视力。距注视点30°以内的范围称为中央视野。30°以外者称为周边视野。现世界卫生组织规定视野小于10°者即使视力正常也属于盲。

许多内障眼病都可引起视野缺损,所以视野检查对许多眼底疾病,特别是有关中枢系统病变,具有十分重要的意义。

（一）对比法

这是一种简单易行不需任何设备的方法。检查时医生与被检者距0.5 m相对而坐,眼位等高。如检查右眼,则遮盖被检者的左眼和医生的右眼,让被检者的右眼与医生的左眼相互注视,医生将手指置于与两人等距离之处,在各方向从外向中央移动,如被检者能在各方向与医生同时看到手指,即可认为视野大致正常。同法检查另一眼。此法简便,有一定的可靠性,但

can be examined with the same method which, though simple, convenient and dependable, is not accurate enough and the result is hard to be recorded for the later references.

1.2.1.2.2 Examination with the Arc Perimeter

The arc perimeter is a quite simple instrument for the dynamic examination of the peripheral vision. In this examination, the patient is asked to put his mandible on the support, with one eye covered and the other eye to be examined placed at the same high level of the 0° position and concentrating on the fixed central point. Then the doctor slowly moves the light visual target from the periphery to the center till the patient can see the light target and the angulation marked on the arc perimeter is recorded. With the arc plate rotated, the examination is continued on the twelve radial lines successively in the same way and the angles of light target of all the twelve radial lines, which are first seen by the patient, are linked to form a line on the visual field form so that the extent of the visual field of the examined eye can be determined.

The extent of visual field may vary with the sizes and colours of the light targets, examining distances, light intensity, height of the patient's nose bridge, sizes of the pupil and palpebral fissure as well as the spiritual and healthy conditions of the patient. The usual visual target is white and 3 mm in diameter and, if the patient's vision is too poor, the visual target of 5 mm or 10 mm in diameter can be used. The colours can be chosen on the basis of diseases, for example, blue or yellow colour for retinapathy and red or green for diseases of optic nerve.

The normal plane extent of visual field（white col-

不够精确,且无法作记录以供参考。

（二）弧形视野计检查法

弧形视野计是比较简单的动态检查周边视野的器械。检查时,令被检查者的下颌放在支架上,遮盖一眼,使受检眼与0°在同一水平线上,并注视中央固定点不动,然后医生将光视标由周边向中央缓缓移动,直到被检查者看见为止,记下弧上所标的角度,旋转弧板,依次查12个径线,将各径线开始看见光视标的角度在视野表上连接画线,即为被检眼的视野范围。

视野的大小,可因视标的大小与颜色、检查的距离、光线的强弱以及被检者鼻梁的高低、瞳孔和睑裂的大小及其精神与健康状况而有所变化。通常用3 mm直径的白色视标,若视力很差,则可改用直径为5 mm或10 mm的视标,并可根据疾病选用不同颜色的视标,如视网膜疾病用蓝色或黄色,视神经疾病用红色或绿色的视标。

正常视野（白色）的平面

our) include the temporal 90°, the paranasal 60°, the lower 70°and the upper 55°. About 10°is successively reduced when the colour is blue, red and green.

1.2.1.2.3 Campimety

The method is mainly used to examine scotoma of the visual field within 30° extent around the visual point. In the examination, the patient is sitting in front of the campimeter in a distance of one meter, with one eye covered and the other one to be examined fixed on the visual point on the front central screen. Then the examiner holds the visual target and moves it slowly along each radial line from the periphery to the center to find out the scale of the scotomata which are marked out first in black dots with a pin and then recorded in the table. All the scotomata in the extent of such visual field are pathogenic except those physiological ones.

1.2.1.2.4 Automatic Perimeter

It is a kind of up-to-date perimeter which, on the basis of the improvement of the above methods, is equipped with a computer and can automatically show the photostimuli from the weak to the strong on each visual field position in accordance with the program. It can print a report according to the patient's positive and negative responses (by means of touching the buttons) when the examination is finished. In the report, the light threshold value of the patient on every position and the difference compared with the normal value of the same age group are recorded in the forms of figure, mark and number so that the extent and depth of total loss of vision and local visual defects are signified.

1. 2. 1. 3 Method of Chromoscopy

Color sense is the faculty of the retina by which vari-

范围,颞侧 90°、鼻侧 60°、下方 70°、上方 55°,蓝、红、绿色视野依次递减 10°左右。

(三）平面视野计检查法

此法主要检查围绕固视点 30° 以内视野范围的暗点。检查时,被检查者坐在平面视野计前 1 m 处,遮盖一眼,受检眼在屏中央的注视点正前方,并注视不动。然后检查者持视标由周边向中央在各子午线上缓慢移动,检查出来的暗点范围先用小黑点大头针作标记,最后描记在记录表上。在此视野范围内,除生理盲点外所出现的任何暗点,皆为病理性暗点。

(四）自动化视野计

此为最新的视野计,在上述改进的基础上配备微机,自动按照程序在视野的各个位点显示由弱到强的光刺激,并根据被检者的应答(以按钮的方式表示看见与否),在检查完毕后打印报告,以图形、记号及数字记录被检者视野中各个位点的光阈值及其与同年龄组正常眼差别,从而给出视野的总丢失量和局限性缺损的范围与深度。

三、色觉检查法

视网膜辨别各种颜色的

ous colors are perceived and distinguished. The pseudois-
ochromatic table (plate), also called color blindness test
cards, is the most commonly used in the chromoscopy.
The examination should be carried out on a fine day, and
both eyes must be examined at the same time. The pseud-
oisochromatic table is placed 0.5 m away from the patient, and the patient is asked to identify the number or
figure in the table in five seconds. If it is difficult for him
to identify or if he makes mistakes or cannot recognize,
the condition can be determined as a certain kind of color
blindness or weakness according to the attached instruc-
tion in the table.

1. 2. 1. 4 Examining Method with Slit-lamp Microscopy

Slit-lamp microscope consists of a slit-lamp system
and a microscope system. It can amplify the pathogenic
changes of the eye to 10 - 16 times under strong light
beams. Of its various operating procedures, six mathods
are often used in clinic because of different ways of illumination and different tissues to be illuminated. They are
the diffuse illumination, the corneoscleral scatter illumination, the direct focal illumination, retro illumination,
specular reflection and indirect illumination. The direct
focal illumination, which is more often applied in clinical
practice, throws light onto the conjunctiva, sclera and iris
to produce a clear illuminated area by the joint of the light
focus and the microscope focus. So lesions in the part can
be observed thoroughly. When the light of the slit-lamp is
thrown onto the transparent cornea or lens, a cream
white optical section will show up. At this time, the examiner can observe the curvature and thickness of the section, find if there is any foreign body or corneal deposit,
and determine the layers and forms of such pathogenic

感觉,称为色觉。检查色觉最
常用的是假同色表。假同色
表,常称色盲本。检查应在晴
天充足的自然光线下进行,两
眼同时进行,方法是将假同色
表放在距被检者眼前 0.5 m
处,让其在 5 秒内读出表内数
字和图案。如果辨认有困难,
读错或不能读出,可按假同色
表内所附说明书判定为何种
色盲或色弱。

四、裂隙灯显微镜检查法

裂隙灯显微镜是由裂隙
灯和显微镜两个系统组成。
可在强光下放大10～16 倍检
查眼部病变。其操作方法很
多,因光线照射的方式以及被
照射组织的不同,临床常用六
种照射方法,即弥散光线照射
法、角巩膜缘分光照射法、直
接焦点照射法、后方反光照射
法、镜面反光带照射法、间接
照射法等。临床常用的是直
接焦点照射法,此法是将灯光
焦点与显微镜焦点联合在一
起,将光线投射在结膜、巩膜
和虹膜上,可见一境界清楚的
射亮区,以便细致地观察该区
的病变。将裂隙光线照在透
明的角膜或晶状体上,则呈一
种乳白色的光学切面,借此可

changes as infiltration, ulcer and necrosis. Then the light is, by regulation, turned into a beam which is thrown onto the anterior chamber to see if there is aqueous flare (also called Tyndall phenomenon), i. e. when the optical density is raised, a cream white band of light will appear between the cornea and lens if protein in the aqueous humur increases or cellular endosmosis exists. Again the focus point is moved backward in order that lesions in the lens and one-third vitreous body can be observed.

1. 2. 1. 5   Examination of Intraocular Pressure

The examination of intraocular pressure includes the methods of digital compression and ophthalmotonometry.

1.2.1.5.1   Digital Compression

This is a very simple and easy examining method of intraocular pressure through which the softness or hardness of the eyeball can be estimated. During the examination, the patient is asked to look downwards as possible as he can, and the examiner places the tips of his two index fingers on the upper margin skin of the patient's superior tarsus and slightly presses his eyeball alternately to estimate the patient's intraocular pressure through the resistance that the finger tips can feel. The symbols used in the method are: Tn indicating normal, T + 1 slightly high, T + 2 very high, and T + 3 extremely high or as hard as a stone. On the other hand, symbols T − 1, T − 2 and T − 3 represent slightly low, very low and extremely low respectively.

1.2.1.5.2   Ophthalmotonometry

1. Schiotz Tonometer

Operational Procedure: The patient takes a supine position with a low headrest and the eye to be measured is

以观察其弯曲度、厚度、有无异物或角膜后沉着物,以及浸润、溃疡、坏死等病变的层次和形态。将光线调成细小光柱射入前房,可检查有无房水闪辉(又称 Tyndall 现象),即在房水中蛋白质增加或有细胞渗入,因而使其光密度增加时,可见角膜与晶状体之间有一乳白色的光带。再将焦点向后移,还可以观察晶状体及前 1/3 玻璃体的病变。

五、眼压检查法

眼压检查,包括指测法及眼压计测定法。

(一)指测法

简单易操作,能估计眼球的软硬度。检查时,嘱患者两眼尽量向下注视,检查者用两手食指尖放在上睑板上缘的皮肤面上,两指尖交替轻压眼球,凭借指尖触知的抵抗力,估计眼压的高低。记录时,以 Tn 表示眼压正常,T + 1 表示眼压轻度增高,T + 2 表示眼压很高,T + 3 表示眼压极高,眼球坚硬如石。反之,则以 T − 1、T − 2、T − 3 分别表示眼压稍低、很低、极低。

(二)眼压计测量法

1. Schiotz 眼压计

操作方法:患者仰卧低枕,被检查眼滴入 0.5% 地卡

dropped two or three times with 0.5% dicaine. Before the measurement, the tonometer is examined on the standard plate so that the needle can point to zero, and then the plate is cleaned with 75% alcohol cotton and dried. The patient is asked to lift his left hand with the index finger as the fixed point and the cornea right on the middle horizontal position. The examiner, holding the tonometer in his right hand, slightly opens with his left thumb and index fingers the patient's eyelids and fixes them on the orbital margin without compressing the patient's eyeball. Then the tonometer plate is vertically placed in the center of the cornea. With a 5.5 weight added, the examiner immediately reads the graduation pointed by the needle and then instantly takes up the tonometer in case the corneal epithelium might be abraded. If the reading is less than 3, a heavier weight is used and another measure is performed. The actual number should be calculated by the conversion of the reading according to the conversion table. When the measure is finished, antibiotic eye drops should be applied to the conjunctival sac. Since the tonometer is of depression type, the reading number is determined by the depression of the cornea under the compression of the tonometer needle, and as the ocular volume may change greatly during the procedure, the reading number is often influenced by the hardness of the eyeball wall. In the case of abnormal hardness of eyeball wall, some slightly high or low incorrect readings may be obtained. Although such errors can be avoided through the measure with two weights and the correct table, the final result is not so accurate as that with an applanation tonometer.

2. Goldmann Applanometer

This is the most accurate international tonometer. It is attached to a slit-lamp microscope to measure intraocular

因2~3次。测前,眼压计先在标准试板上测试,指针指在零度时为正常。用75%酒精棉球擦拭底板待干。测量时嘱患者举起左手伸出食指作为注视点,使角膜恰在水平正中位,检查者右手持眼压计,左手拇指及食指轻轻分开上下睑,固定在眶缘上,不得给眼球施加任何压力。将眼压计底板垂直放在角膜中央,先用5.5砝码,迅速读指针刻度,立即提起眼压计,以免擦伤角膜上皮。如读数小于3,则需要更换较重砝码,再测量。测出的读数查换算表,得出眼压的实际数字。测毕,结膜囊内滴抗生素眼药水。此眼压计为压陷式,其刻度的多少取决于在眼压计压针的压迫下角膜向下凹陷的程度。如果测量时引起眼球容积的变化较大,则测出的数值会受到球壁硬度的影响。在球壁硬度显著异常者会给出偏高或偏低的数据,用两个砝码测量后查表校正可消除球壁硬度造成的误差,但仍不如压平眼压计准确。

2. Goldmann 压平眼压计

这是目前国际通用的最准确的眼压计,它是附装在裂

pressure through the microscope in a sitting position. Since it is a kind of applanation tonometer, the cornea in the measuring process becomes slightly applanated, but without depression and the eyeball volume does not change greatly, avoiding the affection of the hardness of eyeball wall. The Perkin applanation tonometer, which, in principle, is the same as the Goldmann tonometer, is a hand tonometer and has the advantage of operating with the patient either in a sitting position or in a lying position without the need of slit-lamp microscope.

3. Non-contact Applanometer

The principle of the applanometer is to make use of a sort of controlled air pulse, the pressure of which is indicated by the characteristics of linear increase. When the cornea is applanated within a certain area, the monitoring system is applied to receive the light reflected from the corneal surface and the time to applanate the cornea to a certain extent is recorded and calculated in the unit of kPa. The biggest advantage of the applantonometer is that cross infection sometimes caused by using the ophthalmonometry is thoroughly prevented, and the method is applicable to those who are allergic to surface anesthesia while its disadvantage is that the obtained values may be a little lower.

1.2.1.6 Fundus Examination

Fundus examination is always done in a dark room. If it is hard for the speculum examination in the case of stenocoriasis, the patient's pupil is treated with mydriatic agents. Before the mydriatic agents is applied, the depth of the anterior chamber and the width of its angle must be found out, for mydriasis, in a narrow anterior chamber condition, has the potential risk to start angle-closure

隙灯显微镜上,用显微镜观察,坐位测量。它是一种压平眼压计,在测量时仅仅使角膜凸面稍稍变平而不下陷,眼球容积改变很小,所以基本上不受球壁硬度的影响。还有Perkin压平眼压计,原理与Goldmann眼压计相同,其优点是可以手持使用,不需要裂隙灯显微镜,被检者取坐位卧位都可测量。

3. 非接触压平眼压计

其原理是利用一种可控的空气脉冲,其压力具有线性增加的特性,将角膜压平一定面积,再利用监测系统感受角膜表面反射的光线,并将角膜压平到一定程度所需的时间记录下来,换算成眼压的kPa数。它的最大优点是彻底避免了通过眼压计引起的交叉感染,并能应用于对表面麻醉药过敏的患者。其缺点是所得数值可能偏低。

六、眼底检查方法

眼底检查一般在暗室进行,如患者瞳孔小,不易窥入,需用药物放大瞳孔,详查眼底,在点放瞳药之前,必须先了解前房深浅、房角的宽窄,注意窄房角眼放瞳有激发闭角型青光眼发作的潜在

glaucoma.

In the fundus examination, two kinds of ophthalmo-scopes, indirect and direct, are used. With an indirect ophthalmoscope, the examiner can see an inverted image of a larger area amplified four times while, with a direct one, what he sees is an ortho-image of a smaller part amplified about 10 times.

1.2.1.6.1 Fundus Examination with Direct Ophthalmoscope

With his index finger putting on the ophthalmoscope plate for the convenient regulation of the diopter, the examiner holds the ophthalmoscope handle with the other fingers. When examining the right eye, the examiner should stand on the patient's right side with the ophthalmoscope in the right hand to check with the right eye. Likewise, when the left eye is examined, the examiner has to stand on the left side of the patient, with the ophthalmoscope in the left hand to check with the left eye. In the examination, transillumination is used first to find out if there is any cloudiness in the refracting media, then the ophthalmoscope turntable is set at the + 8 to + 10D, and the light is right thrown into the pupil 10 to 20 cm away from the examined eye. In a normal condition, the pupillary area shows the orange-coloured reflection. If cloudiness exists in the cornea, lens or vitreum, there may appear a dark shadow in the red reflection. At this moment, the patient is asked to move his eyeball around and, if the dark shadow turns together with his eyeball, it indicates that the cloudiness is in front of the lens, conversely in the back of the lens, or inside the lens if immovable.

After the transillumination, the turntable is turned back to the "0 to − 3" position and the ophthalmoscope is moved near the eye about 2 cm away to examine the fundus.

危险。

检查眼底用的检眼镜有间接和直接两种。间接检眼镜所见眼底为倒像,放大 4 倍,可见范围大;直接检眼镜所见眼底为正像,放大约 10 倍,可见范围小。

(一)直接检眼镜检查方法

将食指放在检眼镜的盘上,以便随时调整屈光度数,拇指及其余手握住镜柄。检查右眼时,检查者站在被检者右侧,用右手持检眼镜,用右眼检查。检查左眼时,检查者站在被检者左侧,用左手持检眼镜,用左眼检查。检查时,应先用彻照法检查眼的屈光间质有无混浊,用食指将检眼镜转盘拨到 + 8～ + 10D,距受检眼10～20 cm,将检眼镜灯光射入瞳孔,正常者瞳孔区呈橘红色反光,如角膜、晶状体或玻璃体有混浊,则在红色反光中出现黑影。此时嘱患者转动眼球,如黑影转动的方向与眼球一致,则表明混浊位于晶状体前方,反之则位于晶状体后方,如不动,则在晶状体。

彻照完毕后,将转盘拨回到"0～ − 3"处,同时将检眼镜移近受检眼约2 cm处,检查眼

If both the examiner and the patient are of emmetropia, the fundus can clearly be seen. If it can not clearly be seen, the turntable is turned till the fundus can clearly be seen. The patient is asked to look straightly ahead, and the ophthalmoscope light is thrown at the angle of a 15° from the temporal to examine the optic disc. Then the patient is asked to take a round look for the examination of the periphery of the optic disc and finally the macula retinae is examined with the patient's eye fixed on the light of the ophthalmoscope.

The normal optic disc takes an ellipsoid-like shape in a light red colour, clearly bounded, and with excavation in the center, which is also called physiological excavation or cup. At the bottom of this physiological excavation, where some gray dots can be dimly seen, is the cribriform plat.

Normally, the central retinal artery is bright red, its vain dark red and the diametric proportion of the retinal artery and vein is 2∶3. If the artery becomes thinned and the cross points of the artery and vein are broken or blunt, that indicates retinal angiospasm or arteriosclerosis.

The normal retina is transparent with the pigmented epithelium and choroid seen, thus showing an even orange colour or leopard retina. A lot of fundus disorders and general diseases can cause edema, bleeding, exudation, necrosis or pigmental abnormality in the retina.

The macula retina which lies slightly below the temporal optic disc 2PD (disc diameter) away is dark red and has no blood vessels but a reflection point in the center called central fovea reflection. A reflection areola can be seen around the macula of young people and children.

底,如果检查者与被检者都是正视眼,则可看清眼底。如不能看清,可拨动转盘直至看清为止,嘱患者向正前方注视,检眼镜从颞侧约15°处投入光线,以检查视盘,再嘱患者向上下左右各方向注视,以检查周边部。最后嘱患者注视检眼镜灯光,以检查黄斑部。

正常眼底可见视盘略呈椭圆形,浅红色,境界清楚,中央有凹陷,色泽稍淡,称为生理凹陷,亦称为杯。生理凹陷底部隐约可见一些暗灰色小点,该处即为筛板。

视网膜中央动脉色鲜红,静脉色暗红,动静脉管径之比为2∶3,如动脉变细,或动静脉交叉处静脉中断或尖削,则表明有视网膜动脉痉挛或硬化。

视网膜正常时透明,可见下方之色素上皮及脉络膜,故呈均匀橘红色或豹纹状。许多眼底病或全身病都可使视网膜出现水肿、出血、渗出、坏死或色素异常。

黄斑部位于视盘颞侧2PD(视盘直径)稍偏下方,呈暗红色,无血管,其中央有一反光点,称中心凹光反射。青少年黄斑周围可见一反光晕。

1.2.1.6.2   Examination with Indirect Ophthalmoscope

What can be seen in this examination is an inverted image of the larger scale of the fundus amplified four times, but the pupil must be treated with mydriatic agents. At present, the binocular indirect ophthalmoscope is usually used. The frontal mirror is fixed on the doctor's head with the illuminator installed in the headband and the convex lens held in the doctor's left hand. The visual field in the fundus examination by the indirect ophthalmoscope is larger than that by the direct one, so more general conditions of the fundus can be found without missing any pathological changes, particularly in the examination of retinal hole. Besides, since the examination is performed in a quite far distance, operations of blocking and padding the retinal hole and so on can be carried out in an audio-visual way. Indirect ophthalmoscope, therefore, is now the necessary instrument in the examination and treatment of retinal detachment.

1.2.2   Common Syndrome-differentiating Methods in Ophthalmology

1.2.2.1   Differentiating External and Internal Oculopathy

External oculopathy, a general term of pathological changes in the parts of fresh, blood, qi and wind orbiculi (palpebra, canthus, the white and black parts of eye), is usually caused by the six exopathogenic factors (wind, cold, heat, dampness, dryness and fire) or by traumas. It may also be caused by indigestion, noxious dampness and phlegm-fire and is characterized by abrupt onset, rapid changing and obvious external symptoms. The internal

（二）间接检眼镜检查方法

此镜所见的眼底为倒像，放大 4 倍，可见范围较大，但必须放大瞳孔，现多用双目间接眼底镜，用额头固定于头部，光源也装在额带上，左手持一凸透镜。用间接检眼镜检查眼底，所见视野比直接检眼镜大，能比较全面了解眼底情况，不易遗漏眼底的病变，尤其有利于寻找视网膜裂孔，又因其可在较远距离检查眼底，从而使视网膜裂孔的封闭及垫压等操作可以在直观下进行，因此它已成了检查和治疗视网膜脱离的必备仪器。

第二节   眼科常用辨证方法

一、辨外障与内障

外障是肉轮、血轮、气轮与风轮等部位病变的总称。多为外感六淫，或外伤所致。亦有由食滞、湿毒或痰火等引起。其特点为发病突然，变化快，外症较明显。内障眼病泛指水轮疾病，即包括发生于瞳神及其后一切眼内组织的病

oculopathy generally refers to the diseases of pupil（water obiculus）, including the pathological changes occurring in the pupil and all the ocular tissues behind it, often with visual changes. It is often caused by the injury of seven emotions, too much visual work or overwork, or by the dysfunction of viscera, meridian, qi and blood.

1.2.2.2　Differentiating Common Symptoms and Signs

1.2.2.2.1　Differentiating vision

Poor vision, hyperemia of bulbar conjunctiva and nebula are often caused by exopathic wind and heat or by flaming fire of the liver and gallbladder; subjective dim eyesight but normal external conditions of eye is often caused by deficiency of both the liver and kidney as well as fire hyperactivity due to asthenia or by stagnancy of liver qi; sudden diminution of vision without redness and pain in the eye is caused by head-wind and phlegm-fire or by hyperemia due to blood heat or qi disorders; long-term internal oculopathy with blurred vision or light perception is caused by asthenia of both qi and blood; poor eyesight during dawn or twilight and contraction of visual field is caused by deficiency of kidney yang or by impairment of liver-kidney essence; myopia is caused by asthenia of yang; and dizziness after squating is caused by deficiency of essence, qi and blood.

1.2.2.2.2　Differentiating Pain and Itching

Ophthalmalgia caused by external oculopathy with the manifestations of astringing pain, coarse pain and twinge pertains to yang syndrome while ophthalmalgia caused by internal oculopathy with the manifestations of distending pain, referred pain and pain of the deep eyeball pertains to yin syndrome.

Redness and coarse pain of the eye with massive

变。其发病多有视觉方面的改变。内障眼病多为七情所伤、过用目力及劳累过度等，导致脏腑、经络或气血功能失调引起。

二、辨常见症

（一）辨视觉

视物不清，白睛红赤或翳膜遮睛，多外感风热或肝胆火炽；如外眼端好，自觉视物渐昏，多为肝肾两亏，阴虚火旺或肝气郁结；视力骤降，目无赤痛，多属头风痰火，血热妄行或气不摄血；内障日久，视物不见或只辨三光，多属气血两亏；入暮目暗或视野缩小，多属肾阳不足或肝肾精亏；能近怯远，多属阳气虚；坐起生花，多属精气血少。

（二）辨痛痒

外障引起的眼痛多表现为涩痛、碜痛或刺痛，多属阳。内障引起的眼痛常为胀痛、牵拽痛或眼珠深部疼痛，多属阴。

目赤碜痛，眵多粘结，多

mucopurulent secretion is often due to exopathic wind; eyelid hyperemia with pain and swelling accompanied with constipation is usually due to excessive fire in yangming meridian; slight redness and pain of the sclera with a dry and uncomfortable sensation is usually due to deficiency of kidney and blood; dull distending pain of the eyeball is usually due to yang hyperactivity and yin asthenia; severely distending pain of the eyeball is usually due to up-stirring of qi and fire; ocular distension after long time's visual work is usually due to spleen and kidney deficiency which leads to the failure of upward transmission of essence or is due to yang hyperactivity; and pain in the deep eyeball is usually due to stagnation of liver qi or to yin deficiency which leads to fire hyperactivity.

Ocular itching may be caused by pathogenic wind, fire and dampness and by deficiency of blood, but pathogenic wind is often the main cause in clinic. Redness and itching of eye which becomes severe with wind blowing often pertains to the type of exopathic wind-heat; blepharitis marginalis with mucopurulent secretion or swollen granules and itching like insect-moving pertains to the type of damp-heat in the spleen and stomach mingled with pathogeic wind; itching with astringent and uncomfortable sensation occurring now and then pertains to the type of endopathic wind due to blood asthenia; and itching and pain occurring alternatively pertains to the type of invasion of excessive toxin.

1.2.2.2.3 Differentiating Redness and Swelling

Cherry-like swollen eyelid with burning pain often pertains to the type of noxious heat accumulation of spleen and stomach; sudden swelling of eyelid with slight redness and massive tears pertains to the type of exopathic wind; ball-like swelling of eyelid with bright surface and no pain

为外感风热;胞睑赤痛肿硬,大便燥结,多阳明实火;白睛微赤微痛,干涩不舒,多水亏血虚;目珠隐隐胀痛,多阴虚阳亢;目珠胀痛如突,多气火上逆;久视眼胀,多脾肾不足,精不上承或阳亢之象;目珠深处疼痛,多肝郁气滞或阴虚火旺。

目痒可因风、火、湿与血虚引起,但临床上因风邪引起居多。目赤痒,迎风尤甚,多为外感风热;睑弦赤烂,眵泪粘结,或胞内颗粒肥大,痒如虫行,多属脾胃湿热,兼挟风邪;痒涩不舒,时作时止,多血虚生风;痒痛兼作,多邪毒炽盛。

(三) 辨红肿

胞睑红肿如桃,灼热疼痛,多脾胃热毒蕴结;胞睑肿胀骤起,微红多泪,多外感风邪;胞睑肿起如球,皮色光亮,不伴赤痛,多脾胃阳虚,水气

pertains to the type of upward hyperactivity of kidney qi due to yang deficiency of the spleen and stomach; palpebral erosion with watery exudation pertains to the type of fumigation by internal damp-heat accumulation; and livid distension of eyelid pertains to the type of stagnation of qi and blood.

Hyperemia of bulbar conjunctiva with tears and mucopurulent secretion pertains to the type of exopathic wind-heat; flame-like redness of the white of eye pertains to the type of excessive heat of lung meridian; faint redness pertains to the deficient heat of lung meridian; hyperemia of bulbar conjunctiva and photophobia with tears pertains to the type of excessive heat of liver and gallbladder; slight redness and blurred vision with tears pertains to the type of fire hyperactivity due to yin deficiency.

1.2.2.2.4　Differentiating Secretion and Tears

Massive eye secretion is a common concomitant symptom of external oculopathy and often pertains to heat syndrome. Thin eye secretion is due to asthenia heat of lung meridian; massive and hard eye secretion is due to sthenia heat of lung meridian; massive yellow thick secretion is due to excessive noxious heat; and mucopurulent secretion is due to damp-heat.

1.2.2.3　Differentiating Nebula

Nebula refers to the pancorneal opacity or cloudiness occurring on the black part of eye. It may be in the shapes of punctuation, arborization, geography, insect-bite and so on. The terms for nebula vary with its form, colour and depth, but what must first be done in clinic is to determine whether it is a new or an old case and then, in the light of other symptoms, to differentiate its syndrome.

1.2.2.3.1　New Nebula

The category of new nebula is white pancorneal opacity

上泛；胞睑赤烂渗水，多属湿热薰蒸；胞睑青紫肿胀，为气血瘀滞。

白睛红赤，眵泪并作，多外感风热；白睛红赤如火，为肺经实热；白睛隐隐红赤，为肺经虚热；抱轮红赤，羞明流泪，多属肝胆实热；抱轮微红，目昏泪出，多属阴虚火旺。

（四）辨眵泪

眼眵多为外障眼病的一个常见伴发症，多属热。眵稀为肺经虚热；眵多硬结为肺经实热；眵多黄稠为热毒炽盛；眵泪胶粘为湿热。

三、辨翳

起于黑睛上的混浊称为翳，可呈点状、树枝状、地图状或虫蚀状等。根据混浊的形态、色泽、深浅程度不同，翳的名称亦不同，但临床上首先要区别是新翳还是宿翳，然后再结合其他症状进行辨证。

（一）新翳

凡是黑睛混浊，呈灰白

which is obscurely bounded, with coarse surface, the trend to develop and symptoms of ocular redness, pain, photophobia and lacrimation. In most cases, new nebula in the black part of eye is caused by the six exogenous pathogenic factors, progresses easily and often involves the iris and pupil. So syndrome differentiation must be correct in clinic. New nebula in mild case, after recovery, can disappear, but in severe case it may turn into old nebula.

1.2.2.3.2 Old Nebula

The category of old nebula is pancorneal opacity clearly bounded, with smooth surface and no further developing trend and without redness, pain and lacrimation.

It is classified in clinic as cloudiness, spot nebula and cataract according to its thickness.

色,表面粗糙,边界模糊,有发展趋势,伴有不同程度的目赤疼痛、畏光流泪者,统属新翳范畴。黑睛新翳多因外感六淫,亦易传变,常波及黄仁与瞳神,临证须辨清。新翳愈后,轻者可消散,重者则转为宿翳。

(二)宿翳

凡黑睛混浊,表面光滑,边缘清晰,无发展趋势,不伴有赤痛流泪者,统属宿翳范畴。

临床上根据宿翳的厚薄程度,分为云翳、斑翳、白斑。

1.3 Introduction to the Treatment

第三章 治疗概要

1.3.1 Internal Therapies

第一节 内治法

1. 3. 1. 1 Method of Dispersing Pathogenic Wind-heat

一、疏风清热法

This is a method to treat oculopathy caused by pathogenic wind-heat with the diaphoretic drugs pungent in flavour and cool in property to disperse pathogenic wind-heat. It is applicable to ocular diseases due to exopathic wind-heat with the common symptoms such as sudden onset, itching and pain of eye, edema of eyelid, hyperemia of bulba conjunctiva and star-like nebula of cornea as well as the general symptoms of headache, aversion to cold, fever and a floating-rapid pulse.

本法是用具有辛凉解表作用的药物组成方剂,通过疏风散热,解除风热所致眼病的治法,适用于外感风热眼病。常见症状如:病起突然,目痒目痛,胞睑浮肿,白睛红赤,黑睛星翳等。常伴有头痛,恶寒,发热,脉浮数等全身症状。

1. 3. 1. 2 Method of Purging Fire to Remove Toxin

二、泻火解毒法

This is a method to treat oculopathy caused by noxious heat with the drugs cold and cool in property to reduce fire and remove toxin. It is applicable to ocular diseases caused by endopathic heat transformed from exogenous pathogenic factors or by upward invasion of visceral noxious heat with such common symptoms as sudden and severe onset, pain of eye with tenderness, photophobia and burning pain, hot tears, mucopurulent eye secretion, cherry-like swollen eyelid, turbidity of bulbar conjunctiva, ulcer of cornea, hypopyon, miosis and the general

本法是用性质寒凉的药物组成方剂,通过泻火解毒以清除眼病热毒的治法,适用于外感六淫化热入里,或脏腑热毒上攻的眼病。常见症状如:发病急重,眼病疼痛拒按,羞明灼痛,热泪如汤,眵多粘结,胞肿如桃,白睛混赤,黑睛溃陷,黄液上冲,瞳神紧小等。常伴有口渴,便秘,舌红,苔黄

symptoms and signs of dry mouth, constipation, reddish tongue with yellowish coating and so on.

　　The method, with cold-cool actions, may easily damage yang-qi of the spleen and stomach and should avoid long-term use in clinic. It must be used cautiously according to the patient's sickness and constitutional conditions. Besides, in the treatment of corneal diseases and fundus hemorrhage the method must be put into proper use since long-term use of cold and cool drugs can cause stagnancy of qi and blood and may make it difficult for nebular disorders to be cured. Patients with deficient fire should not be treated by this method.

1.3.1.3　Method of Nourishing Yin to Reduce Fire

　　This is a treatment method for the syndrome of fire hyperactivity due to yin deficiency with the drugs which are cold and cool in property and have the action of tonifying yin to reduce pathogenic fire so that the eyesight is improved. The method is applicable to ocular diseases manifesting such common symptoms as dryness of eyeball, slight hyperemia of bulbar conjunctiva, alternative star-like nebula of cornea, miosis or platycoria, high intraocular pressure, blurred vision and the general symptoms and signs of tidal fever with red cheeks, feverish sensation in palms and soles, dizziness and vexation, bitter taste in the mouth and dry throat, red tongue with a scanty coating and thready-rapid pulse.

　　Clinically, there are many different ocular diseases caused by fire hyperactivity due to yin deficiency, so further syndrome differentiation must be carried out when the method is used to treat the specific disease. Redness of canthi, vexation and sleepless, for example, may arise from deficient fire of the heart meridian; slight hyperemia

等全身症状。

　　本法为寒凉直折之法,容易损伤脾胃阳气,故不宜久用,临床上要根据患者病情轻重和体质强弱慎重选择,又因寒凉药久用可致气血凝滞,翳障难消,故对黑睛疾患,眼底出血,用本法必须掌握尺度。虚火者,禁用此法。

三、滋阴降火法

　　本法是用具有寒凉滋润作用的药物组成方剂,通过滋养阴液,清降虚火,解除阴虚火旺的证候而达到明目效果的治法,适用于阴虚火旺的眼病。常见症状如:眼球干涩,白睛微赤,黑睛星翳乍隐乍现,瞳神干缺,或瞳神散大,眼压增高,视物昏朦等。常伴有潮热颧红,手足心热,头晕心烦,口苦口干,舌红少苔,脉细数等全身症状。

　　临床上阴虚火旺的眼病较多,但在具体应用本法时,尚须进一步辨证。如两眦红赤,心烦失眠,属心经虚火;白睛淡红,鼻干咽燥,属肺经虚火;黑睛生翳,抱轮微赤,烦躁

of bulbar conjunctiva and dry nose and throat from deficient fire of lung meridian; and corneal nebula, mild redness of eyelid and irritability from deficient fire of liver
meridian. Therefore, the involved viscera and tissues
should be carefully considered in the selection of recipes
and drugs in treatment.

Since the herbal drugs for the nourishing yin to reduce pathogenic fire are often tonic and greasy in nature,
patients with ophthalmopathy due to exopathogen and
those with spleen and stomach deficiency or unrelieved
pathogenic damp contraindicate the method.

1. 3. 1. 4　Method of Eliminating Dampness

This is a method for the treatment of oculopathy
caused by pathogenic damp with drugs for eliminating
dampness and is applicable to all ocular diseases due to external invasion of pathogenic damp or internal accumulation of dampness, manifesting such common symptoms as
moist ulcer of palpebral margin, severe swelling of eyelid,
eczema papulosum or membranous formation in eyelid,
yellow turbid bulbar conjunctiva, massive mucopurulent
eye secretion, insect-biting corneal nebula, turbidity of
aqueous humor, blurred vision, and the general accompanying symptoms and signs of severe heaviness of the
head, no thirst or thirt without desire for drinking and
weakness of four limbs, poor appetite, abdominal distention, loose stool and greasy tongue coating.

As ophthalmopathy of damp type is obstinate and the
long time's application of damp-relieving drugs may easily
consume body fluids, the drug prescribed in the treatment
must be cautiously selected with the consideration of how
serious the patient is and what kind of constitutional conditions he has, and special attention should be paid to the
cases due to asthenia of yin and blood and to deficiency of

易怒,属肝经虚火等。可结合
脏腑所属,选方用药。

滋阴降火药物性多滋腻,
故外感眼病、脾胃虚弱或湿邪
未化者忌用本法。

四、祛湿法

本法是用祛湿药物组成
方剂,通过祛除湿邪而治疗眼
病的方法,适用于湿邪外侵或
湿浊内蕴所引起的一切眼病。
常见症状如:睑弦湿烂,胞肿
难睁,睑内粟疮或有膜形成,
白睛污黄,眵多胶粘,黑睛有
翳如虫蚀,神水混浊,视瞻昏
渺等。常伴有头重如裹,口不
渴或口渴不欲饮,四肢乏力,
胸闷食少,腹胀便溏,舌苔腻
等全身症状。

湿证眼病比较顽固,祛湿
药久用易耗液伤津,故要根据
病情轻重及患者全身情况慎
重选药。阴虚血少与津液亏
损者,尤宜注意。

body fluids.

1.3.1.5 Hemostasis

This is a method used to treat hemorrhagic oculopathy by prescribing the hemostatic drugs to arrest the bleeding. The method is applicable to ocular hemorrhagic diseases caused by various factors mainly with such common symptoms as suffusion of bulbar conjunctiva, hemorrhage of pupil, retinal hemorrhage, macular hemorrhage, choroidal hemorrhage.

Hemorrhagic symptoms are very common in ophthalmopathy, and the method is an urgent way for acute subordinate symptoms and is applicable to hemorrhagic cases at early stage. If the bleeding is arrested without recurring trend, the treatment method should gradually be changed to activate blood circulation for removing blood stasis so as to improve the absorption of hemorrhage and to avoid leaving blood stasis.

1.3.1.6 Method of Promoting Blood Circulation to Remove Blood Stasis

This is a treatment method by using blood-activating and stasis-eliminating drugs to improve blood circulation and remove accumulation of ocular blood stasis. The method is applicable to the ocular diseases caused by obstruction and sluggishness of blood circulation or by accumulation of blood stasis and is also used to treat eye injuries, manifesting such common symptoms as livid hard swelling of eyelid, hemorrhagic hyperemia of bulbar conjunctiva, bleeding of bulbar conjunctiva, blood stasis of every part of eye, obstruction of retinal vessels, fixed pain of eye with tenderness, and ecchymosis on the tongue.

In addition, the method should be properly applied in the treatment of ocular disorders with blood stasis due to

五、止血法

本法是用具有止血作用的药物组成方剂来中止眼病出血的治法,适用于各种原因引起的以出血症状为主的眼病。常见症状如:白睛溢血,血灌瞳神,视网膜出血,黄斑出血,脉络膜出血等。

眼科出血症状较多常见,本法属急则治标之法,仅适用于出血早期,若出血停止,已无再出血的趋向,应逐渐转向活血化瘀治法,以促进出血的吸收,以免导致留瘀之弊。

六、活血化瘀法

本法是用具有活血化瘀作用的药物组成方剂,以改善血行,消散瘀滞,促进眼部瘀血吸收的方法,适用于各种血脉阻滞,血流不畅,或瘀血停聚的眼病及眼外伤。常见症状如:胞睑青紫肿硬,白睛赤脉粗大,溢血,眼内各个部位的瘀血,视网膜血管阻塞,眼部固定性疼痛拒按,以及舌有瘀斑等。

此外,其他原因引起的眼病在病变的发展过程中若出

other causes in the course of the pathogenic development.

Qi promotes blood circulation, so normal blood circulation depends on qi's activity. Drugs for promoting qi's circulation to remove stagnancy is compatibly used in clinic to increase curative effects.

The method should not be applied for a long time in case the healthy qi be consumed. In the cases with blood stasis of eye and asthenia of qi, it should be cooperated with drugs for nourishing qi. Patients with asthenia of qi and blood as well as pregnant women contraindicate the method.

1.3.1.7 Method of Dispersing Stagnated Liver Qi

This is a treatment method to alleviate depression of the liver or to remove stagnancy of liver qi by using drugs for relieving stagnation of liver qi to regulate qi's activity so that the eyesight can be improved. The method is applicable to all internal and external oculopathy caused by stagnation of liver qi and disorder of qi's circulation. It can be used to treat ocular diseases, no matter whether it is internal or external, so long as it manifests the symptoms of distention of hypochondrium, eructation, chest oppression, irritability, throat-congestion feeling, irregular menstruation of women patients, and a thready pulse and so on. In the cases with stagnant liver causing pathogenic fire, the fire-removing drugs are properly added to remove stagnancy of liver qi. In the cases with stagnant liver plus asthenia of qi and blood, the drugs for tonifying blood and strengthening spleen are used in cooperation with the method.

Since drugs for regulating qi are often pungent in flavour and dryness in property, the method should be ap-

现瘀血证候,在治疗时宜适当配合应用活血化瘀法。

气为血帅,气行则血行,故临床运用时,常配伍行气导滞药物,以提高疗效。

本法不宜久用,以免耗伤正气,对眼部既有瘀滞又见气虚症状者,应用本法需适当配伍补气药物。气血虚弱者及孕妇忌用本法。

七、疏肝理气法

本法是用具有疏肝解郁,调理气机作用的药物组成方剂,以改善或清除肝郁气滞证候而达到明目作用的治法,适用于肝气郁滞,气机不畅,目窍不利的一切内外障眼病。临床无论内外障眼病,只要兼有胁胀,嗳气,胸闷,急躁易怒,咽部似有物阻,妇女月经不调,脉弦等症者,皆可用疏肝理气法治之。肝郁化火者,宜酌加清火之品,以清肝解郁;肝郁兼有气血虚弱者,宜与养血健脾药同用。

理气药物多辛燥,故对阴亏之人须慎用,并注意配伍。

plied cautiously to patients with yin asthenia and attention should be paid to the compatibility of drugs.

1.3.1.8　Method of Nourishing Qi and Blood

The method is used to treat cases due to deficiency of qi and blood with tonic prescriptions to improve eyesight and is applicable to ophthalmopathy as a result of qi and blood asthenia caused by various reasons. In clinic, it is often used to treat chronic internal and external ocular diseases manifesting the general syndrome of deficient qi and blood as well as such common symptoms as sleepy eyes, distention of eye after long visual work, prolonged corneal nebula, gradual dimness of vision and so on.

The spleen and stomach are the acquired foundation of life and the transformation source of qi and blood. When spleen qi is in good order, qi and blood can be constantly transformed and conducted to the eyes. In the tonic treatment method, therefore, attention should also be paid to the regulation of spleen and stomach. In the cases with asthenia and sthenia mingled, purging and tonifying methods can be simultaneously used, or first the purging one, then the tonifying one, or vice versa. Since Qi and blood depend on each other, they should be tonified simultaneously. However, since their deficient extent is always different, particular emphasis in treatment should be paid. For patients with a tendency of qi deficiency and the symptoms of sleepy eyes, a pale tongue and weak pulse, emphasis should be put on tonifying qi. Otherwise, for patients with blood more deficient showing dizziness, poor vision, dreaminess, vexation, insomnia, a pale tongue and thready pulse, emphasis should be put on nourishing blood.

Cases due to pathogenic hyperactivity without deficient signs countraindicate the method.

八、益气养血法

本法是用具有补益气血作用的药物组成方剂,以清除气血虚弱证候而达到明目作用的治法,适用于各种原因引起的气血不足的眼病。临床上多见于慢性内外障眼病,全身兼有气血不足的证候。常见症状如:睁眼乏力,久视眼胀,黑睛翳陷日久不愈,视物渐昏等。

脾胃为后天之本,气血生化之源,脾气健运,气血才能不断上注于目,故补气养血时,还要注意调理脾胃,如属虚实夹杂,则可攻补兼施,或先攻后补,或先补后攻。因气血相依,故益气与养血往往同用,但根据气血偏虚程度的不同,治疗时又有所侧重,偏于气虚者,见眼睁乏力,常欲闭垂,舌淡脉弱,应以益气为主;偏于血虚者,见头昏眼花,不耐久视,多梦易醒,心烦失眠,舌淡脉细,应以养血为主。

本法忌用于邪气亢盛而无虚候者。

1. 3. 1. 9 Method of Invigorating Liver and Kidney

This is a treatment method for the deficiency of liver and kidney with the tonic drugs to invigorate liver and kidney so as to improve the vision. The method is applicable to ophthalmopathy due to deficiency of liver-kidney yin. The common ocular disorders to which the method can be applied include chronic external oculopathy and fundus diseases with mild symptoms, long sick course and repeated occurrence as well as internal oculopathy with retrograde changes. The general symptoms are lassitude in loin and legs, insomnia and amnesia, spermatorrhea for male, irregular menstruation for female, a reddish tongue with a little coating and thready-weak pulse.

The countraindication of the method is ophthalmopathy of sthenia type and it should be applied cautiously to patients with pathogenic dampness remained.

1. 3. 1. 10 Method of Dissipating Mass

This is a method to treat ophthalmopathy by using the drugs with the action to resolve phlegm and dissipate masses. It is applicable to different types of internal and external oculopathy with visible objects caused by phlegm-damp combination and stagnancy of qi and blood. The common symptoms are chalazion, organized cord of eye with old exudation, and nodular projection of bulbar conjunctiva.

In the cases with stagnancy of qi and blood, drugs for regulating qi and blood are compatibly added and, in the cases with phlegm-damp combination, drugs for resolving phlegm and removing dampness are compatibly used.

九、补益肝肾法

本法是用具有补益肝肾作用的药物组成方剂,以消除肝肾亏虚证候而达到明目作用的治法,适用于肝肾不足的眼病。常见症状如:症状较轻,病程较长,易反复发作的慢性外障眼病及眼底病后期,有退行性变化的内障眼病。全身兼有腰膝酸软,失眠健忘,男子遗精,女子月经不调,舌红少苔,脉细无力等,皆可用本法治疗。

本法忌用于实证,湿邪未尽者慎用。

十、软坚散结法

本法是用具有化痰软坚散结作用的方药来治疗眼病的方法。适用于各种内外障眼病中出现痰湿互结,气血凝滞而成为有形之物者。常见症状如:胞睑肿核,眼内机化条索及陈旧性渗出,白睛结节隆起等,可用本法消散之。

属气血凝滞者,须配伍理气活血药物;属痰湿互结者,须配伍祛湿化痰药。

1. 3. 1. 11　Method of Relieving Nebula to brighten eyes prove Visual Acuity

This is a unique ophthalmic method to treat corneal nebula with nebula-relieving drugs so that the vision can be improved. The method is applicable to corneal nebula.

The clinical application of the method should be classified into different stages. For corneal disorders at the beginning which are usually caused by exopathic wind and heat and manifest dispersing stellate nebula, redness and lacrimation, the treatment principle is to dispel wind and remove heat compatibly with some nebula-relieving drugs. When pathogenic wind-heat is being relieved, the treatment should gradually turn to relieving nebula to improve the vision. In the late course of the disease, when the pathogenic factor is removed but the healthy qi is weak and the corneal nebula is remained, consideration must be given to strengthening healthy qi by properly adding some tonic drugs to invigorate qi, blood, liver and kidney according to the patient's condition.

Because the black part of eye (cornea) is related with liver, the treatment method should certainly include the function of removing liver heat and calming liver. Owing to their nebula-removing action, liver-calming drugs can be compatibly used.

For the corneal nebula at the late stage, the treatment should mainly remove the nebula with drugs not too cold and cool in property to avoid having qi and blood stagnated and pathogenic factors retentively accumulated. Otherwise it may be difficult to cure the disease. If, in a long course, the nebula becomes an old one or cataract, it is impossible to cure with drugs. Therefore, time is very important in the treatment of corneal nebula with drugs

十一、退翳明目法

本法是用具有退翳作用的方药以消退黑睛翳障,而达到明目作用的眼科独特治法。适用于黑睛生翳者。

运用本法须有层次,黑睛病初起,属外感风热,表现为星翳散在,红赤流泪,治以疏风清热为主,配伍少量退翳药;若风热渐减,则应逐渐过渡至退翳明目为主,病后期,邪气已退,而正气已虚,黑睛遗留翳障,则须兼顾扶正,结合全身病情,酌加益气养血或补益肝肾之品。

黑睛属肝,不少清肝、平肝、疏肝药物多有退翳作用,故可配伍应用。

黑睛生翳后期,以退翳为主,用药不可过于寒凉,以免气血凝滞,邪气冰伏,翳不易退,若宿翳已久,光滑如瓷,为气血已定,用药则难以消散;故退翳必须抓紧时机,及时辨证用药。

based on the syndrome differentiation.

1.3.2　External Therapies

1.3.2.1　Eye-dropping Method

This is a treatment method by applying drugs directly into the eye to remove redness, swelling, itching and nebula, or for the mydriasis or miosis purposes. It is applicable to the external oculopathy in the parts of eyelids, bulbar conjunctiva, cornea and canthi and to some internal ocular diseases. Eye drops, medicinal powder and ointment are the common agents used in the method.

1.3.2.1.1　Eye Drops

The prescribed drugs are made into a kind of liquid agent. In the application, the patient is advised to look upwards and the doctor, with the dropper or dropping bottle in his right hand, opens the patient's lower lids with his left hand, applies one to two drops of the liquid into the inner canthus or below the cornea, and then, with the lower lids free, lifts the upper lids at the same time so that the liquid can be well-distributed in the eye. Finally, the patient closes his eye for several minutes. The method is applied 3 to 4 times a day, or more times in a very severe case.

1.3.2.1.2　Eye Powder

The prescribed drugs are made into a kind of very fine powder. In the process, the doctor gently opens the patient's eyelids with his fingers and applies into the patient's inner canthus a small amount of the powder (half or one sesame-seed size) which is dipped with the smooth end of a sterilized glass rod soaked in the normal saline. Then the patient is asked to close his eyes with a cool but no irritant sensation as the limit. Finally, the acupoint

第二节　外治法

一、点眼药法

本法是将药物直接点入眼部,用来消红肿,止痛痒,除翳膜,放大或缩小瞳孔。适用于胞睑、白睛、黑睛、两眦部位的外障眼病及部分内障眼病,常用的有眼药水,眼药粉及眼药膏三种。

(一)点眼药水

将药物配成水剂应用,滴时令患者双目上视,医生用左手向下拉开下睑,右手持滴管或滴瓶,将药水滴入大眦角或白睛下方1～2滴,然后轻轻将上睑提起,并同时放松下睑,使药液充分均匀地分布于眼内,轻轻闭目数分钟,一般每日3～4次。对于病情急重者,次数可以增加。

(二)点眼药粉

将药物制成极为细腻的粉末后应用。用时用消毒的小玻璃棒光滑头部沾生理盐水后,再蘸药粉约半粒到一粒芝麻大小,医生用手指轻轻分开患眼胞睑,将药物轻轻放置于大眦角处,令患者闭目,以有清凉而无刺激感为度。点

Yuwei (Extra) is pressed several times by the patient himself so that the circulation of qi and blood is effectively improved. After a few minutes, the patient gently opens his eyes. The method is applied twice or three times a day.

1.3.2.1.3 Eye Ointment

The prescribed drugs are made into a kind of ointment and a small amount of it is squeezed out and applied to the affected part of the eyelid or below the white of the eye and inside the lower lid. Then with the lower eyelid gently raised by the doctor, the patient is asked to close his eye slowly and the eyelid is softly robbed with a cotton ball for 2 to 3 minutes (no robbing in the case of corneal nebula). And the ointment can also be applied with a glass rod, i.e. when the patient is closing his eye, the glass rod with the ointment is slowly drawn out in the canthus direction without touching the black surface of the eye in case the cornea might be injured. The method is performed three times a day or once before sleeping.

1.3.2.2 Fumigation-Washing Method

Fumigation is a treatment method to fumigate the affected part of the eye with the steam of the hot boiled decoction while the washing method is to bath the ill eye with the filtrated liquid of a decoction. Usually the method is applied first by fumigating and then by washing the eye, which, as a whole, is called fumigation-washing method. It is applicable to external oculopathy with symptoms of redness and swelling of eyelid, photophobia and astringing pain, hyperemia of bulbar conjunctiva and massive eye secretion. By using the warm action of the decoction, the method has the function to improve the circulation of qi and blood in the eye so that the pathogenic factors and stagnation can be removed. Besides, because of the direct

毕,患者用手按鱼尾穴数次,以助气血流行。闭目数分钟后,渐渐睁眼即可。一般每日2～3次。

(三) 涂眼药膏

将药物配成膏剂应用。用时将药膏挤出少许,置于胞睑皮肤患处或眼内白睛下方,下睑内面,轻轻拉提下睑后,令患者轻轻闭眼,用棉球轻轻按揉胞睑2～3分钟即可(黑睛生翳者,不用按揉)。也可用玻璃棒点药,在患者闭目时,将玻璃棒徐徐自眦角方向抽出,每日3次或临睡前用1次,抽玻璃棒时,切勿在黑睛表面擦过,以防擦伤黑睛。

二、薰洗法

薰法是用药液煮沸后的热气蒸腾上薰眼部;洗法是将煎剂滤清后淋洗患眼。一般多是先薰后洗,合称薰洗法,适用于胞睑红肿,羞明涩痛,白睛红赤,眵泪较多的外障眼病。本法除利用药液的温热作用,使眼部气血流畅,能疏邪导滞外,还可通过不同的药物,直接作用于眼部,达到疏通经络,退赤消肿,敛泪止痒等效果。

effect of different drugs on the affected part of the eye, it can dredge the meridian to relieve redness and swelling and to arrest tears and itching.

　　Clinically the decoction for fumigation-washing method is prepared, according to the ocular diseases, by decocting the properly prescribed drugs or by boiling again the dregs of an oral decoction. Before the treatment, a cover is made for the medicinal earth-ware pot or the container of the decoction with a hole (two for both eyes) which is the same size of the patient's orbit. When the decoction is ready, the pot or the container is covered with the cover and then the sick eye (or eyes) is fumigated on the hole in the cover. In the cases of eyeball troubles, frequent nictitation is necessary and, in the cases of eyelid diseases, the eye can be closed during the fumigation.

　　During the washing treatment, the eye can be bathed or washed with the antiseptic gauze or sterilized cotton ball soaked with normal saline. Or with his head bowing, the patient first puts his orbit closely on a sterilized eyecup which contains the washing solution, and then raises his head, frequently nictitates and moves the eyeball so that the eye may be thoroughly bathed. The bath is continued for 20 minutes each time and twice or three times a day.

　　The temperature for the fumigation should neither be too high in order to avoid the ocular scald nor too low to lose the treating effect. The washing solution must be filtrated in case the fine drugs enter the eye to cause uncomfortable sensation. At the same time, all the containers, cotton balls, gauze and fingers must be sterilized and, in particular, special attention must be paid to the treatment of ulcerative nebula of cornea. Patients with new bleeding and malignant boils in the eye should not use the treatment.

　　临床上根据不同病情,选择适当的药物煎成药汁,也可将内服药渣再煎水作成薰洗剂。使用前,在煎药锅或盛药液的器皿上作一盖板,盖上开一洞,洞口大小与眼眶范围大小一致,双眼患病可开两个相同的洞,药物煎毕,用盖板覆盖在药锅或盛药器皿口上,将患眼置于洞口薰之。如属眼珠病患,薰时要频频瞬目,使药力达到病所;如胞睑疾患,薰时闭目即可。

　　洗眼时,可用消毒纱布或消毒棉球渍水,不断淋洗眼部;亦可用消毒眼杯盛药液半杯,先俯首,使眼杯与眼窝紧紧靠贴,然后仰首,并频频瞬目,转动眼珠,进行眼浴,每日2～3次,每次20分钟。

　　薰眼蒸气温度不宜过高,以免烫伤,但也不宜过冷而失去治疗作用;洗剂必须过滤,以免药渣入眼,引起不适。同时,一切器皿、棉球、纱布及手指必须消毒,尤其是黑睛有陷翳者,用洗法时更须慎重,眼部有新鲜出血或患有恶疮者,忌用本法。

1.3.2.3 Irrigation Method

1.3.2.3.1 Irrigation of Conjunctival Sac

This is a method directly to irrigate the conjunctival sac with clean water or the liquid of a decoction in order to remove the secretion, foreign bodies and chemical substances in the conjunctival sac. It is applicable to diseases of bulbar conjunctiva with foreign bodies and massive secretion and can be used for preoperative preparation and emergency treatment of chemical injury of the eye.

Procedure: The irrigation is done with an undine or a piece of rubber tube attached to a pendent bottle loaded with normal saline or medicinal liquid. If the patient takes a sitting position, he is asked to hold his head a little backward and the water or drug container closely touches his cheek and, if he takes a lying position, he is ordered to divert his head a little to the sick eye and the container closely touches the front part of his ear. Then the eyelids are gently opened and the irrigation starts slowly from the lower eyelid to the intraocular part. At the same time, the patient is asked to open his eyes and moves the eyeball so as to enlarge the irrigation area. In the cases of massive eye secretion or with a foreign body on the conjunctiva, the eyelids are turned up to expose the inner part of the upper lid and the conjunctiva part of the superior fornix for a thorough irrigation. When the irrigation is finished, the eye is dried with the antiseptic gauze and the container is taken away.

1.3.2.3.2 Irrigation of Lacrimal Passage

This is a method to irrigate the lacrimal passage with the normal saline or medicinal lotion and is often used to detect the lacrimal condition and remove the accumulated secretion in the lacrimal sac. It is applicable to epiphora, chronic dacryocystitis and the routine preparation of intraocular

三、冲洗法

（一）结膜囊冲洗法

用水或中药药液直接冲洗结膜囊，其目的是除去结膜囊内的眼眵、异物和化学性物质等。适用于结膜囊异物、眵泪较多的白睛疾患，术前准备及眼化学伤的急救措施等。

方法：用盛有生理盐水或药液的洗眼壶或吊瓶的胶管来冲洗，冲洗时，患者如是坐位，头稍后仰，将受水器紧贴颊部；如患者取卧位，令头稍偏向患眼侧，将受水器紧贴耳前皮肤，轻轻拉开胞睑，冲洗液渐渐由下睑皮肤移到眼内，嘱患者睁眼及转动眼珠，以扩大冲洗范围，眼分泌物较多者或结膜有异物者，应翻转上下胞睑，暴露上睑内面及上穹隆部结膜，彻底冲洗。冲洗完毕，用消毒纱布揩干眼周围，然后除去受水器。

（二）泪道冲洗法

是用生理盐水或药液冲洗泪道的方法。它多用来探测泪道是否通畅及清除泪囊中积存的分泌物，适用于泪溢症、慢性泪囊炎及内眼手术前

operation.

　　Procedure：A short cotton stick dipped with the 0.5% to 1% dicaine is inserted between the inner canthi, or the eye is dropped with the 0.5% to 1% dicaine twice. After 2 to 3 minutes, the patient is ordered to hold his head backward and the doctor draws the patient's lower eyelid downwards with his index finger and fixes it on the orbital margin to expose the lower lacrimal punctum. If it is too small, the lacrimal punctum is dilated with a canaliculus dilator. Then the doctor holds in his right hand a syringe which contains 5 to 10 ml normal saline and has a No. 5 or 6 syringe needle curved nearly to a right angle and vertically inserts the needle into the lacrimal punctum 1.5 mm deep, then the needle is turned inward 90° to a horizontal level and pushed towards the nasal side 3 to 5 mm, the irrigating lotion is slowly injected. If there is resistance, the needle should not be inserted with great force.

　　If the lacrimal passage is free, the irrigating lotion may flow from the passage into the nose and out of the nostrils; if the passage is obstructed, the lotion may be totally refluent in the upper and lower lacrimal punctums; if mucopurulent secretion is refluent out from the small lacrimal punctum, chronic lacryocystitis can be decided; if the lacrimal duct is obstructed, the lotion may flow out from the upper lacrimal punctum; if it is a stenosis case of the nasolacrimal duct, there may be some resistance during the irrigation, and most lotion may be refluent from the upper punctum with a little through and drops out of the nostrils.

1.3.2.4　Sickling-washing Method

　　This is a treating method gently to prick or scale the affected part with a filiform needle or materials with the

的常规准备。

　　方法：用蘸有0.5%～1%地卡因溶液的短棉签，夹在大眦头，或用0.5%～1%地卡因液点眼 2 次，约 2～3 分钟后，嘱患者头向后仰，医生左手食指将下睑往下拉，固定于下眶缘部，暴露下泪点。若泪点较小，可先用泪点扩张器扩张之，右手持装有 5～10 ml 生理盐水的注射器，将磨成钝头并弯成近直角的 5～6 号注射针头，垂直插入下泪点约 1.5 mm深，然后向内转 90°成水平位，沿泪小点缓慢向鼻侧推进，再进针 3～5 mm 时，缓缓注入冲洗液，若有阻力，不可用力强行通过。

　　如泪道通畅，冲洗液从泪道流入鼻内，从两侧鼻孔流出；如鼻泪管阻塞，冲洗液全部从上、下泪点返流；若从泪小点返流出黏液脓性分泌物，则为慢性泪囊炎；如泪总管阻塞，冲洗液从上泪点返流；如鼻泪管狭窄，冲洗时有一定阻力，大部分冲洗液从上泪点返流，仅少量冲洗液通过，鼻孔流出水液呈滴状。

四、蔺洗法

　　本法是用锋针或表面粗糙之器物轻刺或轻刮患部然

coarse surface and then to irrigate the wound with normal saline. It can directly remove blood stasis and stagnation of the sick part to relieve noxious pathogen and improve qi and blood circulation. The method is applicable to ocular granular troubles with blood stasis in the eyelids such as granular trachoma, conjunctival folliculosis and follicular conjunctivitis.

Procedure: After the local surface anesthesia by dropping 0.5% to 1% dicaine, the eyelids are turned up and the blood stasis or big rough granules is pricked or scaled with the sterilized filiform needle or materials like cuttlebone rod specially prepared till mild bleeding occurs. Then the eye is dropped with normal saline or anti-inflammatory eye drops to irrigate the blood stasis. The method can be performed again in two to three days. But caution is that the method should not be used in such condition as hyperemia of bulbar conjunctiva, massive mucopurulent eye secretion and new nebula of the cornea.

后用水冲洗的治法,具有直接对病患处祛瘀消滞,散邪泄毒,疏通气血的作用。适用于胞睑内面有瘀积或有粗糙颗粒的疾患,如沙眼、结膜滤泡症、滤泡性结膜等。

方法:局部滴0.5%～1%地卡因溶液作表面麻醉后,翻转胞睑,以消毒后的锋针或特制的海螵蛸棒之类器物轻刺或轻刮睑内的瘀积或粗大颗粒,以微出血为度,剌毕用生理盐水或消炎眼药水点眼冲洗瘀血,隔2～3日可再施行1次。但要注意,如为白睛暴赤,眵多稠结,黑睛新翳者,不用此法。

1.3.3 Common Oral Drugs in Ophthalmology

第三节 眼科常用内服药

1.3.3.1 Drugs for Removing Wind

一、祛风药

Drugs for removing wind have the effect to dispel pathogenic wind from the body surface to relieve swelling, stop pain and itching, arrest tears and remove nebula, so they are widely used in ophthalmology, especially in the treatment of external oculopathy at the beginning stage.

The common wind-removing drugs in ophthalmology are of two kinds, diaphoretics pungent in flavour and cool in property and diaphoretics pungent in flavour and warm in property.

祛风药具有祛风解表,消肿止痛,止痒敛泪及退翳作用,故在眼科运用较为广泛,尤其是外障眼病的初期。

眼科常用的祛风药有辛凉解表药与辛温解表药两类。

1.3.3.1.1　Diaphoretics Pungent in Flavour and Cool in Property

Drugs of this kind are chiefly indicated for ophthal-mopathy due to pathogenic wind-heat and the common drugs used in clinic are Sangye (*Folium Mori*), Juhua (*Flos Chrysanthemi*), Bohe (*Herba Menthae*), Gegen (*Radix Puerariae*), Chantui (*Periostracum Cicadae*), Chaihu (*Radix Bupleuri*), Manjingzi (*Fructus Viticis*) and so on. All these drugs can expel pathogenic wind-heat to stop itching and pain and remove swelling and redness. Sangye and Juhua have the effect to remove pathogenic wind-heat and liver heat to improve the vision. They are often compatibly used to treat ocular diseases caused by pathogenic wind-heat of liver meridian; Bohe is a common drug to treat oculopathy due to pathogenic wind and heat, and Gegen which acts on the yangming meridian to re-move wind and heat in the meridian is often used to treat oculopathy with pain in the forehead; Chantui can remove pathogenic wind-heat to relieve nebula and arrest itching, so it is often used to treat corneal nebula, blepharitis mar-ginalis and other obvious itching symptoms of eye; Chaihu has the effect of reducing fever, soothing the depressed liver and invigorating the spleen yang, so when compati-bly used with other different drugs, it is often applied to treat corneal nebula due to pathogenic wind-heat or liver heat, ptosis of upper eyelid due to deficiency of the middle energizer, or various internal and external oculopathy due to stagnancy of liver qi.

1.3.3.1.2　Diaphoretics Pungent in Flavour and Warm in Property

Drugs of this kind are chiefly indicated for ophthal-mopathy due to pathogenic wind-cold and the common drugs used in clinic are Jingjie (*Herba Schizonepetae*), Qianghuo (*Rhizoma seu Radix Notopterygii*), Fangfeng

（一）辛凉解表药

该类药主治风热眼病。常用药有桑叶、菊花、薄荷、葛根、蝉蜕、柴胡、蔓荆子等。此类药有疏散风热，止痒止痛，清利头目，消肿退赤的作用。桑叶，菊花能疏散风热，清肝明目，二者配伍常应用于肝经风热眼病；薄荷为治疗风热眼病的常用要药，葛根入阳明经，能清阳明经风热，常用于风热眼病兼有前额头痛者；蝉蜕散风热，退翳止痒，故常用于黑睛翳障，睑弦赤烂等目痒症状较明显者；柴胡有解热、疏肝、升提与退翳等作用，故可以通过不同配伍，广泛应用于风热或肝热所致的黑睛翳障，或中气不足所致的上睑下垂及肝气郁结所致的多种内外障眼病。

（二）辛温解表药

该类药主治风寒眼病。常用药有荆芥、羌活、防风、藁本、细辛、白芷等。此类药有发散风寒，消肿止痛，止痒退

(*Radix Ledebouriae*), Gaoben (*Rhizoma et Radix Ligustici*), Xixin (*Herba Asari*), and Baizhi (*Radix Angelicae Dahuricae*). These drugs have the effect of dispersing pathogenic wind-cold to subdue swelling, stop pain and itching and remove nebula. The drugs Jingjie, Qianghuo and Fangfeng can be very effective in dispersing wind to stop pain and itching and removing nebula and are often used compatibly to treat ophthalmalgia, headache, unbearable itching of eye and conjunctivitis caused by exopathic wind-cold; Qianghuo has a better effect in treating ophthalmagia due to pathogenic wind-dampness; Gaoben, the action of which is to disperse pathogenic wind and cold and can reach the vertex, is often used together with other wind-eliminating drugs to treat the cases due to exopathic wind and cold with pain in the vertex; Xixin, with a very strong effect of stopping pain, is often used to treat ophthalmopathy due to pathogenic wind-cold with severe ophthalmolgia and headache but its application should not last long; Baizhi, pertaining to yangming meridian, can relieve pain and lacrimation and is usually used to treat the cases due to exopathic wind and cold with headache and massive tears.

1.3.3.2 Heat-clearing Drugs

Heat-clearing drugs which are cold or cool in property have the effect to relieve swelling and pain by removing redness and detoxicating and are chiefly used to treat various ophthalmopathy of heat types caused by noxious heat and pathogenic fire which invade the eye. The common drugs for heat-removing are classified as heat-clearing and detoxicating drugs, heat-clearing and fire-purging drugs, viscera-purging and heat-clearing drugs, heat-clearing and vision-improving drugs and heat-clearing and blood-cooling drugs.

翳的作用。荆芥,羌活,防风的祛风止痛和止痒退翳作用强,三药常配伍应用于外感风寒所致的目痛头痛、目痒难忍、目赤生翳、羌活更擅长于风湿眼痛;藁本发散风寒,善达头顶,故对外感风寒眼病兼头顶痛者,常以之与其他祛风药配伍同用效果更好;细辛止痛作用尤强,故风寒眼病,头目疼痛剧烈者,常用本药祛风止痛,但不宜久用;白芷入阳明经,有镇痛止泪作用,多用于外感风寒而头痛多泪者。

二、清热药

清热药性寒凉,具有退赤解毒,消肿止痛作用,适用于热毒火邪上攻于目所引起的各种热证眼病。常用的清热药分为清热解毒药,清热泻火药,通腑泄热药,清热明目药和清热凉血药等。

1.3.3.2.1 Heat-clearing and Detoxicating Drugs

Drugs of this kind are chiefly indicated for ophthalmopathy of the excessive heat type due to all sorts of pathogenic noxious heat. The common drugs used in clinic are Jinyinhua（*Flos Lonicerae*）, Lianqiao（*Fructus Forsythiae*）, Daqingye（*Folium Isatidis*）, Banlangen（*Radix Isatidis*）, Zihuadiding（*Herba Violae*）, Pugongying（*Herba Taraxaci*）and so on.

1.3.3.2.2 Heat-clearing and Fire-purging Drugs

Drugs of this kind are mainly indicated for ophthalmopathy due to excessive pathogenic heat. The common drugs used in clinic include Longdancao（*Radix Gentianae*）, Huanglian（*Rhizoma Coptidis*）, Huangqin（*Radix Scutellariae*）, Huangbai（*Cortex Phellodendri*）, Shanzhizi（*Radix Dittospori*）, Shigao（*Gypsum Fibrosum*）, Zhimu（*Rhizoma Anemarrhenae*）, Sangbaipi（*Cortex Mori*）, Danzhuye（*Herba Lophatheri*）and so on. Among them, Longdancao, which can remove excessive pathogenic heat of the liver and spleen, is often used to treat corneal disorders due to fire hyperactivity of the liver; Huanglian purges heart fire and irritability and is used to treat blepharitis angularis or canthal redness; Huangqin and Sangbaipi can purge lung fire and are used to treat hyperemia of bulbar conjunctiva; Huangbai purges kidney fire, disperses deficient fire and controls ministerial fire, and it is often used compatibly with Zhimu to treat ophthalmopathy caused by yin deficiency and fire hyperactivity, and together with Huanglian and Huangqin to treat ophthalmopathy due to pathogenic damp-heat; Shanzhizi can purge the fire of sanjiao (triple energizer) and is applicable to all types of ophthalmopathy due to excessive heat when combined with other heat-clearing drugs; Shi-

（一）清热解毒药

该类药主治一切热毒引起的实热证眼病。常用药有金银花、连翘、大青叶、板蓝根、紫花地丁、蒲公英等。

（二）清热泻火药

该类药主治邪热炽盛的眼病。常用药有龙胆草、黄连、黄芩、黄柏、山栀子、石膏、知母、桑白皮、淡竹叶等。其中龙胆草清肝胆实热，常用于肝火上炎所致的黑睛疾患；黄连泻心火，清心除烦，可用于眦帷赤肿痛或两眦红赤；黄芩、桑白皮泻肺火，多用于白睛红赤；黄柏泻肾火，可用于清虚火，制相火，临床常用黄柏与知母配伍以清虚热、滋肾阴，治疗阴虚火旺眼病，与黄连、黄芩配伍治疗湿热眼病；山栀子泻三焦之火，与其他清热药相配，可用于各种实热眼病；石膏、知母泻胃火，可用于胞睑红肿与黄液上冲；淡竹叶清心火，利小便，用于胬肉红赤，两眦红赤等。

gao and Zhimu purge stomach fire and are used to treat palpebral edema and hypopyon; Danzhuye can remove heart fire and induce diuresis and is used to treat pterygium and canthal redness.

1.3.3.2.3 Viscera-Purging and Heat-clearing Drugs

Drugs of this kind is chiefly indicated for redness, swelling and pain of eye and tears with mucopurulent secretion due to sthenia of yangming fu-organ and internal heat affection of the eye. The common drugs are Dahuang (*Radix et Rhizoma Rhei*) and Mangxiao (*Natrii Sulphas*) and so on.

1.3.3.2.4 Heat-clearing and Vision-improving Drugs

The common drugs of this kind are Xiakucao (*Spica Prunellae*), Juemingzi (*Semen Cassiae*), Qingxiangzi (*Semen Celosiae*), Mimenghua (*Flos Buddlejae*), Muzeicao (*Herba Equiseti Hiemalis*) and so on. Xiakucao reduces stagnant fire from the liver and gallbladder, applicable to the treatment of ocular redness, swelling and pain due to hyperactivity of liver-fire. Combined with Xiangfu, it can treat pain of the eye due to liver stagnation. Qingxiangzi and Juemingzi clear the liver and improve eyesight. Mimenghua expels wind-heat, nourishes the liver and moistens dryness. They can be used to treat eye disorders of both deficiency and excess syndromes, especially the disorder caused by heat resulting from deficiency of the liver and kidney. Muzeicao disperses wind-heat, removes cataract and improves eyesight.

1.3.3.2.5 Heat-clearing and Blood-cooling Drugs

Drugs of this kind are mainly indicated for ophthalmopathy caused by heat invasion of blood, especially for bleeding due blood heat and sudden diminution of vision.

（三）通腑泻热药

该类药主治阳明腑实，里热上攻引起的目赤肿痛，眵泪胶粘。常用药有大黄、芒硝等。

（四）清热明目药

常用药有夏枯草、决明子、青葙子、密蒙花、木贼草等。夏枯草泻肝胆郁火，用于肝火所致目赤肿痛，眼底出血，配伍香附还可治肝郁目痛；决明子、青葙子清肝明目；密蒙花祛风热，养肝润燥，不论虚实眼病皆可用，肝肾阴亏有热者更为适宜；木贼草能疏风热，退翳明目。

（五）清热凉血药

该类药主治热入营血所致的眼病，尤其是血热妄行，视力骤降者。常用药有生地

The common drugs used clinically are Shengdihuang (*Radix Rehmanniae*), Mudanpi (*Cortex Moutan Radicis*), Xuanshen (*Radix Scrophulariae*), Chishaoyao (*Radix Paeoniae Rubra*), Zicao (*Radix Arnebiae seu Lithospermi*) and so on. The drugs Mudanpi and Chishaoyao can remove heat by cooling blood and activate blood circulation to relieve blood stasis; Shengdihuang and Xuanshen remove heat by cooling blood and nourish yin to promote body-fluid production; Zicao is better for heat-clearing and blood-cooling.

1.3.3.3 Tonic Drugs

Since most ophthalmopathy cases of asthenia types are usually caused by deficiency of qi and blood or of the liver and kidney, the common ophthalmic tonic drugs are clinically classified as qi and blood tonics, and liver and kidney tonics.

1.3.3.3.1 Qi and Blood Tonics

1. Qi Tonics

Drugs of this kind are applicable to sleepy eyelids and chronic nebula. The common drugs used in clinic are Huangqi (*Radix Astragali seu Hedysari*), Baizhu (*Rhizoma Atractylodis Macrocephalae*), Dangshen (*Radix Codonopsis Pilosulae*), Shanyao (*Rhizoma Dioscoreae*) and so on.

2. Blood Tonics

Drugs of this kind are applicable to dry sensation of eye, dizziness and night blindness due to deficiency of blood. The common drugs used in clinic are Shudihuang (*Radix Rehmanniae Praeparata*), Baishaoyao (*Radix Paeoniae Alba*), Danggui (*Radix Angelicae Sinensis*), Heshouwu (*Radix Polygoni Multiflri*), Sangshenzi (*Fructus Mori*), Ejiao (*Colla Corii Asini*), Guiyuanrou (*Arillus Longan*) and so on.

黄、牡丹皮、玄参、赤芍药、紫草等。牡丹皮、赤芍药清热凉血,活血化瘀;生地黄、玄参清热凉血,养阴生津;紫草偏于凉血解毒。

三、补益药

眼病之虚证,多属气血不足或肝肾不足,眼科补益药中以益气养血及补益肝肾药较为常用。

(一)益气养血药

1. 益气药

该类药适用于气虚所致的胞睑乏力,常欲闭垂及陷翳不愈等症。常用药有黄芪、白术、党参、山药等。

2. 养血药

该类药适用于血虚所致的眼干涩昏花,夜盲等。常用药有熟地黄、白芍药、当归、何首乌、桑椹子、阿胶、桂圆肉等。

1.3.3.3.2 Liver and Kidney Tonics

Drugs of this kind are applicable to internal and external oculopathy due to asthenia of the liver and kidney. The common drugs used in clinic are Gouqizi (*Fructus Lycii*), Nüzhenzi (*Fructus Ligustri Lucidi*), Tusizi (*Semen Cuscutae*), Chushizi (*Frucuts Broussonetiae*), Duzhong (*Cortex Eucommiae*), Hanliancao (*Herba Ecliplae*), Fupenzi (*Fructus Rubi*), Shudihuang (*Radix Rehmanniae Praeparata*) and so on. Among them, Gouqizi, which nourishes the liver and kidney and replenishes vital essence to improve eyesight, is widely used to treat internal and external oculopathy caused by deficiency of the liver and kidney; Nüzhenzi, nourishing liver and kidney yin, is good at treating internal heat due to yin asthenia and is often used compatibly with Hanliancao to treat ocular bleeding at the early stage because of their joint action of cooling blood and stopping bleeding; Tusizi tonifies the liver and kidney to improve the vision; Chushizi reinforces liver and kidney to improve eyesight; Fupenzi tonifies the liver and kidney to reinforce vital essence to improve the vision; Duzhong, which nourishes the liver and kidney to strengthen bones and muscles, is widely used in a compatible way to treat internal oculopathy caused by asthenia of the liver and kidney with lassitude in loins and legs or listlessness and weakness; Shudihuang has a stronge action of nourishing yin and is often used to treat internal ocular diseases due to yin deficiency but should cautiously be applied to the cases with asthenia of the spleen and stomach, for it is moist and greasy in nature.

1.3.3.4 Drugs for Eliminating Dampness

Ophthalmopathy caused by pathogenic dampness is quite common in clinic. Drugs for eliminating dampness

(二) 补益肝肾药

该类药适用于肝肾不足之内外障眼病。常用药有枸杞子、女贞子、菟丝子、楮实子、杜仲、旱莲草、覆盆子、熟地黄等。枸杞子滋补肝肾,益精明目,广泛用于肝肾不足引起的内外障眼病;女贞子滋养肝肾之阴,善治阴虚内热,与旱莲草配伍,滋阴凉血止血,常用于眼内出血的早期;菟丝子补益肝肾,明目;楮实子平补肝肾,养肝明目;覆盆子补肝肾,固精明目;杜仲补肝肾,强筋骨,通过配伍可以广泛用于肝肾不足内障眼病兼有腰膝酸痛或萎软无力者;熟地黄滋阴力较强,故阴虚内障眼病常用之。

熟地黄滋腻,脾胃虚弱者当慎用。

四、祛湿药

湿邪所致眼病较为多见,祛湿药能收湿敛疮,退肿去翳

can astringe pathogenic dampness to treat ulcer, swelling and nebula and are widely used in ophthalmic treatment. However, they must be cautiously applied to the cases due to deficiency of yin and blood or consumption of body fluids. The common drugs of this group include two kinds: aromatic drugs for resolving dampness and drugs for inducing diuresis and excreting dampness.

1.3.3.4.1　Aromatic Drugs for Resolving Dampness

　　Drugs of this kind are applicable to ophthalmopathy caused by internal retention of pathogenic dampness. The common drugs used in clinic are Huoxiang (*Herba Agastachis*), Peilan (*Herba Eupatorii*), Cangzhu (*Rhizoma Atractylodis*), Shichangpu (*Rhizoma Acori Craminei*), Baidoukou (*Semen Amomi Rotundus*), Sharen (*Fructus Amomi*) and so on. The drugs Huoxiang and Peilan, which can relieve dampness by diaphoretic and regulate the middle energizer to resolve turbidity, are often used together to treat internal and external oculopathy caused by exopathic dampness or damp obstruction of spleen and stomach; Cangzhu astringes dampness by invigorating spleen and is used to treat palpebral ulcer, nebula and retinal edema, and it can treat nyctalopia due to liver asthenia when decocted with pig liver; Shichangpu which is aromatic can remove dampness and improve vision by resuscitation; Baidoukou and Sharen have the effect of regulating qi, drying dampness and warming the middle energizer and are often used to treat ocular disorders due to damp retention in the spleen and stomach.

1.3.3.4.2　Drugs for Inducing Diuresis and Excreting Dampness

　　Drugs of this kind are used for the treatment of ocular troubles resulting from the upward attack of dampness

明目,故在眼科应用也很广泛,但阴虚血少或津液已伤当慎用。常用的祛湿药有芳香化湿药与利水渗湿药两类。

（一）芳香化湿药

　　该类药适用于湿浊内阻所致的眼病。常用药有藿香、佩兰、苍术、石菖蒲、白豆蔻、砂仁等。藿香、佩兰发表祛湿以和中化浊,两药往往同用,治疗外感湿邪或湿困脾胃所致的内外障眼病。苍术燥湿健脾,用于胞睑赤烂,翳膜遮睛,视网膜水肿等,与猪肝同煮,可治肝虚雀目;石菖蒲芳香化浊,开窍明目;白豆蔻、砂仁有理气燥湿温中作用,常用于眼病兼有湿邪阻滞脾胃证候者。

（二）利水渗湿药

　　该类药适用于水湿上泛或湿热薰蒸所致的眼病。常

or pathogenic damp-heat. The common drugs used in clinic include Fuling (*Poria*), Zhuling (*Polyporus*), Zexie (*Rhizoma Alismatis*), Cheqianzi (*Semen Plantaginis*), Yiyiren (*Semen Coicis*), Huashi (*Talcum*), Chixiaodou (*Semen Phaseoli*), Mutong (*Caulis Aristolochiae Manshuriensis*) and so on. Among the drugs, Fuling and Yiyiren excrete dampness and induce diuresis by invigorating spleen and are used to treat ophthalmopathy caused by excessive dampness due to spleen asthenia; Zhuling, with the stronger effect of inducing diuresis and excreting dampness, can treat ocular edema, especially severe retinal edema when compatibly used with Fuling; Zexie, besides its effect of inducing diuresis and excreting dampness, can purge the pathogenic damp-heat of kidney and bladder and is compatibly used with Cheqianzi and Zhuling to treat ophthalmopathy due to damp retention or pathogenic damp-heat; Cheqianzi, which also has the effect of removing liver heat to improve eyesight, is compatibly used with other liver-heat-removing drugs to treat ocular redness, swelling and nebula due to hepatical heat; Huashi, which induces diuresis, excretes dampness and removes pathogenic heat and summer-heat, is used to treat ocular diseases due to pathogenic damp-heat; Chixiaodou, inducing diuresis to remove swelling and detoxicating to evacuate pus, can not only treat retinal edema but also cure ocular ulcer and furuncle when it is compatibly used with other heat-clearing and detoxicating drugs; Mutong can remove heat and induce diuresis and is good at removing the pathogenic heat of heart and small intestine, so it is compatibly used with Zhuye, Huanglian and Shengdihuang to treat ophthalmopathy due to dampness and heat manifesting canthal redness, aphthous stomatitis, yellowish urine and a reddish tip of the tongue.

用药有茯苓、猪苓、泽泻、车前子、薏苡仁、滑石、赤小豆、木通等。茯苓、薏苡仁健脾渗湿利水,用于脾虚湿泛眼病;猪苓淡渗利湿作用较强,可与茯苓配伍应用,用于眼部组织水肿,尤其是视网膜水肿严重者;泽泻利水渗湿,且能泄肾与膀胱之湿热,与车前子、猪苓配伍,可用于水湿滞留或湿热眼病;车前子还能清肝明目,故凡肝热所致红肿翳膜,亦可用车前子配伍其他清肝药同用;滑石利水渗湿,清热解暑,一般用于湿热眼病;赤小豆利水消肿,解毒排脓,既可用于视网膜水肿,亦可配伍清热解毒药治疗胞睑疮疖;木通清热利湿,擅长于清利心与小肠邪热,故湿热眼病,有两眦部红赤、口舌生疮、尿黄、舌尖红等现象者,可用木通配竹叶、黄连、生地黄等药。

1.3.3.5 Blood-regulating Drugs

Drugs of this kind are used for the treatment of oph-thalmopathy caused by suffusion, blood stasis, blood heat and blood asthenia. For suffusion cases, the treatment should be to arrest bleeding, for blood stasis to activate blood circulation, for blood heat to cool blood, and for blood asthenia to tonify blood. As blood-cooling drugs and blood tonics are mentioned in the heat-clearing and tonic drugs above, hemostatic drugs and drugs for promoting blood circulation and removing blood stasis are to be dis-cussed here.

1.3.3.5.1 Hemostatic Drugs

These drugs are applicable to hemorrhagic ophthal-mopathy. Since their hemostatic effects are different by cooling, by astringing and by removing stasis, the com-mon hemostatics in ophthalmology should be carefully cho-sen in clinic according to the hemorrhagic causes.

Cooling Hemostatics: They are used to treat hemor-rhagic syndromes of bleeding due to blood heat, and the common drugs are Daji (*Herba seu Radix Cirssi Japoni-ci*), Xiaoji (*Herba Cephalanoploris*), Cebaiye (*Cacumen Biotae*), Baimaogen (*Rhizoma Imperatae*), Diyu (*Radix Sanguisorbae*), Huaihua (*Flos Sophorae*) and so on.

Astringing Hemostatics: They are used to treat oph-thalmopathy with new hemorrhagia and traumatic bleed-ing, and the common drugs are Baiji (*Rhizoma bletel-lae*), Xueyutan (*Crinis Carbonisatus*), Xianhecao (*Herba Agrimoniae*), Oujie (*Nodus Netamoinis Rhizo-matis*) and so on.

Stasis-removing Hemostatics: They are used to treat the cases of bleeding due to blood-stasis and the common drugs are Sanqi (*Radix Notoginseng*), Puhuang (*Pollen Typhae*), Qiancao (*Radix Rubiae*), Huaruishi (*Ophi-

五、理血药

该类药适用于因血溢、血瘀、血热、血虚所致的眼病。血溢者宜止血,血瘀者宜活血,血热者宜凉血,血虚者宜补血。凉血药和补血药在清热药和补益药中已有介绍,这里仅介绍止血药和活血化瘀药。

(一) 止血药

该类药适用于出血性眼病。眼科常用的止血药,其作用有凉血止血,收敛止血和祛瘀止血的不同,故临证时当根据出血原因选择使用。

凉血止血药:适用于血热妄行的出血证。常用药有大蓟、小蓟、侧柏叶、白茅根、地榆、槐花等。

收敛止血药:适用于眼病的新出血及外伤出血。常用药有白及、血余炭、仙鹤草、藕节等。

化瘀止血药:适用于血瘀而致出血者。常用药有三七、蒲黄、茜草、花蕊石等。

calcitum) and so on.

1.3.3.5.2 Drugs for Promoting Blood Circulation and Removing Blood Stasis

Drugs of this kind are used to treat ophthalmopathy caused by stagnancy of qi and blood and are often applied together with drugs to promote qi circulation. The common drugs are Taoren (*Semen Persicae*), Honghua (*Flos Carthami*), Danshen (*Radix Salviae Miltiorrhizae*), Chuanxiong (*Rhizoma Ligustici Chuangxiong*), Liujilu (*Herba Artemisiae Anomalae*), Zelan (*Herba Alismatis*), Wangbuliuxing (*Semen Vaccariae*), Ruxiang (*Resina Olibani*), Moyao (*Myrrha*), Chishaoyao (*Radix Paeoniae Rubra*), Mudanpi (*Cortex Moutan Radicis*), Sumu (*Lignum Sappan*), Jixueteng (*Caulis Spatholobi*) and so on.

1.3.3.6   Drugs for Regulating Qi

Drugs of this kind are used to treat ophthalmopathy caused by disorder of qi, most of which are pungent in flavour and warm in property, can easily consume qi and yin and should be cautiously used in the case of yin asthenia syndromes. The common drugs for regulating qi are classified into two groups: the drugs for relieving liver and regulating qi and the drugs for promoting qi circulation to remove stagnancy.

1.3.3.6.1   Drugs for Relieving Liver and Regulating Qi

Drugs of this kind are used to treat ophthalmopathy due to stagnancy of liver qi. The common drugs used in clinic are Chaihu (*Radix Bupleuri*), Xiangfu (*Rhizoma Cyperi*), Qingpi (*Pericarpium Citri Reticulatae Viride*), Chuanlianzi (*Fructus Meliae Toosendan*), Yujin (*Radix Curcumae*), Foshou (*Fructus Citri Sarcodactylis*) and so on.

（二）活血化瘀药

该类药适用于气滞血瘀所致的眼病,常与行气药同用。常用药有桃仁、红花、丹参、川芎、刘寄奴、泽兰、王不留行、乳香、没药、赤芍药、牡丹皮、苏木、鸡血藤等。

六、理气药

该类药适用于气机失调所致眼病。理气药多辛温发散,易耗气伤阴,故阴虚者慎用。常用的理气药有疏肝理气药与行气导滞药两种。

（一）疏肝理气药

该类药适用于肝气郁结的眼病。常用药有柴胡、香附、青皮、川楝子、郁金、佛手等。

1.3.3.6.2　Drugs for Promoting Qi Circulation to Remove Stagnancy

Drugs of this kind are used to treat ophthalmopathy caused by qi stagnancy of spleen and stomach. The common drugs used in clinic are Chenpi (*Pericarpium Citri Reticulatae*), Muxiang (*Radix Auklandiae*), Zhishi (*Fructus Aurantii Immaturus*), Houpo (*Cortex Magnoliae Officinalis*), Wuyao (*Radix Linderae*), Binglang (*Semen Arecae*), Chenxiang (*Lignum Aquilariae Resinatum*) and so on.

1.3.3.7　Drugs for Dissipating Mass

Drugs of this kind have the effect of removing blood stasis and mass or removing stagnant food to improve appetite. In the course of ocular disorders, they can compatibly used to treat lumps, nodules and scars caused by stagnancy of qi and blood and by accumulated phlegm. The common drugs in clinic are Kunbu (*Thallus Laminariae*), Haizao (*Sargassum*), Walengzi (*Concha Arcae*), Xiakucao (*Spica Prunellae*), Beimu (*Bulbus Fritillariae*), Muli (*Concha Ostreae*), Sanleng (*Rhizoma Sparganii*), Ezhu (*Rhizoma Zedoariae*), Haigeke (*Concha Meretricis seu Cyclinae*), Haifushi (*Pumex*) and so on.

1.3.3.8　Drugs of Removing Nebula to Improving Vision

Drugs of this kind can dispel wind and heat, remove hepatical heat, calm liver and relieve nebula to improve the vision. The common drugs used in clinic are Chantui (*Periostracum Cicadae*), Qinpi (*Cortex Fraxini*), Gujingcao (*Flos Eriocauli*), Muzeicao (*Herba Equiseti Hiemalis*), Mimenghua (*Flos Buddlejae*), Shijueming (*Concha Haliotidis*), Baijili (*Fructus Tribuli*), Qingxiangzi (*Semen Celosiae*), Zhenzhumu (*Concha Marga-*

（二）行气导滞药

该类药适用于脾胃气滞的眼病。常用药有陈皮、木香、枳实、厚朴、乌药、槟榔、沉香等。

七、软坚散结药

该类药具有祛瘀软坚或消导积滞的作用，凡在眼病过程，出现气血凝滞，痰瘀互结的肿块，结节及瘢痕等，均可配伍软坚散结药。常用药有昆布、海藻、瓦楞子、夏枯草、贝母、牡蛎、三棱、莪术、海蛤壳、海浮石等。

八、退翳明目药

该类药具有疏散风热，清肝平肝，退翳明目作用。常用药有蝉蜕、秦皮、谷精草、木贼草、密蒙花、石决明、白蒺藜、青葙子、珍珠母、蛇蜕、海螵蛸等。

ritifera Usta）, Shetui（*Periostracum Serpentis*）, Hai-
piaoxiao（*Os Sepiella seu Sepiae*）and so on.

　　Chantui, Qinpi, Gujingcao and Mimenghua are applicable to nebula due to pathogenic wind and heat, and Shijueming, Baijili, Zhenzhumu and Qingxiangzi are applicable to nebula due to hepatical heat. When compatibly
used, they are all used widely in clinic to treat various
new and old nebulas.

　　蝉蜕、秦皮、谷精草、密蒙
花,宜用于风热翳障;石决明、
白蒺藜、珍珠母、青葙子宜用
于肝热翳障。退翳药通过配
伍,可以广泛用于各种新
老翳。

2 Discussion of Specific Diseases

2.1 Eyelid Disorders

各 论

第一章　胞睑
疾病

2.1.1 Hordeolum

[Introduction]

Hordeolum is a kind of acute inflammatory infection of the glands of the eyelids. If the infection occurs in the eyelid glands, it is called internal hordeolum and, if in the eyelash follicle or in the appendix glands of Moll or Zeis, it is called external hordeolum. Clinically the disease mainly manifests the symptoms of swelling, pain and induration in the infected part of the eyelids. It is common in children and young people and attacks repeatedly.

In most cases, hordeolum is caused by Staphylococcus aureus.

From its clinical manifestations, the disease should pertain to Zhenyan (needle eye) in traditional Chinese medicine. Its exopathic cause is the invasion of pathogenic wind-heat, and it is internally associated with the heat accumulation in spleen and stomach or with the weak and debilitated physique. The main pathogenesis of the disease is that the pathogenic factor invades the eyelid causing qi and blood to stagnate in the eye.

[Main Diagnostic Points]

1. External Hordeolum

At the early stage, redness, swelling and pain occur

第一节　麦粒肿

【概述】

麦粒肿是一种常见的眼睑腺急性化脓性炎症。如为眼睑腺感染,称为内麦粒肿;如为睫毛毛囊或其附属腺体 Moll 或 Zeis 腺感染,则称为外麦粒肿。本病主要临床表现为眼睑患部皮肤红肿、疼痛、有硬结。本病多见于青少年,易反复发作。

本病多为金黄色葡萄球菌感染。

根据本病的临床表现,当属于中医学"针眼"范畴。其外因为风热外邪的侵入,内因与脾胃积热、素体虚弱有关。主要病机为邪气上攻胞睑,气血壅滞。

【诊断要点】

1. 外麦粒肿

初起睑缘部皮肤红肿疼

in the skin of the palpebral margin with obvious tenderness, and induration in shape of a ripe wheat-seed may be palpated. If the condition is mild, all the symptoms may disappear themselves in a few days. If the condition is severe, there may appear in 3 to 5 days a yellow pus head. When the pus head ruptures by itself, the pain may be alleviated, and the soreness and swelling will soon subside.

2. Internal Hordeolum

The clinical manifestations of internal hordeolum are not so severe as those of external one. Severe symptoms of the external canthus, however, may lead to ocular chemosis or even give rise to the prominence of bulbar conjunctiva out of the palpebral fissure. The surface of the palperbral conjunctiva is red or purple and prominent, with a yellow and white pus head in the middle. When the pus head ruptures itself from the conjunctiva and the pus is excreted, the condition of the disorder may be eased.

[Syndrome Differentiation and Treatment]

The treatment of the disease, in principle, is to remove, with the pus being immature, heat and swelling so as to relieve or dissipate pus while, with the pus being mature, the treatment should be to accelerate the pus to rupture itself or excrete it by operation. For patients with the remaining pathogens unrelieved, spleen and stomach being weak, and pathogenic qi invading the eyelid, the principle of the treatment is to remove the remaining pathogens, strengthen spleen and nourish qi.

1. Syndrome of Pathogenic Wind-heat Invasion of Eyelid

Main Symptoms and Signs　Local slight redness, swelling and itching of the eyelid with a palpable induration at the initial stage, often accompanied by headache and fever; thin yellowish tongue coating and floating-rapid pulse.

痛,压痛明显,在近睑缘部可触及硬结,形似麦粒。轻者数日内可自行消散,重者3～5日后,局部出现黄色脓点,脓头可自行溃破排脓,疼痛缓解,红肿消退。

2. 内麦粒肿

其临床表现不如外麦粒肿严重。外眦部的重症内麦粒肿可引起球结膜水肿,甚至突出于睑裂之外。睑结膜面呈红色或紫红色隆起,中心部有黄白色脓点,脓头自结膜面自行溃破后脓液排出,症状减轻。

【辨证论治】

对本病的治疗,原则上未成脓者,应退热消肿,促其消散;已成脓者,当促其溃脓或切开排脓。对于余邪未清,脾胃虚弱而邪气客胞睑者,可清余热,健脾益气治之。

1. 风热客睑证

主要证候　病初起,胞睑局部微有红肿痒痛,可触及硬结。常伴有头痛、发热、舌苔薄黄,脉浮数。

Therapeutic Method　Removing pathogenic wind-heat.

Recipe　The Modified Yinqiaosan Decoction：Jinyin-hua（*Flos Lonicera*）10 g, Lianqiao（*Fructus Forsythiae*）10 g, Bohe（*Herba Methae*, decocted later）6 g, Jingjie（*Herba Schizonepetae*）10 g, Lugen（*Rhizoma Phragmitis*）15 g, Zhuye（*Folium Phyllostachydis henonis*）10 g, and Gancao（*Radix Glycyrrhizae*）3 g.

Modification　For cases with severe pathogenic wind, 10 g of Sangye（*Folium Mori*）and 10 g of Juhua（*Flos Chrysanthemi*）are added；for cases with severe pathogenic heat, Jingjie is removed and more Jinyinhua and Lianqiao are applied plus 10 g of Huangqin（*Radix Scutellariae*）；if the infection is in the canthus, 6 g of Huanglian（*Rhizoma Coptidis*）is used；and if the pain is serious, 6 g of Zhiruxiang（*Rhizoma Olibani*）and 6 g of Moyao（*Myrrha*）are added.

2. Syndrome of Pathogenic Heat Invasion of Eye

Main Symptoms and Signs　Local redness, swelling and severe pain in the eyelid, larger palpebral induration with a burning sensation, tender pain and a visible yellow-white pus head, often accompanied with fever, thirst, constipation and yellowish urine；yellowish tongue coating and rapid pulse.

Therapeutic Methods　Removing noxious heat and purging fire.

Recipe　The modified Huanglian Jiedu Decoction：Huanglian（*Rhizoma Coptidis*）6 g, Huangqin（*Radix Scutellariea*）10 g, Huangbai（*Cortex Phellodendri*）10 g, Pugongying（*Herba Taraxaci*）15 g, Zihuadiding（*Herba Violae*）15 g, Danggui（*Radix Angelicae Sinensis*）10 g, and Mudanpi（*Cortex Moutan Radicis*）10 g.

Modification　In the cases with constipation, 6 g of Dahuang（*Radix et Rhizoma Rhei*）is added；for cases

治　法　清热祛风。

方　药　银翘散加减。常用药：金银花 10 g，连翘 10 g，薄荷（后下）6 g，荆芥 10 g，芦根 15 g，竹叶 10 g，甘草 3 g。

加　减　风重者，加桑叶 10 g，菊花 10 g；热重者，去荆芥，重用金银花、连翘，加黄芩 10 g；位于眦部者，加黄连 6 g；疼痛较重者，加制乳香 6 g，没药 6 g。

2. 热毒攻目证

主要证候　胞睑局部红肿，疼痛剧烈，睑硬结较大，灼热疼痛拒按，可见黄白色脓点。常伴有发热、口渴、便秘、溲黄、苔黄、脉数等症。

治　法　清热泻火解毒。

方　药　黄连解毒汤加减。常用药：黄连 6 g，黄芩 10 g，黄柏 10 g，蒲公英 15 g，紫花地丁 15 g，当归 10 g，牡丹皮 10 g。

加　减　大便干结者，加大黄 6 g；口渴欲饮者，加天花

with thirsty feeling, 10 g of Tianhuafen (*Radix Trichosandis*) is added; 6 g of Zhiruxiang (*Resina Olibani*) and 6 g of Moyao (*Myrrha*) are applied in the cases with the local eyelid being purple and dark; and if the pus is not ruptured, 10 g of Chuanshanjia (*Squama Manitis*) and 6 g of Zaojiaoci (*Spina Gleditsiae*) are used.

3. Syndrome of Latent Pathogenic Heat in Spleen and Stomach

Main Symptoms and Signs　Mild redness, swelling and pain in the eyelid and a small induration which does not rupture for a long time or ruptures without any healing.

Therapeutic Method　Strengthening healthy qi to eliminate pathogen.

Recipe　The modified Tuoli Xiaodusan Decoction: Huangqi (*Radix Astragali seu Hedysari*) 15 g, Chuangxiong (*Rhizoma Ligustici Chuanxiong*) 10 g, Danggui (*Radix Angelicae Sinensis*) 10 g, Baizhu (*Rhizoma Atractylodis Macrocephalae*) 10 g, Fuling (*Poria*) 10 g, Zaojiaoci (*Spina Gleditsiae*) 6 g, Jinyinhua (*Flos Lonicerae*) 10 g, Huangqin (*Radix Scutellariea*) 10 g, Fangfeng (*Radix Ledebouriellae*) 6 g, and Shenggancao (*Radix Glycyrrhizae*) 3 g.

Modification　If the redness and swelling is obvious, 15 g of Pugongying (*Herba Taraxaci*) and 10 g of Lianqiao (*Fructus Forsythiae*) are added.

4. Syndrome of Asthenia of Spleen and Stomach

Main Symptoms and Signs　Common attack in children with redness, swelling and mild pain of the eyelid, a small induration and easy recurrence, accompanied by dim complexion, hypodynamia, anorexia and loose stool; pale tongue and thin pulse.

Therapeutic Methods　Strengthening the spleen and nourishing qi with pathogen-removing adjuvants.

粉10 g;局部紫暗者,加制乳香6 g,没药6 g;有脓未溃者,加穿山甲10 g,皂角刺10 g。

3. 脾胃伏热证

主要证候　胞睑红肿疼痛较轻,硬结较小,久不溃破或溃后久不敛口。

治　法　扶正祛邪。

方　药　托里消毒散加减。常用药:黄芪15 g,川芎10 g,当归10 g,白术10 g,茯苓10 g,皂角刺6 g,金银花10 g,黄芩10 g,防风6 g,生甘草3 g。

加　减　红肿明显者,加蒲公英15 g,连翘10 g。

4. 脾胃虚弱证

主要证候　多见于小儿,胞睑红肿,疼痛轻微,硬结较小,但易反复。常伴面色少华,乏力纳呆,大便不实,舌淡脉细。

治　法　健脾益气,佐以祛邪。

Recipe The Modified Shenling Baizhusan Decoction: Dangshen (*Radix Codonopsis Pilosulae*) 10 g, Baizhu (*Rhizoma Atractylodis Macrocephalae*) 10 g, Fuling (*Poria*) 10 g, Chenpi (*Pericarpium Citri Reticulatae*) 10 g, Shanyao (*Rhizoma Dioscoreae*) 10 g, Yiyiren (*Semen Coicis*) 15 g, Fangfeng (*Radix Ledebouriellae*) 6 g, Danggui (*Radix Angelicae Sinensis*) 10 g, Jingjie (*Herba Schizonepetae*) 6 g, Lianqiao (*Fructus Forsythiae*) 10 g, and Jinyinhua (*Flos Lonicerae*) 10 g.

Modification For the dyspeptic cases, Shenqu (*Massa Fermentata Medicinalis*) 10 g, Shanzha (*Fructus Crataegi*) 10 g, Maiya (*Fructus Hordei Germinatus*) 10 g and Jineijin (*Endothelium Corneum Gigeriae Galli*) 6 g are added and, for those with stagnant pathogenic heat, 10 g of Zhimu (*Rhizoma Anemarrhenae*) and 10 g of Huangqin (*Radix Scutellariea*) are added.

[Other Treatments]

1. Chinese Patent Drugs

(1) Yinqiao Jiedu Tablet 4 tablets each time, three times a day and applicable to the syndrome of pathogenic wind-heat invasion of eyes.

(2) Yiqing Capsule 2 capsules each time, three times a day and applicable to the syndrome of noxious heat invasion of eyelid.

(3) Huanglian Shangqing Pill 6 g each time, twice a day and applicable to the syndrome of stagnation of pathogenic wind-heat and noxious fire.

(4) Xiangsha Liujun Pill 6 g each time, twice a day and applicable to the syndrome of asthenia of spleen and stomach.

2. Simple and Proved Recipes

(1) 9 g powder of Shengnanxing (*Rhizoma Arisaematis*) and 15 g of Xianshengdihuan (*Radix Rehmanniae*) are pounded into the plastic form which is pasted on

方　药　参苓白术散加减。常用药：党参10 g，白术10 g，茯苓10 g，陈皮6 g，山药10 g，薏苡仁15 g，防风6 g，当归10 g，荆芥6 g，连翘10 g，金银花10 g。

加　减　消化不良者，加神曲10 g，山楂10 g，麦芽10 g，鸡内金6 g；兼郁热者加知母10 g，黄芩10 g。

【其他疗法】

1. 中成药

（1）银翘解毒片　每服4片，每日3次。适用于风热客睑证。

（2）一清胶囊　每服2片，每日3次。适用于热毒攻目证。

（3）黄连上清丸　每服6 g，每日2次。适用于风热火毒壅滞证。

（4）香砂六君丸　每服6 g，每日2次。适用于脾胃虚弱证。

2. 单验方

（1）生南星末9 g，鲜生地黄15 g。共捣烂为膏，贴太阳穴。适用于早期麦粒肿。

the acupoint of Taiyang (*EX-HN*15). The method is applicable to hordeolum at the initial stage.

(2) The decoction consists of 30 g of Jinyinhua (*Flo Lonicerae*) and 60 g of Pugongying (*Herba Taraxaci*), both of which are decocted with water for 15 to 30 minutes. The decocted solution is orally taken in the morning and evening. Then the dregs of the decoction are put into 500 ml water and heated till it is boiling. Finally the hot decoction is used to fume and wash the infectious eye several times every day. The method is applicable to hordeolum patients with severe redness, swelling and pain.

(3) Pugongying (*Herba Taraxaci*) 60 g and Yejuhua (*Flos chrysanthemi Indici*) 15 g, both drugs are decocted with water one dose a day. The first decocted solution is taken orally and the second one is used to fume and wash the sick eye several times every day. The method is applicable to the symptoms of pain, redness and swelling of the eyelid caused by hordeolum.

(4) The beverage includes the drugs of Jinyinhua (*Flos Lonicerae*) 12 g, Juhua (*Flos Chrysanthemi*) 15 g, Zihuadiding (*Herba Violae*) 10 g, Pugongying (*Herba Taraxaci*) 10 g, Lianqiao (*Fructus Forsythiae*) 10 g, and Baizhi (*Radix Angelicae Dahuricae*) 10 g, all of which are decocted with water one dose a day. The decoction is applicable to the syndrome of noxious heat invasion of the eye.

3. External Therapies

(1) Damp-heat Compress: For initial hordeolum or cases without suppuration, this hot-moistening compress is applied to the affected eye with hot water or the hot solution from the dregs of the oral decoction.

(2) The infectious eye is frequently smeared with the realgar powder mixed with vinegar.

（2）金银花30 g,蒲公英60 g。煎15～30分钟,将药液分2次服。再次药渣加500 ml水煮沸,待温后薰洗患眼,每日数次。适用于麦粒肿红肿、疼痛较甚者。

（3）蒲公英60 g,野菊花15 g。水煎服,每日1剂,头煎内服,第二煎薰洗患眼,每日数次。适用于本病眼睑疼痛、红肿。

（4）金银花12 g,菊花15 g,紫花地丁10 g,蒲公英10 g,连翘10 g,白芷10 g。水煎服,每日1剂。适用于本病心脾热毒上攻证。

3. 外治法

（1）湿热敷疗法：适用于早期或未酿脓者,可用热水或内服药渣再煎水作湿热敷。

（2）醋调雄黄粉频涂患部皮肤。

（3）For hordeolum at the initial stage, a proper amount of Pugongying (*Herba Taraxaci*) is pounded and compressed on the sick part of the eye.

（4）Xiedu Plaster for External Dressing　The plaster is made up of following drugs: Chuandahuang (*Radix et Rhizoma Rhei*) 90 g, Muxiang (*Radix Aucklandiae*) 30 g, Xuanshen (*Radix Scrophulariae*) 60 g, Bailian (*Radix Ampelopsis*) 60 g, Shegan (*Rhizoma Belamcandae*) 60 g and Mangxiao (*Natrii Sulphas*) 60 g. All the drugs are ground to powder which is made into plastic form with the egg white. The plaster is compressed on the hordeolum and changed when it is dry.

（5）The Chinese patent drug Zijinding, when mixed with vinegar, is compressed on the affected part.

2.1.2　Blepharitis

[Introduction]

Blepharitis is a kind of chronic inflammation of the lid-margins. Clinically, it shows the manifestations of hyperemia of the lid-margins, scales or tiny scattering pustules at the lash roots, and is characteristically classified into three kinds: blepharitis squamosa, blepharitis ulcerosa and blepharitis angularis. In most cases, both eyes are attacked and it is rather difficult to cure. The case may recur and become severe and mild alternately.

The cause of squamous blepharitis, though uncertain at present, is concerned with the functional hypersecretion of the tarsal glands, for, in the affected part of the lid-margins, oval furfuraceous bacillus can be often found, which may decompose the lipid substances into an irritable fatty acid. Ametropia, anthenopia, malnutrition, and a long-time use of unqualified cosmetics may be the predisposing cause of

（3）鲜蒲公英适量,捣烂后敷在患处,适用早期麦粒肿。

（4）协毒膏外敷:川大黄90 g,木香30 g,玄参、白敛、射干、芒硝各60 g。以上诸药共研为散,以鸡子白调如膏状,敷贴眼睑长麦粒肿处,药干即换之。

（5）紫金锭醋调敷患部。

第二节　睑缘炎

【概述】

睑缘炎是发生在眼睑边缘部分的一种慢性炎症。临床主要表现为睑缘充血潮红,睫毛根部附有鳞屑或散在小脓疱。按其临床特点可分为鳞屑性、溃疡性和眦部睑缘炎三种。多为双眼发病,病情较为顽固,时轻时重,或易反复发作。

鳞屑性睑缘炎的病因尚不十分清楚,与睑板腺分泌功能过度旺盛有关,患部常可找到卵圆皮屑芽胞菌,它可能把脂类物质分解为有刺激性的脂肪酸。屈光不正、视疲劳、营养不良或长期使用劣质化

the disease. Ulcerative blepharitis, an acute or subacute suppurative inflammation of the ciliary follicles and their accessory glands, is usually caused by the infection of the golden staphylococci or transformed from squamous blepharitis having been infected. Angulary blepharitis is a chronic inflammation mainly occurring in the canthi, and it is usually caused by the inflection of Morax-Axenfeld bacillus or is associated with the deficiency of riboflavin.

Clinically all the conditions of the disease is separately called in traditional Chinese medicine "Jianxuan Chilan", "Lanxuanfeng", and "Ziwei Chilan". The cause of the disease is closely related with the pathogenic wind, dampness and heat. Internally, the pathogenic dampness and heat is accumulated in spleen and stomach, and externally there is the invasion of pathogenic wind. The combat and combination of both the internal and external pathogenic fators gives rise to the stagnation of wind, dampness and heat in the lid-margins, thus causing the disease. The onset of angulary blepharitis is also associated with internal hyperactivity of heart fire and pathogenic wind-fire which burns and damages the lid-margins and canthi. Since wind hyperactivity can give rise to itching, damp hyperactivity to ulceration, and heat hyperactivity to redness, the disease is clinically characterized with itching, ulceration and redness.

[Main Diagnostic Points]

1. Clinical Manifestations

Local itching, ulceration, redness and pain of the lid-margin are basic characteristics of the disease. Nevertheless, it shows different types because its main symptoms and affected parts are different.

(1) Blepharitis squamsa Hyperemia of palpebral

妆品等也可能是本病的诱因。溃疡性睑缘炎是睫毛毛囊及其附属腺体的慢性或亚急性化脓性炎症,多由金黄色葡萄球菌感染所致;亦可由鳞屑性睑缘炎遭受感染后转变而成。眦部睑缘炎是一种主要侵犯眦部睑缘的慢性炎症,多由莫-阿双杆菌感染所致,或与核黄素缺乏有关。

根据本病的临床表现,当属于中医学"睑弦赤烂"、"烂弦风"、"眦帷赤烂"等病范畴。其病因常与风、湿、热三邪关系密切。内因脾胃湿热蕴积,外因风邪侵袭,内外合邪,以致风、湿、热三邪搏结,郁滞于睑弦发为本病。眦部睑缘炎的发病还与心火内盛,风火上炎,灼伤睑眦有关。风胜则痒,湿胜则烂,热胜则赤,所以该病以痒、烂、红赤为特征。

【诊断要点】

1. 临床表现

睑缘局部以痒、烂、红、痛为基本特征。又因主症与部位的不同,故有不同的类型。

(1) 鳞屑性睑缘炎 睑

margin, adherent squamae at the eyelash base, easy loss and regeneration of eyelash.

(2) Blepharitis ulcerosa Hyperemia of palpebral margin, yellow crusts at the eyelash base, ulceration or bleeding or pyorrhea of the palpebra margin after the crusts being removed, easy loss of eyelash without regeneration because of the base injury.

(3) Blepharitis angularis Hyperemia, swelling and erosion of the outer canthus with a strong subjective itching; at severe stages, the whole canthus being involved.

2. Laboratory Examination

Usually diagnosis can be decided according to clinical manifestations, and the staphylococcus aureus or Morax-Axenfeld bacillus found in the Bacteriological examination may be helpful for the diagnosis.

[**Syndrome Differentiation and Treatment**]

In clinical practice, the disease is classified as the syndromes of severe wind-heat pathogenic factor, severe damp-heat and hyperactivity of heart fire. The basic treatment of the disease should be put on relieving wind, heat and dampness, accompanied by the external applications of eye lotions and ointments.

1. Syndrome of Severe Wind-heat

Main Symptoms and Signs Redness and swelling of the palpebral margin with urticant and burning sensation, tightened and unsmooth lid-margin which is serious when confronting with wind, chaff-like desquamation at the ends of eyelash; thin whitish or thin yellowish tongue coating and floating rapid pulse.

Therapeutic Method Removing wind and heat to arrest itching.

Recipe The modified Siwu Decoction: Lianqiao (*Fructus Forsythiae*) 10 g, Bohe (*Herba Men thae*, to be decocted later) 5 g, Jingjiesui (*Spica Schizonepetae*)

缘充血,睫毛根部有鳞屑附着,睫毛易脱落但可再生。

（2）溃疡性睑缘炎 睑缘充血,睫毛根部有黄色痂皮,清除痂皮后,可见睑缘溃烂,或出血,或溢脓,因睫毛根部破坏,故睫毛易落,且不能再生。

（3）眦部睑缘炎 外眦睑缘充血、肿胀、糜烂,自觉奇痒。严重时内外眦皆可波及。

2. 实验室检查

通常根据临床表现可以作出诊断,若进行细菌学检查,可以查到金黄色葡萄球菌或莫-阿双杆菌。

【辨证论治】

本病临床主要分为风热偏重证、湿热偏重证、心火上炎证。治疗以祛风、清热、除湿为基本治法,并可内外兼治,配合药水洗眼及眼膏涂擦。

1. 风热偏重证

主要证候 睑弦红赤,刺痒灼热,睑弦紧涩见风尤甚,睫毛根部有糠皮样脱屑。舌苔薄白或薄黄,脉浮数。

治 法 祛风清热止痒。

方 药 加减四物汤加减。连翘10 g,薄荷(后下)5 g,荆芥穗10 g,防风10 g,牛

10 g, Fangfeng (*Radix Ledebouriellae*) 10 g, Niubangzi (*Fructus Arctii*) 10 g, Shengdihuang (*Radix Rehmanniae*) 10 g, Tianhuafen (*Radix Trichosanthes*) 15 g, Kushen (*Radix Sophorae Flavescentis*) 10 g, Chuanxiong (*Rhizoma Ligustici Chuanxiong*) 6 g, Danggui (*Radix Angelicae Sinensis*) 10 g, and Chishaoyao (*Radix Paeoniae Rubra*) 10 g.

Modification For cases with severe moist ulceration of palpebral margin, 10 g of Difuzi (*Fructus Kochiae*) and 10 g of Baixianpi (*Cortex Dictamni Radicis*) are added; for those with severe red lid-margin, 10 g of Jinyinhua (*Flos Lonicerae*) and 15 g of Pugongying (*Herba Taraxaci*) are added.

2. Syndrome of Severe Damp-heat

Main Symptoms and Signs Redness and ulceration of lid-margins with a bleeding of yellow liquid or purutant blood, crust piling, tears with mucopurulent secretion, alternate pain and itching, sometimes with trichiasis and loss of eyelash; reddish tongue with yellowish and greasy coating and soft-rapid pulse.

Therapeutic Method Removing heat and damp.

Recipe The modified Chushi Decoction: Huangqin (*Radix Scutellariea*) 10 g, Huanglian (*Rhizoma Coptidis*) 5 g, Huashi (*Talcum*) 10 g, Cheqianzi (*Semen Plantaginis*, bagged) 15 g, Mutong (*Caulis Aristolochiae Manshuriensis*) 6 g, Fuling (*Poria*) 12 g, Lianqiao (*Fructus Forsythiae*) 10 g, Fangfeng (*Radix Ledebouriellae*) 10 g, Jingjie (*Herba Schizonepetae*) 10 g, Zhike (*Fructus Aurantii*) 10 g, Chenpi (*Pericarpium Citri Reticulatae*) 10 g, and Gancao (*Radix Glycyrrhizae*) 3 g.

Modification For cases with bleeding, 10 g of Chishaoyao (*Radix Paeoniae Rubra*) and 10 g of Mudanpi (*Cortex Moutan Radicis*) are added; if the itching is se-

蒡子10 g,生地黄10 g,天花粉15 g,苦参10 g,川芎6 g,当归10 g,赤芍药10 g。

加　减　睑弦湿烂甚者,加地肤子10 g,白鲜皮10 g;睑弦红赤重者,加金银花10 g,蒲公英15 g。

2. 湿热偏重证

主要证候　睑弦红赤溃烂,黄水溢出或脓血交加,痂块堆积,眵泪胶粘,痒痛并作,或见倒睫,睫毛脱落。舌质红,苔黄腻,脉濡数。

治　法　清热除湿。

方　药　除湿汤加减。黄芩10 g,黄连5 g,滑石10 g,车前子(包煎)15 g,木通6 g,茯苓12 g,连翘10 g,防风10 g,荆芥10 g,枳壳10 g,陈皮10 g,甘草3 g。

加　减　伴有出血者,加赤芍药10 g,牡丹皮10 g;痒甚者,加苦参10 g,地肤子10 g,

rious, 10 g of Kushen (*Radix Sophorae Flavescentis*), Difuzi (*Fructus Kochiae*) and Baixianpi (*Cortex Dictamni Radicis*) are added respectively.

3. Syndrome of Hyperactivity of Heart Fire

Main Symptoms and Signs　Swelling and pain of the canthal margins with a burning and unbearable itching which is relieved by rubbing, bleeding and erosion of the canthus in a serious condition accompanied by small vesicles in the mouth and tongue sometimes; reddish tongue with yellowish coating and a rapid pulse.

Therapeutic Method　Removing pathogenic heart fire.

Recipe　The modified Daochi Powder and Huanglian Jiedu Decoction: Shengdihuang (*Radix Rehmanniae*) 10 g, Mutong (*Caulis Akebiae*) 5 g, Zhuye (*Folium Phyllostachydis Henonis*) 10 g, Gancaoshao (*Apex Radicis Glycyrrhizae*) 3 g, Huangqin (*Radix Scutellariae*) 10 g, Huanglian (*Rhizoma Coptidis*) 5 g, Huangbai (*Cortex Phellodendri*) 10 g, and Shanzhizi (*Fructus Gardeniae*) 10 g.

Modification　If the canthal itching is severe, 10 g of Baijili (*Fructus Tribuli*) and 10 g of Baizhi (*Radix Angelicae Dahuricae*) are added; if the canthal redness and ulceration is severe, 10 g of Chishaoyao (*Radix Paeoniae Ruba*) and 10 g of Mudanpi (*Cortex Moutan Radicis*) are added; if erosion and itching of the canthus is severe, 10 g of Difuzi (*Fructus Kochiae*), Baixianpi (*Cortex Dictamni Radicis*) and Tufuling (*Rhizoma Smilacis Glabrae*) are added respectively.

［Other Treatments］

1. Chinese Patent Drugs

（1）**Huanglian Shangqing Bolus**　6 g each time, twice every day and applicable to the syndrome of severe wind-heat.

白鲜皮10 g。

3. 心火上炎证

主要证候　眦部眼睑红赤疼痛,灼热奇痒,喜揉擦,甚者眦部睑弦破裂出血、糜烂,兼见口舌生疱,小便赤热。舌红,苔黄,脉数。

治　法　清心泻火。

方　药　导赤散合黄连解毒汤加减。生地黄10 g,木通5 g,竹叶10 g,甘草梢3 g,黄芩10 g,黄连5 g,黄柏10 g,山栀子10 g。

加　减　眦部发痒甚者,加白蒺藜10 g,白芷10 g;眦部赤烂甚者,加赤芍药10 g,牡丹皮10 g;眦角糜烂、发痒甚者,加地肤子10 g,白鲜皮10 g,土茯苓10 g。

【其他疗法】

1. 中成药

（1）**黄连上清丸**　每服6 g,每日2次。适用于风热偏重证。

(2) Xiaofeng Granule   10 g each time, twice every day and applicable to the syndrome of severe wind-heat.

(3) Fangfeng Tongsheng Pill   6 g each time, twice every day and applicable to the syndrome of severe wind-heat.

(4) Sanmiao Pill   5 g each time, twice every day and applicable to the syndrome of severe damp-heat.

(5) Daochi Pill   3 g each time, twice every day and applicable to the syndrome of hyperactivity of heart fire.

2. Simple and Proved Recipes

(1) Yejuhua (*Flos Chrysanthemi Indici*) 15 g and Huanglian (*Rhizoma Coptidis*) 5 g, both of the drugs, when double bagged with gauze, are boiled in 500 ml water for 30 minutes and the liquid is filtered. The decoction dregs are boiled again with water for 30 minutes and the second liquid is filtered. The mixture of the first and second liquids is filtered several times, with the clear liquid concentrated to 300 ml for later use. The affected part of the eye is first washed with cotton by absorbing the concentrated liquid and then applied with the liquid for 20 minutes three times every day. The method is applicable to the syndrome of severe damp-heat pathogen.

(2) Yiyiren (*Semen Coicis*) 24 g, Huangqin (*Radix Scutellariae*) 10 g, Caozhizi (*Fructus Gardeniae*) 10 g, all the drugs are decocted with water twice and the decoction is orally taken in the morning and evening. The recipe is applicable to the syndrome of severe damp-heat.

(3) The white of an egg, when thoroughly mixed, is smeared on the affected part with a writing brush, 5 to 6 times every day. The method can remove heat and pathogenic toxin to stop itching and is applicable to the syndrome of severe wind-heat pathogen.

（2）消风冲剂　每服10 g,每日 2 次。适用于风热偏重证。

（3）防风通圣丸　每服6 g,每日 2 次。适用于风热偏重证。

（4）三妙丸　每服5 g,每日 2 次。适用于湿热偏重证。

（5）导赤丸　每服3 g,每日 2 次。适用于心火上炎证。

2. 单验方

（1）野菊花15 g,黄连5 g。将野菊花与黄连放在两层纱布做的袋内,加水500 ml,煮沸半小时,取出药液,过滤。药渣再加水煮沸半小时,滤出药液,将两次药液混合,反复过滤几次,取澄清液,再浓缩到300 ml待用。用棉花蘸药液洗患处,后作湿敷,每日 3 次,每次湿敷 20 分钟。适用于湿热偏重证。

（2）薏苡仁 24 g,黄芩10 g,炒栀子10 g。水煎 2 次取汁,每日 2 次,口服,上、下午各服 1 次。适用于湿热偏重证。

（3）鸡蛋 1 个,轻轻敲开一个小洞,将蛋清取出,充分搅拌,然后用毛笔蘸蛋清涂擦患处,每日5～6 次。可以清热解毒、止痒退肿。适用于风热偏重证。

3. External Therapies

(1) Eye-washing Lotions a. The affected part is washed and fumed twice a day with the liquid by boiling dregs of the oral decoction. Before the washing and fuming, the local crusts and purulence should be cleaned. b. Qianliguang (*Herba Senecionis Scandentis*) 10 g, Baixianpi (*Cortex Dictamni Radicis*) 10 g, Yejuhua (*Flos Chrysanthemi Indici*) 10 g, Pugongying (*Herba Taraxaci*) 15 g, Fangfeng (*Radix Ledebouriellae*) 10 g, Jingjie (*Herba Schizonepetae*) 10 g, all the drugs are decocted with water and, with the decocted liquid, the affected part is washed and fumed twice every day. Before the washing and fuming, the local crusts and purulence should be cleaned. The method is applicable to the syndrome of severe damp-heat.

(2) Eye Ointments The affected part of the eye, with the local crusts and purulence being cleaned, is smeared three times every day with the following mixtures or ointments: a. the ointment made of egg and butter, which is applicable to all kinds of blepharitis ciliaris; b. Verdigris Ointment, which is applicable to all kinds of blepharitis ciliaris; c. the mixture of Babao Eye Ointment and Chlorotetracycline Eye Ointment, which is applicable to all kinds of blepharitis ciliaris; d. Coptidis Ointment, which is applicable to the blepharitis ulcerosa and blepharitis angularis due to hyperactivity of heart fire; e. Ointment of Fel Uris, which is applicable to the blepharitis ulcerosa due to severe damp-heat.

3. 外治法

（1）药水洗眼 ① 内服药渣煎水薰洗，每日薰洗 2 次。薰洗前应清除局部的痂皮或脓液。② 千里光10 g，白鲜皮10 g，野菊花10 g，蒲公英15 g，防风10 g，荆芥10 g。煎水薰洗，每日薰洗 2 次。薰洗前应清除局部的痂皮或脓液。适用于湿热偏重证。

（2）眼膏涂擦 ① 鸡蛋黄油膏涂擦眼睑患部，每日 3 次。涂眼膏前应清除局部的痂皮及脓液。适用于各类型睑缘炎。② 铜绿膏涂擦眼睑患部，每日 3 次。涂眼膏前应清除局部的痂皮及脓液。适用于各类型睑缘炎。③ 八宝眼药加金霉素眼膏，调匀后涂患处。涂眼膏前应清除局部的痂皮及脓液。适用于各类型睑缘炎。④ 黄连膏涂擦眼睑患部，每日 3 次。涂眼膏前应清除局部的痂皮及脓液。适用于心火上炎所致溃疡性睑缘炎、眦角性睑缘炎。⑤ 熊胆眼膏擦眼睑患部，每日 3 次。涂眼膏前应清除局部的痂皮及脓液。适用于湿热偏重之溃疡性睑缘炎。

2.1.3 Trachoma

[Introduction]

Trachoma is a chronic inflammatory ocular disease of conjunctiva and cornea caused by a strain of bacteria Chlamydia trachomatis. In clinic, it mainly shows the symptoms of papillary hyperplasia of palpebral conjunctiva, follicle formation and pannus above the cornea. Its spread has much to do with the patients' health habits, living environment, nutritional and medical conditions, and so on. According to WHO's statistics, trachoma has made 0.36 billion of people in the globe suffering from various visual disorders and at least 2 millions of them have become blindness because of trachoma.

Since the disease is caused by Chlamydia trachomatis, its antigens are the types of A, B, C and Ba.

Clinically, the disease pertains to "Jiaochuang" (*trochomata*) in traditional Chinese medicine. Its exopathic cause is ocular filth and invasion of pathogenic wind-heat, and the endopathic cause is accumulation of pathogenic heat in the spleen and stomach. The key pathogenesis of the disease is that the combination of interior pathogenic heat and toxin accumulates up to the eyelid, which gives rise to stagnated meridians and disorder of qi and blood. Wind, heat and blood stasis form the pathological nature of the disease. Although it occurs in the eyelid, the disease is associated with the conditions of spleen and stomach.

[Main Diagnostic Points]

1. Clinical Manifestation

The uncomfortable feeling is not obvious at the initial stage, and the disease can only be found through somato-

第三节　沙眼

【概述】

沙眼是沙眼衣原体感染引起的一种结膜和角膜的慢性炎症性眼病。临床主要表现为睑结膜乳头增生,滤泡形成,角膜上方有血管翳。其传播与患者的卫生习惯、居住环境、营养状况、医疗条件等因素密切相关。据 WHO 统计,沙眼使世界上约 3.6 亿人发生视力障碍,其中至少有 200 万人因之失明。

本病的病因是由沙眼衣原体感染所致,其抗原型为 A、B、C 或 Ba。

根据本病的临床表现,当属于中医学"椒疮"范畴。外因多为眼部不洁,风热邪毒袭入所致;内因与脾胃蕴热有关。主要病机为内热与邪毒相结,上壅胞睑,脉络瘀滞,气血失和。病理性质为风、热、瘀。病位在胞睑,与脾胃相关。

【诊断要点】

1. 临床表现

早期可无明显不适感觉,仅于体检时才被发现。多数

scopy. In most cases, the subjective symptoms are mild with itching, unsmooth, burning, dry and foreign body sensations in the eye. In a few severe cases, there may appear obvious symptoms of irritability and injury of eyesight to some degrees when accompanied by blepharelosis, trichiasis and corneal ulcer.

2. Ocular Examinations

(1) **Chronic inflammatory changes of conjunctiva** Diffuse congestion of palpebral conjunctiva, hyperplasia and hypertrophy of papillae, formation of follicles and scars (papillae and follicles are the basic injury of trachoma, indicating there exist active pathogenic changes, and the scar is the result of repairing); red and small papillae in clusters, yellowish red or dark red follicles which are large, not transparent, and different in size; and filiform or reticular scars.

(2) **Corneal pannus** Stretching from above the cornea to the superficial transparent area of cornea, the pannus is in the form of curtain-falling which can often be found at the initial stage of trachoma. For the late severe trachoma, neogenetic blood vessels surround the cornea and invade it, even covering the whole cornea. This may greatly affect the vision of a patient.

It is easy to diagnose a typical case of trachoma, but a mild and early one is difficult to determine and can be easily confused with the other corneal disorders because papillae and follicles are not the specific changes of trachoma. According to the Ophthalmology Association of China Association of Medicine, the diagnostic evidences of trachoma should be: a. Obscure vessel congestion of the superior fornix and of the upper palpebral conjunctiva, and papillary hyperplasia or follicular formation, or both of the

沙眼其自觉症状轻微,有痒涩感,异物感,烧灼感或干燥感等症状。少数严重的沙眼,合并有睑内翻,倒睫,角膜溃疡等并发症时,则出现明显刺激症状,视力也可不同程度的受损。

2. 眼部检查

(1) 结膜慢性炎症病变 弥漫性睑结膜充血,乳头增生肥大,滤泡形成及瘢痕。乳头和滤泡为沙眼的基本损害,表示有活动性病变,瘢痕为修复的结果。乳头呈红色、较小而群集。滤泡色黄红或暗红,较大,不透明,形状大小不一。瘢痕为线状或网状。

(2) 角膜血管翳　常由角膜上方伸入角膜透明区,呈垂帘状,位于角膜浅层,且这种改变在沙眼早期就可出现。晚期严重沙眼,其新生血管从角膜四周包围伸入角膜,甚至遍及全角膜,而严重影响视力。

典型的沙眼在临床上容易诊断,轻型早期病例则较困难,易与其他结膜病相混淆,因为乳头滤泡并不是沙眼的特异性改变。中华医学会眼科学会决定,沙眼的诊断依据为: ① 上穹窿部和上睑结膜血管模糊充血,乳头增生或滤泡形成,或二者兼有。② 用

two; b. Cornea pannus in the magnifier or slip-lamp examination; c. Scars in the superior fornix or in the upper palpebral conjunctiva; d. Chlamydi trachomatis on the scaling section of the conjunctiva.

On the basis of the first item, trachoma can be diagnosed if one of the other items exists.

3. Clinical Stages of Trachoma

The Ophthalmology Association of China Association of Medicine classifies trachoma into three stages: Ⅰ. active pathogenic changes (obscure vessel congestion, papillary hyperplasia or follicular formation) in the superior fornix and in the upper eyelid conjunctiva; Ⅱ. active lesions in the conjunctiva and occurrence of scars; Ⅲ. no active lesions, only scars in the conjunctiva. Trachoma at the first and second stages is again divided into mild, moderate and severe cases. In mild cases, the active lesion takes up less than a third of the upper conjunctiva and, in moderate cases, it covers a third to two thirds, and more than two thirds in severe cases.

The diagnosis of trachoma, therefore, should involve the course of the disease and the degrees of the pathogenic changes. Trachoma Ⅰ⁺⁺, for example, means the condition of the disease is a moderate case at the first stage.

[Syndrome Differentiation and Treatment]

In clinical practice, trachoma is classified as the syndromes of wind and heat invasion of eyelid, excessive heat in spleen and stomach, and stagnation of blood heat. Its treatment should include both internal and external meth-

放大镜或裂隙灯显微镜检查可见角膜有血管翳。③上穹窿部或上睑结膜出现瘢痕。④结膜刮片找到沙眼包涵体。

在第一项的基础上,兼有其他三项中之一者可以诊断为沙眼。

3. 沙眼的临床分期

中华医学会眼科学会将沙眼分为三期。第Ⅰ期:上穹窿部和上睑结膜有活动病变(结膜血管模糊充血,乳头增生,滤泡形成)。第Ⅱ期:结膜有活动病变,同时出现瘢痕。第Ⅲ期:结膜仅有瘢痕,而无活动病变。第Ⅰ、Ⅱ期沙眼按病变严重程度又分为轻、中、重三级。轻度者即活动病变占上睑结膜总面积1/3以下。中度者活动病变占上睑结膜面积的1/3~2/3范围。重度者其活动病变占上睑结膜2/3以上。

所以沙眼的诊断应包括其病程的长短及病变的轻重程度。如沙Ⅰ⁺⁺即沙眼的第Ⅰ期中度。

【辨证论治】

本病临床主要分为风热客睑证、脾胃热盛证、血热壅滞证。治疗当内外兼施。轻症可以局部点药为主,重症则

ods. In mild cases, local eye-dropping is the main method while, in severe cases, the basic treatment method, besides the eye-dropping, is the internal therapy of removing pathogenic wind and heat, activating blood circulation and dredging meridian. If necessary, operation should be needed.

除点眼药外,宜配合内治,以疏风清热,活血通络为基本治法。必要时,还可配合手术治疗。

1. Syndrome of Wind and Heat Invasion of Eyelid

Main Symptoms and Signs　Slight itching of the eye with uncomfortable and unsmooth sensation, little dry eye secretion, photophobia, lacrimation, light redness in the conjunctiva with a few red granules, obscure general symptoms; thin tongue coating and floating pulse.

Therapeutic Method　Removing pathogenic wind and heat.

Recipe　The modified Yinqiaosan Decoction: Lianqiao (*Fructus Forsythiae*) 10 g, Jinyinhua (*Flos Lonicerae*) 10 g, Jiegeng (*Radix Platycodi*) 6 g, Niubangzi (*Fructus Arctii*) 10 g, Jingjiesui (*Spica Schizonepetae*) 10 g, Bohe (*Herba Menthae*, to be decocted later) 5 g, Dandouchi (*Semen Sojae Praeparatum*) 10 g, Lugen (*Rhizoma Phragmitis*) 10 g, Zhuye (*Folium Phyllostachydis Henonis*) 10 g, Fangfeng (*Radix Ledebouriellae*) 10 g, Baizhi (*Radix Angelicae Dahuricae*) 10 g, Huangqin (*Radix Scutellariae*) 10 g, Chishaoyao (*Radix Paeoniae Rubra*) 10 g, and Shenggancao (*Radix Glycyrrhizae*) 3 g.

1. 风热客睑证

主要证候　眼部微痒不适,干涩眵少,羞明流泪,睑内微红,有少量红赤颗粒,全身兼症不明显。舌苔薄,脉浮。

治　法　疏风清热。

方　药　银翘散加减。连翘10 g,金银花10 g,桔梗6 g,牛蒡子10 g,荆芥穗10 g,薄荷(后下)5 g,淡豆豉10 g,芦根10 g,竹叶10 g,防风10 g,白芷10 g,黄芩10 g,赤芍药10 g,生甘草3 g。

2. Syndrome of Excessive Heat in Spleen and Stomach

Main Symptoms and Signs　Dry itching and pain of the eye with profuse tears and gum, redness in the conjunctiva with more granules, constipation; reddish tongue with a yellowish coating and a rapid pulse.

Therapeutic Method　Clearing the spleen to disperse pathogenic wind and heat.

2. 脾胃热盛证

主要证候　眼涩痒痛,眵泪胶粘,睑内红赤,颗粒较多,大便秘结。舌红苔黄,脉数。

治　法　清脾泻热,疏风散邪。

Recipe The modified Chufeng Qingpi Decoction: Chenpi (*Pericarpium Citri Reticulatae*) 6 g, Lianqiao (*Fructus Forsythiae*) 10 g, Fangfeng (*Radix Ledebouriellae*) 10 g, Zhimu (*Rhizoma Anemarrhenae*) 10 g, Mangxiao (*Natrii Sulphas*) 10 g, Huangqin (*Radix Scutellariae*) 10 g, Xuanshen (*Radix Scrophulariae*) 10 g, Huanglian (*Rhizoma Coptidis*) 5 g, Jingjie (*Herba Schizonepetae*) 10 g, Dahuang (*Radix et Rhizoma Rhei*) 5 g, Jiegeng (*Radix Platycodi*) 6 g, and Shengdihuang (*Radix Rehmanniae*) 10 g.

Modification In the cases of pathogenic dampness, Kushen (*Radix Sophorae Flavescentis*), Difuzi (*Fructus Kochiae*) and Cangzhu (*Rhizoma Atractylodis*), respective 10 g of each, are added.

3. Syndrome of Stagnation of Blood Heat

Main Symptoms and Signs Stabbing pain in the eye with burning and unsmooth sensation, photophobia, lacrimation, profuse tears and gum, hard swelling eyelid with a heavy falling sensation and difficult to open, obvious redness of the conjunctiva covered with rough granules, trachomatous pannus of cornea, vexation and dryness in the mouth; reddish tongue with yellowish coating and a rapid pulse.

Therapeutic Method Dissipating stasis by cooling blood.

Recipe The modified Guishao Honghuasan Decoction: Danggui (*Radix Angelicae Sinensis*) 10 g, Dahuang (*Radix et Rhizoma Rhei*) 5 g, Shanzhizi (*Fructus Gardeniae*) 10 g, Huangqin (*Radix Scutellariae*) 10 g, Honghua (*Flos Carthomi*) 6 g, Chishaoyao (*Radix Paeoniae Rubra*) 10 g, Baizhi (*Radix Angelicae Dahuricae*) 10 g, Fangfeng (*Radix Ledebouriellae*) 10 g, Shengdihuang (*Radix Rehmanniae*) 10 g, Lianqiao (*Fructus Forsythiae*) 10 g, and Gancao (*Radix Glycyr-

方 药 除风清脾饮加减。陈皮6 g,连翘10 g,防风10 g,知母10 g,芒硝10 g,黄芩10 g,玄参10 g,黄连5 g,荆芥10 g,大黄5 g,桔梗6 g,生地黄10 g。

加 减 兼湿邪者,加苦参10 g,地肤子10 g,苍术10 g。

3. 血热壅滞证

主要证候 眼内灼热刺痛,沙涩羞明,眵多流泪,胞睑肿硬,眼睑重坠难开,睑内红赤明显,颗粒累累,粗糙不平,黑睛赤膜下垂,心烦口干。舌红苔黄,脉数。

治 法 凉血散瘀。

方 药 归芍红花散加减。当归10 g,大黄5 g,山栀子10 g,黄芩10 g,红花6 g,赤芍药10 g,白芷10 g,防风10 g,生地黄10 g,连翘10 g,甘草3 g。

rhizae) 3 g.

[Other Treatments]

1. Chinese Patent Drugs

(1) **Yinqiao Jiedu Tablet**　4 tablets each time, three times a day and applicable to the syndrome of wind and heat invasion of the eyelid.

(2) **Xiaofeng Granule**　10 g each time, twice a day and applicable to the syndrome of wind and heat invasion of the eyelid.

(3) **Huanglian Shangqing Pill**　6 g each time, twice a day and applicable to the syndrome of excessive heat in the spleen and stomach.

(4) **Fangfeng Tongsheng Pill**　6 g each time, twice a day and applicable to the syndrome of excessive heat in the spleen and stomach plus pathogenic wind.

2. Simple and Proved Recipes

Both of 15 g of Gujingcao (*Flos Eriocauli*) and 7 Jujubes are decocted with water for oral administration, one dose a day, which is applicable to the syndrome of wind and heat invasion of the eyelid.

3. External Therapies

(1) **Eye Drops**　a. Coptis and Watermelon-Frost Eye Drops. The eye is dropped three or four times every day for trachoma in mild cases. b. Huatiedan Eye Drops. The eye is dropped three times every day for trachoma in mild and severe cases. c. Xihuangsan Eye Drops. The eye is dropped once or twice every day for trachoma of various syndromes.

(2) **Rubbing Therapy**　The cuttle-bone-rod-rubbing therapy can be used to treat trachoma in severe cases with papillae, follicles and granules of the conjunctiva. Procedure: cut the cuttle-bone with a knife into the duck-billed rod. After sterilizing it in the boiling decoction of coptis

【其他疗法】

1. 中成药

（1）银翘解毒片　每服4片，每日3次。适用于风热客睑证。

（2）消风冲剂　每服10 g，每日2次。适用于风热客睑证。

（3）黄连上清丸　每服6 g，每日2次。适用于脾胃热盛证。

（4）防风通圣丸　每服6 g，每日2次。适用于脾胃热盛兼杂风邪证。

2. 单验方

谷精草15 g，大枣7枚。水煎服，每日1剂。适用于风热客睑证。

3. 外治法

（1）点眼药　① 黄连西瓜霜眼药水点眼，每日点眼3～4次。适用于沙眼轻症者。② 化铁丹眼药水点眼，每日点眼3次。适用于沙眼轻症及重症者。③ 犀黄散点眼，每日点眼1～2次，点于内眦部。适用于沙眼各证。

（2）磨擦法　用海螵蛸棒磨擦法治疗沙眼重症，睑结膜乳头、滤泡较多、颗粒累累者。

方法：将海螵蛸用小刀削

root, take it out and dry up for later use. If Dengxincao (*Medulla Junci*) is used, first cut it to small pieces and sterilize with the above method. In the operation, grip the piece with a pair of tweezers. After the surface anesthesia of the eye to be operated on with 0.5% to 1% of dicaine and the cleaning of the conjunctival sac, turn the upper and lower eyelids from inside out with the operator's left hand to let the fornix be fully exposed, and then, with the operator's right hand holding the cuttle-bone-rod, gently and swiftly rub the part of palpebral conjunctiva covered with granules back and forth for many times till punctate hemorrhage appears. When the rubbing is finished, wash the conjunctival sac with normal saline or antibiotic. Finally smear the eye with some eye ointment. The operation should be performed once every five days, or more times depending on the conditions of the disease.

During the operation, special attention must be paid to the sterilization and the gentle maneuver in order that the cornea might not be injured. If the lesion is severe and extensive, the rubbing therapy is divided into different treatment courses or stages.

(3) Sickle-washing Therapy The sterilized filiform needle is used. Or dried clean Longxucao (*Culmus et Folium Poae Sphondylodis*), soaked for 24 hours in 10% of boiled decoction of coptis root, is prepared for later use. When operating, first drop 0.5% to 1% of dicaine into the eye, then turn with the operater's left hand the upper and lower eyelids from inside out to expose the affected fornix. Stab the granules with the tip of the needle till blood is slightly exuding. Finally drop the eye with some antibiotics when the operation is finished.

Attention must be paid to the sterilization and the

磨成一端成鸭嘴形的小棒。用黄连水煮沸消毒,取出待干备用(若用灯心草,先剪成小段,制法同上,术时用小镊子夹持操作)。术眼点0.5%～1%地卡因液进行表面麻醉,并清洁结膜囊后,用左手分别翻开上、下眼睑,充分暴露穹窿部,右手持海螵蛸棒,以轻快手法来回多次磨擦睑内面颗粒密集处,以点状出血为度。磨擦后用生理盐水或抗生素眼液冲洗结膜囊,并涂眼膏。每隔5日1次,根据病情,可以多次重复进行。

操作时应注意消毒,磨擦时手法不可太重,切不可损伤角膜。病变严重而且广泛时,可以分期分段进行磨擦。

(3) 劆洗法 用消毒之小锋针(或用洗净晒干的龙须草,先于10%黄连液中浸泡1日后晾干贮存备用)。术时,术眼点0.5%～1%地卡因,操作者左手分别翻转上、下眼睑,暴露睑结膜病变处,用小锋针之针锋刺破颗粒,以微微渗血为度,术毕用抗生素眼药水点眼。

操作时须注意消毒,勿损

injury of the cornea should be avoided. If the lesion area is too large, the therapy can be divided into several treatment courses or stages.

伤角膜,病变范围较广时,可以分期分段进行。

2.2 Diseases of Canthi

第二章　两眦
疾病

2.2.1 Epiphora

第一节　泪溢

[Introduction]

Epiphora is a kind of lacrimation disorder which is caused by the condition that the drainage of tears is blocked and tears cannot flow into the nasal cavity. Clinically, the disease mainly shows, in the absence of obvious swelling and pain, constant or intermittent weeping with cold and thin tears and pertains to cold lacrimation disorders. It is classified, according to the clinical features, as the irritated epiphora with cold wind and the constant epiphora.

Mostly, the disease arises as a result of anomaly of the palpebral margins and the obstruction or functional inefficiency of the lacrimal pathway.

From the clinical manifestations, the disease pertains to the "lacrimation troubles" in traditional Chinese medicine. Etiologically and pathogenically, deficiency of liver blood, abnormal thin dacryon and invasion of external pathogenic wind cause the irritated epiphora with cold tears, or the restraining failure of tears due to insufficiency of qi and blood or to deficiency of both liver and kidney gives rise to the constant weeping of cold tears, or the perpetuating trachoma which has the dacryon invaded by pathogenic toxin leads to the stricture or obstruction of the lacrimal passage so that the tears overflow instead of osmosing downwards. Most cases of cold lacrimation are of deficient syndrome while most of irritated epiphora

【概述】

泪溢是指泪道排出泪液受阻所引起的泪液不能流入鼻腔而出现的流泪症状。临床主要表现为眼无明显的红赤肿痛,而泪液经常溢出,泪水清冷稀薄,属冷泪范畴。根据其临床特征,又分为迎风冷泪与无时冷泪。

本病病因多为睑缘位置异常,泪道系统阻塞或功能不全所引起。

根据本病的临床表现,当属于中医学"流泪症"范畴。病因病机常由肝血不足,泪窍不密,风邪外引而致迎风泪出;或因气血不足或因肝肾两虚,不能约束其液,而致冷泪常流;或椒疮日久,邪毒侵入泪窍,导致排泪窍道狭窄或阻塞,泪不下渗而外溢。冷泪多虚证,迎风冷泪多窍虚招邪,属轻症;无时冷泪者多脏腑自虚所致,较为严重。后者大多从前者演变而来。

with cold tears are due to deficiency of eye and invasion of pathogenic factors, and both are of the mild conditions. On the other hand, constant weeping of cold tears mainly due to the visceral deficiency is of severe one. The latter often develops from the former.

[Main Diagnostic Points]

1. Irritated Epiphora with Cold Wind

Usually, the affected eye suffers from no redness, swelling and pain, and from no weeping, too. But lacrimation occurs when the eye encounters the cold wind. Or, irritated by the winter and early spring wind, the eye is weeping with excessive cold tears. When being washed, the lacrimal passage is perfect in function or functioning but not perfectly.

2. Constant Epiphora

The patient is always weeping all the year round and the condition is severe when meeting with wind. With the lacrimal sac being pressed, no mucus overflows from the dacryon. The lacrimal passage, when being washed, may be of constricture or blocked, or the eversion of the dacryon may exsist.

[Syndrome Differentiation and Treatment]

In clinic, the disease is classified into three syndromes: deficiency of liver blood, deficiency of both qi and blood, and deficiency of both liver and kidney. The treatment of irritated epiphora with cold tears should be mainly to nourish blood and remove pathogenic wind and, for the cases of constant weeping with excessive cold tears, the treatment should be put on the restoration of qi. If the dacryon or lacrimal pathway is blocked, operation may be needed.

1. Syndrome of Deficiency of Liver Blood Affected Repeatedly by Exopathogen

Main Symptoms and Signs　Weeping of the affect-

【诊断要点】

1. 迎风流泪

平素患眼无赤肿痛，亦不流泪，但遇风则引起流泪，无风则止。或仅在冬季或春初时遇寒风刺激即泪出汪汪，冲洗泪道时，泪道通畅或通而不畅。

2. 无时冷泪

患者不分春夏秋冬，无风有风，不时泪下，迎风尤甚。挤压泪囊部，并无黏液自泪点溢出。冲洗泪道时，泪道可有狭窄或不通。或有泪点外翻现象。

【辨证论治】

本病临床可分为肝血不足证、气血不足证、肝肾两虚证。治疗上，迎风冷泪者以养血祛风为主；无时冷泪者，治宜补虚为主。如排泪窍道已经阻塞者，可进行手术治疗。

1. 肝血不足，复感外邪证

主要证候　患眼无赤痛，

ed eye with cold wind, no redness and pain, dizziness, dim complexion; pale tongue with whitish thin coating and a weak thready pulse.

Therapeutic Methods Tonifying the liver and nourishing blood to relieve wind and arrest weeping.

Recipe The modified Zhilei Bugansan Decoction: Danggui (*Radix Angelicae Sinensis*) 10 g, Shudihuang (*Radix Rehmanniae Praeparata*) 10 g, Baishaoyao (*Radix Paeoniae Alba*) 10 g, Chuanxiong (*Rhizoma Ligustici Chuanxiong*) 10 g, Baijili (*Fructus Tribuli*) 10 g, Fangfeng (*Radix Ledebouriellae*) 6 g, Muzeicao (*Herba Equiseti Hiemalis*) 10 g, and Xiakucao (*Spica Prunellae*) 10 g.

2. Syndrome of Deficiency of Qi and Blood Causing Dysfunctional Drainage of Tears

Main Symptoms and Signs Constant weeping of thin and cold tears of the affected eye, no redness and pain, dim complexion, mental tiredness and physical fatigue, amnesia and severe palpitation; pale tongue with thin coating and weak thready pulse.

Therapeutic Methods Benefiting qi and nourishing blood to restore lacrimal draining function and arrest weeping.

Recipe The modified Bazhen Decoction: Dangshen (*Radix Codonopsis Pilosulae*) 10 g, Baizhu (*Rhizoma Atractylodis Macrocephalae*) 10 g, Baishaoyao (*Radix Paeoniae Alba*) 10 g, Danggui (*Radix Angelicae Sinensis*) 10 g, Shudihuang (*Radix Rehmanniae Praeparata*) 10 g, Fuling (*Poria*) 10 g, Chuanxiong (*Rhizoma Ligustici Chuanxiong*) 5 g, and Zhigancao (*Radix Glycyrrhizae Praeparata*) 3 g.

Modification In the cases of weeping with excessive tears, 10 g of Fangfeng (*Radix Ledebouriellae*) and 10 g of Baizhi (*Radix Angelicae Dahuricae*) are added;

迎风流泪,兼头晕目眩,面色少华。舌质淡,苔薄白,脉细无力。

治　法　补肝养血,祛风止泪。

方　药　止泪补肝散加减。当归10 g,熟地黄10 g,白芍药10 g,川芎10 g,白蒺藜10 g,防风6 g,木贼草10 g,夏枯草10 g。

2. 气血不足,收摄失司证

主要证候　患眼不红不痛,流泪频频,泪水清冷稀薄,兼面色少华,神疲体倦,健忘怔忡。舌淡苔薄,脉细无力。

治　法　益气养血,收摄止泪。

方　药　八珍汤加减。党参10 g,白术10 g,白芍药10 g,当归10 g,熟地黄10 g,茯苓10 g,川芎5 g,炙甘草3 g。

加　减　迎风泪多者,加防风10 g,白芷10 g;冬月泪多,有畏寒、肢冷、苔白腻者,

2 g of Xixin (*Herba Asari*) and 6 g of Guizhi (*Ramulus Cinnamomi*) are added in the cases of severe lacrimation in winter, aversion to cold, cold limbs and a whitish greasy tongue coating.

3. Syndrome of Deficiency of Both Liver and Kidney Causing Tear Drainage out of Control

Symptoms and Signs　Constant or intermittent weeping with excessive thin and cold tears, dizziness, tinnitus and lassitude in loin and legs; pale tongue with whitish thin coating and weak thready pulse.

Therapeutic Method　Nourishing live and kidney to restore the draining function and arrest weeping.

Recipe　The modified Zuogui Beverage: Shudihuang (*Radix Rehmanniae Praeparata*) 10 g, Shanzhuyu (*Fructus Corni*) 10 g, Gouqizi (*Fructus Lycii*) 10 g, Shanyao (*Rhizoma Dioscoreae*) 10 g, Fuling (*Poria*) 10 g, and Gancao (*Radix Glycyrrhizae*) 3 g.

Modification　In the cases of aversion to cold and cold limbs due to deficiency of kidney yang, Bajitian (*Radix Morindae Officinalis*), Roucongrong (*Herba Cistanchis*) and Sangpiaoxiao (*Oötheca Mantidis*), respective 10 g each, are added; in the cases of severe irritated epiphora with cold wind, 10 g of Fangfeng (*Radix Ledebouriellae*) and 10 g of Baizhi (*Radix Angelicae Dahuricae*) are added.

[Other Treatments]

1. Chinese Patent Drugs

(1) **Mingmu Dihuang Pill**　6 g each time, twice a day and applicable to the syndrome of deficiency of both the liver and kidney.

(2) **Qiju Dihuang Pill** (*Oral Drink*)　6 g (8 *concentrated pills or* 10 ml *of oral drinking*) each time, twice a day and applicable to the syndrome of deficiency of both the liver and kidney.

加细辛2 g,桂枝6 g。

3. 肝肾两虚,约束无权证

主要证候　眼泪常流,拭之又生,泪水清冷而稀薄,兼头昏耳鸣,腰膝酸软。舌质淡,苔薄白,脉细弱。

治　法　养肝益肾,固摄止泪。

方　药　左归饮加减。熟地黄10 g,山茱萸10 g,枸杞子10 g,山药10 g,茯苓10 g,甘草3 g。

加　减　伴有畏寒、肢冷等肾阳虚者,加巴戟天10 g,肉苁蓉10 g,桑螵蛸10 g;流泪迎风尤甚者,加防风10 g,白芷10 g。

【其他疗法】

1. 中成药

(1) 明目地黄丸　每服6 g,每日2次。适用于肝肾两虚证。

(2) 杞菊地黄丸(口服液)　每服6 g(浓缩丸每服8粒,口服液每服10 ml),每日2次。适用于肝肾两虚证。

(3) Shihu Yeguang Pill 6 g each time, twice a day and applicable to the syndrome of deficiency of both the liver and kidney.

2. Simple and Proved Recipes

(1) Longyanrou Porridge The porridge is prepared by boiling together 15 g of Longyanrou (*Arillus Longan*), 3 to 5 Jujubes and 60 g of rice fruit and is taken as porridge. It is applicable to patients with epiphora due to deficiency of the heart and spleen.

(2) Xianren Porridge The ingredients of the porridge are 30 to 60 g of Zhiheshouwu (*Radix Polygoni Multiflori*), 3 to 5 Jujubes, 60 g of rice fruit and a proper amount of brown sugar. The Zhiheshouwu is first concentrated by boiling to a thick solution with the dregs removed. The thick solution, rice fruit and Jujubes are decocted with water into porridge. When the brown sugar or cristal sugar is added for taste into the porridge, the porridge is ready after being again decocted for one or two boiling times. This porridge is applicable to epiphora due to deficiency of both the liver and kidney.

3. External Therapies

(1) Eye Drops a. Babao Eye Drops: The eye drops is applicable to irritated epiphora with cold wind and is applied once or twice every day. b. Red-Eye Drops: The drops is applicable to irritated epiphora with cold wind and is applied once or twice every day. c. Anti-Epiphora Drops: The drops is applicable to irritated epiphora with cold wind and is used once or twice every day.

(2) Probing Exploration Therapy If the lacrimal passage is extremely constrictive or blocked, the probing of the passage is first performed with the types of probing needles gradually thicker so that the passage may be expanded.

(3) Operation If the lacrimal passage, after having been explored with probes, can not drain tears or keep

（3）石斛夜光丸 每服 6 g,每日 2 次。适用于肝肾两虚证。

2. 单验方

（1）龙眼肉粥 龙眼肉 15 g,大枣 3～5 枚,粳米 60 g, 共煮为粥,顿食之。适用于泪溢心脾两虚患者。

（2）仙人粥 制何首乌 30～60 g,粳米 60 g,大枣 3～5 枚,红糖适量。先将制何首乌煎取浓汁,去渣,同粳米、大枣同入砂锅内煮粥。粥将成时,放入红糖或冰糖少许以调味,再煮一二沸即可服食。适用于泪溢肝肾不足患者。

3. 外治法

（1）点眼药 ① 八宝眼药:每日点眼 1～2 次。适用于迎风流泪者。② 红眼药:每日点眼 1～2 次。适用于迎风流泪者。③ 止泪散:每日点眼 1～2 次。适用于迎风流泪者。

（2）探通法 如泪道高度狭窄或阻塞者,可先行泪道探插,并逐步增粗探针以扩张之。

（3）手术治疗 如探插仍不通或通畅难以长久维持

permanently unobstructed, operation should be considered if necessary, such as lacrimal dilatation and canaliculo-rhinostomy.

2.2.2 Acute Dacryocystitis

[Introduction]

Acute dacryocystitis is a kind of acute phlegmon of the lacrimal sac and the surrounding tissues. The clinical symptoms of the infection are redness, swelling and a heat sensation in the sac area.

The cause of the disease is usually due to the virulent infection of bacteria. It is usually the transformation of chronic dacryocystitis, and it may sometimes arise all of a sudden without the history of epiphora.

Clinically, the disease pertains to "Loujingchuang" (dacryocystitis) in traditional Chinese medicine. The etiology and pathogenesis of the disease is often described in TCM as: Accumulation of pathogenic heat in the heart meridian or habitual dacryocystitis, internal accumulation of excessive pathogenic heat with repeated affection of pathogenic wind, all these factors cause the hyperactivity of internal fire so that pathogenic wind and heat combat and stagnate in the inner canthus; or the addiction to pungent and fried foods leads to excessive pathogenic heat to stagnate in heart and spleen, which invades the dacryon and gives rise to stagnation of qi and blood, causing the disease. At the beginning, most cases are excessive in nature, but in the perpetual course it may change to deficient types.

[Main Diagnostic Points]

1. Clinical Manifestations

（1）The disease often attacks suddenly with the

者,可根据具体情况,考虑手术治疗。如泪道扩张术,泪小管吻合术和泪囊鼻腔吻合术等。

第二节　急性泪囊炎

【概述】

急性泪囊炎为泪囊及其周围组织的急性蜂窝织炎。临床主要表现为泪囊区红肿热痛。

其病因为毒力较强的细菌感染所致。多由慢性泪囊炎转变而来,亦有无泪溢史而突然发作者。

根据本病的临床表现,当属于中医学"漏睛疮"范畴。病因病机多为心经蕴热或素有漏睛,热毒内蕴,复感风邪,引起内火,风热搏结于内眦;或素嗜辛辣炙煿,心脾热毒壅盛,上攻泪窍,气血瘀滞,结聚成疮而致。初起多实,日久亦可致虚。

【诊断要点】

1. 临床表现

（1）发病较急,泪囊部红

symptoms of redness, swelling and a heat sensation of the sac and obvious local tenderness. In severe cases, the upper and lower lids and the dorsum of the nose may be involved.

(2) The submaxillary and pre-auricular lymph nodes become swollen, accompanied by fever and other general symptoms.

(3) In the course of a few days, the redness and swelling are localized and pus is formed which is soft and white-yellow in colour. When the pus is discharged, the inflammation disappears promptly. Sometimes the rupture of the sore which cannot heal in a long course may cause the formation of lacrimal fistula.

(4) The history of chronic dacryocystitis can often be seen in some cases.

2. Laboratory Examination

Leukocytosis is found in the blood routine examination.

[Syndrome Differentiation and Treatment]

The onset of the disease often begins suddenly and violently and must be treated instantly. In clinic, the disease is classified into the syndromes of ocular invasion of pathogenic wind and heat, excess of toxic heat, and asthenia of healthy qi and retention of pathogenic qi. In principle, the treatment methods of the disease should be: In the cases of the pus being immature to dispel and resolve the pathogenic factors mainly with internal therapies, in the cases of the invasion of pathogenic wind and heat at the initial stage to subdue swelling and mass by expelling wind and heat, in the cases of excess of toxic heat to remove blood stasis and swelling through clearing away toxic heat, and in the cases of pathogenic qi superior to health qi causing the stagnation of pathogenic qi to increase healthy qi and remove pathogenic factors with the

肿热痛,压痛明显,严重时可波及上下眼睑及鼻梁。

(2) 颌下及耳前淋巴结肿大,可伴体温增高等全身症状。

(3) 数日后,红肿局限,逐渐成脓,质软皮薄,隐见黄白色,继之破溃出脓,炎症迅速消退。亦常见疮口久不愈合,脓汁常流而成瘘管。

(4) 常有慢性泪囊炎史

2. 实验室检查

血常规检查示白细胞数增加。

【辨证论治】

本病起病急骤,来势较猛,必须及时治疗。临床主要分为风热上攻证、热毒炽盛证、正虚邪留证。原则上未成脓时宜内治,以消散为主。初起风热上攻,治宜疏风散热,消肿散结;若热毒炽盛者,治宜清热解毒,祛瘀消肿;如正不胜邪,邪气留恋者,则宜扶正祛邪,托里排毒。亦可配合外治疗法。

toxin eliminating manipulation. Sometimes external methods may be applied as the accessory treatment.

1. Syndrome of Ocular Invasion of Pathogenic Wind and Heat

Main Symptoms and Signs Redness, swelling and pain of the affected part with projection, profuse tears, headache, aversion to cold and fever; thin yellowish tongue coating and floating rapid pulse.

Therapeutic Method Dispelling pathogenic wind and heat to remove swelling and mass.

Recipe The modified Qufeng Sanre Decoction: Lianqiao (*Fructus Forsythiae*) 10 g, Niubangzi (*Fructus Arctii*) 10 g, Qianghuo (*Rhizome seu Radix Notopterygii*) 6 g, Bohe (*Herba Menthae*, decocted later) 6 g, Dahuang (*Radix et Rhizoma Rhei*) 5 g, Chishaoyao (*Radix Paeoniae Rubra*) 10 g, Fangfeng (*Radix Ledebouriellae*) 6 g, Dangguiwei (*Radix Angelicae Sinensis*) 10 g, Chuanxiong (*Rhizoma Ligustici Chuanxiong*) 10 g, Shanzhizi (*Fructus Gardeniae*) 10 g, and Gancao (*Radix Glycyrrhizae*) 3 g.

Modification In the cases of normal stool, Dahuang is removed and 3 g of Huanglian (*Rhizoma Coptidis*) is added.

2. Syndrome of Excess of Toxic Heat

Main Symptoms and Signs Redness, swelling and unbearable pain of the affected part with hard tender projection which spreads along the lid and down the cheek, feverish body, vexation, thirst, preferring to drink and constipation; reddish tongue with dry yellowish coating and full rapid pulse.

Therapeutic Method Removing toxic heat to resolve swelling and mass.

Recipe The modified Huanglian Jiedu Decoction: Huanglian (*Rhizoma Coptidis*) 3 g, Huangbai (*Cortex*

1. 风热上攻证

主要证候　患处红肿疼痛高起,泪多,头痛,恶寒发热。苔薄黄,脉浮数。

治　法　疏风清热,消肿散结。

方　药　驱风散热饮子加减。连翘10 g,牛蒡子10 g,羌活6 g,薄荷(后下)6 g,大黄5 g,赤芍药10 g,防风6 g,当归尾10 g,川芎10 g,山栀子10 g,甘草3 g。

加　减　大便通畅者,去大黄,加黄连3 g。

2. 热毒炽盛证

主要证候　患处红肿高起,坚硬拒按,疼痛难忍,红肿漫及面颊胞睑,身热心烦,口渴思饮,大便燥结。舌质红,苔黄燥,脉洪数。

治　法　清热解毒,消肿散结。

方　药　黄连解毒汤加减。黄连3 g,黄柏10 g,黄芩

Phellodendri) 10 g, Huangqin (*Radix Scutellariae*) 10 g, Shanzhizi (*Fructus Gardeniae*) 10 g, and Dahuang (*Radix et Rhizoma Rhei*) 6 g.

Modification In the cases of excessive pathogenic heat, 10 g of Jinyinhua (*Flos Lonicerae*) and 15 g of Pugongying (*Herba Taraxaci*) are added while, in the cases of serious swelling and pain, 10 g of Chuanshanjia (*Squama Manitis*, prepared) and 10 g of Zaojiaci (*Spina Gleditiae*) are added.

3. Syndrome of Asthenia of Health Qi and Retention of Pathogenic Qi

Main Symptoms and Signs Frequent onsets of the affected part with slight redness and swelling, a little tenderness, no diabrosis or diabrosis difficult to heal, small amount of pus which is constantly flowing, a whitish pale complexion, mental tiredness and fatigue; pale tongue with thin coating and weak pulse.

Therapeutic Method Dispelling pathogenic factor with toxin-eliminating manipulation.

Recipe The modified Qianjin Tuolisan Decoction: Dangshen (*Radix Codonopsis Pilosulae*) 10 g, Shenghuangqi (*Radix Astragali seu Hedysari*) 10 g, Fuling (*Poria*) 10 g, Gancao (*Radix Glycyrrhizae*) 3 g, Danggui (*Radix Angelicae Sinensis*) 10 g, Shaoyao (*Radix Paeoniae Alba*) 10 g, Chuanxiong (*Rhizoma Ligustici Chuanxiong*) 10 g, Jiegeng (*Radix Platycodi*) 3 g, Jinyinhua (*Flos Lonicerae*) 10 g, Baizhi (*Radix Angelicae Dahuricae*) 6 g, Fangfeng (*Radix Ledebouriellae*) 6 g, and Maimendong (*Radix Ophiopogonis*) 10 g.

[Other Treatments]

1. Chinese Patent Drugs

(1) **Yinqiao Jiedu Tablet** 4 tablets each time, three times a day and applicable to the syndrome of ocular invasion of pathogenic wind and heat.

10 g,山栀子10 g,大黄6 g。

加　减　热甚者,加金银花10 g,蒲公英15 g;肿痛甚者,加穿山甲(炮制)10 g,皂角刺10 g。

3. 正虚邪留证

主要证候　患处时有小发作,微红微肿,稍有压痛,但不溃破或溃后漏口难敛,脓汁少而不绝,面色㿠白,神疲乏力,舌淡苔薄,脉弱无力。

治　法　托里排毒。

方　药　千金托里散加减。党参10 g,生黄芪10 g,茯苓10 g,甘草3 g,当归10 g,芍药10 g,川芎10 g,桔梗3 g,金银花10 g,白芷6 g,防风6 g,麦门冬10 g。

【其他疗法】

1. 中成药

(1) 银翘解毒片　每服4片,每日3次。适用于风热上攻证。

(2) Huanglian Shangqing Pill 6 g each time, twice a day and applicable to the syndrome of ocular invasion of pathogenic wind and heat.

(3) Yiqing Capsule 2 capsules once, three times a day and applicable to the syndrome of excess of toxic heat.

(4) Niuhuang Jiedu Pills (Tablet) 3 g (2 tablets) each time, twice or three times a day and applicable to the syndrome of excess of toxic heat.

(5) Niuhuang Xiaoyan Pills 10 pills each time, three times a day and applicable to the syndrome of excess of toxic heat.

2. External Therapies

(1) External treatment with drugs a. Moist-hot compress: In the cases of the pus not yet being formed, the moist-hot compress of the affected area is applied for 20 to 30 minutes with hot water or the liquid by boiling the dregs of an oral decoction twice or three times a day. b. Of the following herbs—fresh Furongye (*Folium Hibisci*) 30 g, Yejuhua (*Flos Chrysanthemi Indici*) 20 g, Machixian (*Herba Portulacae*) 30 g, Baihuasheshecao (*Herba Hedyodis Diffusae*) 30 g, fresh pugongying (*Herba Taraxaci*) 30 g, one or two, after being washed and cleaned, are selected and pounded into pulp for the compress of the affected part. The method is applicable to the cases of immature pus. c. External Compress of Xiedu Plaster: Dahuang (*Radix et Rhizoma Rhei*) 90 g, Muxiang (*Radix Aucklandiae*) 30 g, Xuanshen (*Radix Scrophulariae*) 60 g, Bailian (*Radix Ampelopsis*) 60 g, Shegan (*Rhizoma Belamcandae*) 60 g, Mangxiao (*Natrii Sulphas*) 60 g, all these drugs are smashed to powder which is fixed with the white of egg to form a kind of paster. The paster is compressed on the affected part with a change when it is dry. The method is applicable to the

（2）黄连上清丸　每服 6 g,每日 2 次。适用于风热上攻证。

（3）一清胶囊　每服 2 粒,每日 3 次。适用于热毒炽盛证。

（4）牛黄解毒丸(片)　每服3 g(片剂每服 2 片),每日 2～3 次。适用于热毒炽盛证。

（5）牛黄消炎丸　每服 10 粒,每日 3 次。适用于热毒炽盛证。

2. 外治法

（1）药物外治　① 湿热敷疗法:用热水或内服药渣再煎水作湿热敷,每次敷20～30分钟,每日敷2～3次。适用于本病未酿脓者。② 新鲜芙蓉叶30 g,野菊花20 g,马齿苋30 g,白花蛇舌草30 g,鲜蒲公英30 g,用其中一二味洗净,捣烂后敷在患处。适用于本病未酿脓者。③ 协毒膏外敷:大黄90 g,木香30 g,玄参、白蔹、射干、芒硝各60 g。以上诸药共研为散,以鸡子白调如膏状,敷贴红肿处,药干即换之。适用于本病未酿脓者

cases of immature pus.

(2) Operation　a. When the pus is mature, it is drained by incision and the drain line is placed. Or the medicated thread Jiuyidan (*Nine-one Dan*) which is made of the drugs of 27 g of Duanshigao (*Calcined Gypsum Fibrosum*) and 3 g of Shengdan (*Hydrargyrum Oxide*) is applied and dressing change is done once a day. Till the pus is up, the thread is removed so that the wound can heal. b. If fistula is formed, operation should be considered, such as dacryocystectomy plus fistulectomy.

（2）手术治疗　① 已成脓者,应切开排脓,并放置引流条。亦可掺用九一丹(煅石膏27 g,升丹3 g)药捻。每日换药,待脓尽,除去引流条,使切口愈合。② 若已成漏者,可考虑手术治疗。如泪囊摘除加瘘管摘除术。

2.3 Disorders of Bulbar Conjunctiva

2.3.1 Acute Catarrhal Conjunctivitis

[Introduction]

Acute catarrhal conjunctivitis is a common ocular disease as a result of bacterial infection. Clinically it manifests mainly the symptoms of obvious congestion of the conjunctiva, purulent and mucous secretion and a tendency of natural cure. The disease is very infective and often epidemic in the warm seasons of a year.

The most common pathogens of the disease are Koch-Week's bacillus, Diplococcus pneumoniae, staphylococci and bacillus influenzae.

From the clinical manifestations, the disease should pertain to "Baofeng Kere" (pseudomembranous conjunctivitis) in traditional Chinese medicine. Externally, it mainly arises as the sudden invasion of pathogenic wind and heat from outside, and internally due to the interior pathogenic heat and excessive yang. The chief pathogensis of the disease is that the pathogenic wind and heat combine with each other externally and internally, which invades the eye and causes the sudden onset of the disease.

[Main Diagnostic Points]

1. Clinical Manifestations

(1) The symptoms in mild cases include itching and uncomfortable feeling of the affected eye as if caused by a

第三章 白睛疾病

第一节 急性卡他性结膜炎

【概述】

急性卡他性结膜炎是常见的细菌感染性眼病。临床主要表现为眼部结膜明显充血,脓性或黏液性分泌物,有自愈趋势。本病传染性强,常在温暖季节流行。

本病的致病菌最常见的有 Koch - Weeks 杆菌、肺炎双球菌、葡萄球菌和流行性感冒杆菌等。

根据本病的临床表现,当属于中医学"暴风客热"范畴。外因多为风热之邪,突从外袭,内因为内热阳盛。主要病机为风热内外相合,上攻白睛,以致猝然发病。

【诊断要点】

1. 临床表现

(1) 轻者患眼瘙痒不适和异物感,重者羞明灼热,眼睑

foreign body. In severe cases, there is photophobia with a burning fever and heavy sensation of the eyelid. Sometimes, because of hypersecretion, the vision becomes blurring but can restore when the secretion is cleared.

（2）Congestion occurs in the palpebral conjunctiva and fornix in mild cases and; in severe cases, the congestion of the bulbar conjunctiva is obvious, even with chemosis, swelling of the lid and large amount of mucous and purulent secretion in the conjunctival sac. In some cases, there may be petechial and patchy hemorrhage.

（3）The disease is usually of bilateral type - simutaneous binocular onset or one eye after another. Usually, a mild start comes to its utmost in 3 to 4 days and relieves in 8 to 14 days. Cases due to Diplococcus pneumoniae arrive to the worst in 8 to 10 days and then turn back to recovery while cases owing to Koch-Week's bacillus, which are serious, need two to four weeks and then back to recovery.

2. Laboratory Examination

Koch-Week's bacillus, Diplococcus pneumoniae, staphylococci or bacillus influenzae can often be found in the secretion culture of the conjunctival sac. These bacteria multiples quickly during the onset of the first 3 to 4 days and can not easily be found at the later stage or after the administration of medicine.

[Syndrome Differentiation and Treatment]

Generally, the disease is mostly caused by the pathogenic wind and heat in the lung meridian. In clinic, it is classified into the syndromes of wind exceeding heat, heat exceeding wind and excess of both wind and heat. In principle, the treatment should focus on diffusing lung - qi to dispel wind and removing pathogenic heat and fire. Also it should be clearly differentiated whether the key pathogenic factor is wind or heat or both together. If wind is the

沉重。也可因为分泌物过多而视物不清,但拭去分泌物后即可恢复视力。

（2）轻者仅睑结膜及穹窿部结膜充血,重者还有明显的球结膜充血,甚至结膜水肿,眼睑肿胀,结膜囊内大量黏液或脓性分泌物。部分患者球结膜有点片状出血。

（3）本病多为双侧型,双眼同时或先后发病。轻症通常3～4日内发展到最高峰,8～14日消退。肺炎双球菌引起者,8～10日到达极限,而后立即好转。Koch - Weeks 杆菌引起者较重,约需2～4星期方可痊愈。

2. 实验室检查

结膜囊分泌物培养多可找到 Koch - Weeks 杆菌、肺炎双球菌、葡萄球菌或流行性感冒杆菌。这些细菌在发病3～4日内繁殖旺盛,晚期或临床用药之后即不易找到。

【辨证论治】

本病总属肺经风热为患,临床主要分为风重于热证、热重于风证、风热并重证。治疗以宣肺疏风,清热泻火为原则,并辨清其风重、热重或风热并重,风重以祛风为主,热重以清热为主,风热并重宜祛风清热。

main factor, the treatment should be chiefly dispelling the wind, if heat is the main factor, the treatment should be removing the heat, and if both wind and heat are the main pathogenic factors, the treatment should be dispelling the wind and removing the heat.

1. Syndrome of Pathogenic Wind Exceeding Pathogenic Heat

Main Symptoms and Signs　Slight swelling of the lid, mild redness of the bulbar conjunctiva with itching and unsmooth feeling, photophobia and delacrimation, headache and stuffy nose, fever and aversion to wind; thin and whitish or light yellowish tongue coating and floating pulse.

Therapeutic Method　Expelling wind with diaphoresis plus heat-removing drugs.

Recipe　The modified Qianghuo Shengfeng Decoction: Qianghuo (*Rhizoma seu Radix Notopterygii*) 10 g, Fangfeng (*Radix Ledebouriellae*) 10 g, Duhuo (*Radix Angelicae Pubescentis*) 10 g, Jingjie (*Herba Schizonepetae*) 6 g, Chaihu (*Radix Bupleuri*) 6 g, Baizhu (*Rhizoma Atractylodis Macrocephalae*) 10 g, Bohe (*Herba Menthae*, to be decocted later) 6 g, Baizhi (*Radix Angelicae Dahuricae*) 6 g, Chuanxiong (*Rhizoma Ligustici Chuanxiong*) 6 g, Zhike (*Fructus Aurantii*) 6 g, Huangqin(*Radix Scutellariae*) 10 g, Jiegeng (*Radix Platycodi*) 6 g, Qianhu (*Radix Peucedani*) 6 g, and Gancao (*Radix Glycyrrhizae*) 3 g.

Modification　In the cases of less pathegenic wind, Qianghuo and Duhuo are removed while in the cases of obvious pathogenic heat, 10 g of Jinyinhua (*Flos Lonicerae*), Lianqiao (*Fructus Forsythiae*) and Sangbaipi (*Cortex Mori*) and 6 g of Juhua (*Flos Chrysanthemi*) are added respectively.

1. 风重于热证

主要证候　胞睑微肿,白睛红赤轻,痒涩兼作,羞明多泪,头痛鼻塞,恶风发热。舌苔薄白或微黄,脉浮数等。

治　法　疏风解表,兼以清热。

方　药　羌活胜风汤加减。羌活10 g,防风10 g,独活10 g,荆芥6 g,柴胡6 g,白术10 g,薄荷(后下)6 g,白芷6 g,川芎6 g,枳壳6 g,黄芩10 g,桔梗6 g,前胡6 g,甘草3 g。

加　减　风邪不盛者,去羌活、独活;热象较明显者,加金银花10 g,连翘10 g,桑白皮10 g,菊花6 g。

2. Syndrome of Pathogenic Heat Exceeding Pathogenic Wind

Main Symptoms and Signs Serious redness and swelling of the bulbar conjunctiva with hot tears and mucopurulent secretion, palpebral swelling, restlessness and thirst, yellowish urine and constipation; red tongue with yellowish coating and rapid strong pulse.

Therapeutic Method Removing pathogenic heat and fire accompanying dispelling wind.

Recipe The modified Xiefei Beverage: Shigao (*Gypsum Fribrosum*, to be decocted first) 20 g, Huangqin (*Radix Scutellariae*) 10 g, Sangbaipi (*Cortex Mori*) 10 g, Lianqiao (*Fructus Forsythiae*) 10 g, Shanzhizi (*Fructus Gardeniae*) 10 g, Chishaoyao (*Radix Paeoniae Rubra*) 10 g, Zhike (*Fructus Aurantii*) 6 g, Mutong (*Caulis Akebiae*) 6 g, Jingjie (*Herba Schizonepetae*) 6 g, Fangfeng (*Radix Ledebouriellae*) 6 g, Baizhi (*Radix Angelicae Dahuricae*) 6 g, Qianghuo (*Rhizoma seu Radix Notopterygii*) 6 g, and Gancao (*Radix Glycyrrhizae*) 3 g.

Modification In the cases of excessive toxic heat, Qianghuo and Baizhi are removed, and 10 g of Jinyinhua (*Flos Lonicerae*) and 15 g of Pugongying (*Herba Taraxaci*) and 15 g of Yuxingcao (*Herba Houttuyniae*) are added; in the cases of serious constipation, 5 g of Dahuang (*Radix et Rhizoma Rhei*) and 6 g of Mangxiao (*Natrii Sulphas*) are added.

3. Syndrome of Severe Pathogenic Wind and Heat

Main Symptoms and Signs Redness and swelling of the lid and bulbar conjunctiva, alternate pain and itching, photophobia with a burning sensation, hot tears and mucopurulent secretion, fever and aversion to cold, constipation and yellowish urine; red tongue with yellowish coating and rapid strong pulse.

2. 热重于风证

主要证候　白睛红赤肿胀较甚,眵多粘结,热泪如汤,胞睑红肿,烦躁口渴,溺黄便秘。舌红苔黄,脉数有力。

治　法　清热泻火,兼以疏风。

方　药　泻肺饮加减。石膏(先煎)20 g,黄芩10 g,桑白皮10 g,连翘10 g,山栀子10 g,赤芍药10 g,枳壳6 g,木通6 g,荆芥6 g,防风6 g,白芷6 g,羌活6 g,甘草3 g。

加　减　热毒炽盛者,去羌活、白芷,加金银花10 g,蒲公英15 g,鱼腥草15 g;大便秘结甚者,加大黄5 g,芒硝6 g。

3. 风热并重证

主要证候　胞睑、白睛红赤肿胀,痛痒交作,灼热羞明,热泪如汤,眵多粘结,恶寒发热,便秘溲黄,口渴思饮。舌红苔黄,脉数有力。

Therapeutic Methods Dispelling pathogenic wind externally and removing pathogenic fire-heat internally.

Recipe The modified Fangfeng Tongshengsan Decoction: Fangfeng (*Radix Ledebouriellae*) 10 g, Jingjie (*Herba Schizonepetae*) 10 g, Jiegeng (*Radix Platycodi*) 6 g, Bohe (*Herba Menthae*, to be decocted later) 6 g, Lianqiao (*Fructus Forsythiae*) 10 g, Shanzhizi (*Fructus Gardeniae*) 10 g, Huangqin (*Radix Scutellariae*), Huashi (*Talcum*) 10 g, Chuanxiong (*Rhizoma Ligustici Chuanxiong*) 10 g, Danggui (*Radix Angelicae Sinensis*) 10 g, Baishaoyao (*Radix Paeoniae Alba*) 10 g, Dahuang (*Radix et Rhizoma Rhei*) 6 g, and Gancao (*Radix Glycyrrhizae*) 3 g.

[Other Treatments]

1. Chinese Patent Drugs

(1) **Yinqiao Jiedu Tablet** 4 tablets each time, three times a day and applicable to the syndrome of heat exceeding wind.

(2) **Huanglian Shangqing Pill** 6 g each time, twice a day and applicable to the syndrome of heat exceeding wind.

(3) **Sanhuang Pill** 6 g each time, three times a day and applicable to the syndrome of heat exceeding wind.

(4) **Qingning Pill** 6 g each time, twice or three times a day and applicable to the syndrome of heat exceeding wind.

(5) **Fangfeng Tongsheng Pill** 6 g each time, twice a day and applicable to the syndrome of excess of both wind and heat.

(6) **Mingmu Shangqing Pill** 6 g each time, twice a day and applicable to the syndrome of excess of both wind and heat.

2. Simple and Proved Recipes

(1) Mangxiao (*Natrii Sulphas*), Huangdan (*Mini-*

治 法 外散风邪,内泻火热。

方 药 防风通圣散加减。防风10 g,荆芥10 g,桔梗6 g,薄荷(后下)6 g,连翘10 g,山栀子10 g,黄芩10 g,滑石10 g,川芎10 g,当归10 g,白芍药10 g,大黄6 g,甘草3 g。

【其他疗法】

1. 中成药

(1)银翘解毒片 每服4片,每日3次。适用于热重于风证。

(2)黄连上清丸 每服6 g,每日2次。适用于热重于风证。

(3)三黄丸 每服6 g,每日3次。适用于热重于风证。

(4)清宁丸 每服6 g,每日2~3次。适用于热重于风证。

(5)防风通圣丸 每服6 g,每日2次。适用于风热并重证。

(6)明目上清丸 每服6 g,每日2次。适用于风热并重证。

2. 单验方

(1)芒硝、黄丹、乳香、没

um）, Ruxiang（*Resina Olibani*）, Moyao（*Myrrha*）, 6 g of each, and 3 g of Xionghuang（*Realgar*）, all these herbs are ground into powder for the nasal insufflation with water. The method can be applied to all the syndromes of the disease.

(2) Hezi（*Fructus Chebulae*）, Chuanxiong（*Rhizoma Ligustici Chuanxiong*）, Shanzhizi（*Fructus Gardeniae*）, respective 3 g of each, and 4 g of Honghua（*Flos Carthomi*）, all are ground, screened and completely mixed. 3 g of the mixed powder is boiled once with 30 ml water for a few minutes. The affected eye is steamed with the hot decoction three times a day. When it is cool, a small amount of the decoction is stored in a cup for the slight rubbing and washing of the upper and lower conjunctivas with a cotton stick, and the rest is orally taken. The decoction is effective on all the syndromes of the disease.

(3) Huanglian（*Rhizoma Coptidis*）6 g, Bingpian（*Borneolum*）3 g, Zanghonghua（*Stigma Croci Sativi*）2 g, Xiongdan（*Fel Ursi*）2 g, all are ground, screened and completely mixed. The mixed powder are filled with 500 ml normal saline, and the solution, which is kept stationary for 7 days, is first filtered and then sealed for the later washing of the affected eye 3 to 5 times a day. This method can be applied to all the syndromes of the disease.

(4) Shengdihuang（*Radix Rehmanniae*）10 g, Rendongteng（*Caulis Lonicerae*）10 g, Lianqiao（*Fructus Forsythiae*）10 g, Shanzhizi（*Fructus Gardeniae*）5 g, Bohe（*Herba Menthae*, to be decocted later）5 g, Zhimu（*Rhizoma Anemarrhenae*）6 g, Shigao（*Gypsum Fribrosum*, to be decocted first）5 g, Fangfeng（*Radix Ledebouriellae*）5 g, Jingjie（*Herba Schizonepetae*）5 g. All the ingredients are decocted with water. The decoc-

药各6 g,雄黄3 g。共研细末,含水吹鼻。适用于本病各证。

（2）河子3 g,川芎3 g,山栀子3 g,红花4 g。研碎成细末,过筛、混匀即得。每日3次,每次3 g,以30 ml水煎数分钟,用热气薰患眼,温后将少许汤倒入其他器具内,用棉签沾药汁轻轻擦洗患眼上下睑结膜,余下药汁凉后全部服下。适用于本病各证。

（3）黄连6 g,冰片3 g,藏红花2 g,熊胆2 g。研碎成细末,过筛、混匀即得。装入生理盐水溶液500 ml中,静置7日,过滤取汁,密闭备用。每日3~5次,冲洗患眼。适用于本病各证。

（4）生地黄10 g,忍冬藤10 g,连翘10 g,山栀子5 g,薄荷(后下)5 g,知母5 g,石膏(先煎)5 g,防风5 g。荆芥5 g。水煎服,每日1剂。适用于风热并重证。

tion is taken orally one dose a day and is applicable to the syndrome of both pathogenic wind and heat.

(5) Shigao (*Gypsum Fribrosum*, to be decocted first) 20 g to 25 g, Shengdihuang (*Radix Rehmanniae*) 20 g, Zhimu (*Rhizoma Anemarrhenae*) 10 g, Jingjie (*Herba Schizonepetae*) 5 g, Fangfeng (*Radix Ledebouriellae*) 5 g, Niubangzi (*Fructus Arctii*) 5 g. All the drugs are decocted with water. The decoction is orally taken one dose every day and is applicable to the syndrome of both pathogenic wind and heat.

(6) Dangguiwei (*Radix Angelicae Sinensis*) 15 g, Chishaoyao (*Radix Paeoniae Rubra*) 15 g, Bohe (*Herba Menthae*, to be decocted later) 15 g, Huanglian (*Rhizoma Coptidis*) 15 g, Muzcicao (*Herba Equiseti Hiematis*) 20 g, Huangqin (*Radix Scutellariae*) 10 g, Baijili (*Fructus Tribuli*) 20 g, Shijueming (*Concha Haliotidis*, to be decocted first) 15 g, Caojueming (*Semen Haliotidis*) 15 g, Gancao (*Radix Glycyrrhizae*) 15 g, and Baijuhua (*Flos Chrysanthemi*) 15 g, all the drugs are decocted with water for oral taking and fumigating. The decoction is applicable to the syndrome of excessive pathogenic heat.

(7) Longdancao (*Radix Gentianae*) 10 g, Jinyinhua (*Flos Lonicerae*) 15 g, and Chengliu (*Cacumen Tamaricis*) 15 g, all the herbs are decocted with water one dose a day and is orally taken or used for fumigation three times every day. Three days make up a course of treatment. The decoction is applicable to the syndrome of excessive pathogenic heat.

3. External Therapies

(1) **Eye Drops**　a. Eye Drops of Coptis and Watermelon Frost: The eye is dropped 3 to 4 times a day, which is applicable to the mild cases of the disease. b. Qianli Guang Eye Drops: The eye is dropped 3 to 4

（5）石膏（先煎）20～25 g,生地黄20 g,知母10 g,荆芥5 g,防风5 g,牛蒡子5 g。水煎服,每日1剂。适用于风热并重证。

（6）当归尾15 g,赤芍药15 g,薄荷（后下）15 g,黄连15 g,木贼草20 g,黄芩10 g,白蒺藜20 g,石决明（先煎）15 g,草决明15 g,甘草15 g,白菊花15 g,煎服并薰洗。适用于热邪偏盛者。

（7）龙胆草10 g,金银花15 g,柽柳15 g。水煎服,每日1剂,分3次服,3日为1个疗程。适用于热邪偏盛者。

3. 外治法

（1）点眼药　①黄连西瓜霜眼药水:每日点眼3～4次。适用于本病轻症者。②千里光眼药水:每日点眼

times a day, which is applicable to the mild condition of the disease. c. Danzhi Erlian Ointment: The ointment is smeared on the eye before sleep and is applicable to the mild cases of the disease. d. Xiongdan Eye Drops: The eye is dropped 3 to 4 times a day, which is applicable to all syndromes of the disease.

(2) Fumigation-washing Method 20 g of fresh Yejuhua (*Flos Chrysanthemi Indici*) and respective 60 g of Pugongying (*Herba Taraxaci*), Cheqiancao (*Herba Plantaginis*), Zihuadiding (*Herba Violae*), all the ingredients are decocted with water for the fumigation and washing of the eye once or twice every day. It is applicable to the severe cases of the disease.

2.3.2 Epidemic Keratoconjunctivitis

[**Introduction**]

Epidemic keratoconjunctivitis is a highly infectious ocular disease characterized by an abrupt and severe onset. In clinic, it mainly manifests the symptoms of acute follicular or pseudomembranous congenstion and subepithelial infiltration of the cornea which occurs later. The disease may appear in scattered cases or attacks epidemically. Epidemic once all over the world, it is often found in scattered cases at present.

The pathogen of the disease is adenovirus, including types 8, 19, 29 and 37 (subgroup D of human adenovirus), but type 8 is usually found and often gives rise to the fulminant epidemic of the disease. The other types are often seen in scattered cases.

Clinically, the disease pertains to "Tianxing Chiyan Baoyi" (epidemic keratoconjunctivity) in traditional Chi-

3~4 次。适用于本病轻症者。
③ 胆汁二连膏：每晚临睡前涂眼。适用于本病轻症者。
④ 熊胆眼药水：每日点眼3~4 次。适用于本病各证。

（2）薰洗法　用新鲜野菊花20 g,蒲公英30 g,车前草30 g,紫花地丁30 g煎水薰洗患眼。每日1~2 次。适用于本病重症者。

第二节　流行性角膜结膜炎

【概述】

流行性角膜结膜炎是一种传染性强,发病急剧的眼病。临床主要表现为急性滤泡性或伪膜性结膜充血,以及随后发生的角膜上皮下浸润。本病可散发,亦可流行,曾在全世界广泛流行,目前以散发病例较多见。

本病的病原体是腺病毒,可由腺病毒 8、19、29 和 37 型（人类腺病毒亚组 D）所引起。其中腺病毒 8 型最多见,常引起暴发流行,其他型者多为散在病例。

根据本病的临床表现,当属于中医学"天行赤眼暴翳"

nese medicine. Its exopathic cause is the affection of epidemic and noxious pathogenic factors, and the endopathic one is the hyperactivity of lung fire. The pathogenesis of the disease is that the combination of external and internal pathogenic factors invades both the liver and lung, which makes the pathogenic qi of liver and lung attack upwards the eye. This leads to the formation of the disease.

[Main Diagnostic Points]

1. Clinical Manifestations

(1) The affected eye, with a foreign body and burning sensation, suffers from photophobia, dacryorrhea and watery secretion; and dim vision occurs in the later course.

(2) The lid becomes edematous; the palpebral and bulbar conjunctiva are obviously congested with chemosis and; two or three days after the onset of the disease, folliculi occur in the palpebral conjunctiva and the fornix, sometimes with local bleeding beneath the conjunctiva.

(3) The lymphoglandulae auriculares anteriores of the affected side get swollen and tender to compression.

(4) Eight to ten days after the onset, the inflammation of the conjunctiva gradually relieves, and there arises the spotty infiltration (0.5 to 0.7 mm in diameter caused by adenovirus type 8). The lesion is largely concentrated in the middle of the cornea without ulceration and pannus. The corneal damage may leave the round superficial cloudiness on the cornea, which may disappear in a few months or years.

(5) The incubation period of the disease is about 5 to 12 days with 8 days in most cases. The disease often starts in both eyes successively.

2. Laboratory Examination

Adenovirus can be isolated from the secretion culture

范畴。外因为外感疫疠毒邪，内因为肺火亢盛。病机为内外合邪，侵及肝肺，肝肺二经邪气上攻于目所致。

【诊断要点】

1. 临床表现

（1）患眼异物感，灼热感，畏光流泪，有水样分泌物，后期视物模糊。

（2）眼睑水肿，睑球结膜充血明显，球结膜水肿，发病2～3日内睑结膜及穹窿部结膜出现滤泡，有时结膜下有小片出血。

（3）患侧耳前淋巴结肿大，有压痛。

（4）发病8～10日后，结膜炎症逐渐减轻，角膜上皮下出现较大点状浸润，腺病毒8型所致者直径可达0.5～0.7 mm。病变主要集中在角膜中央区，但不形成溃疡，亦无角膜血管翳。角膜损害可遗留圆形浅层云翳，持续数月或数年后可消失。

（5）潜伏期约5～12日，以8日为多，常双眼先后发病。

2. 实验室检查

部分病例可在结膜囊分

of conjunctival sac in some cases.

[Syndrome Differentiation and Treatment]

In clinic, the disease is usually classified into the syndromes of initial affection of epidemic and noxious pathogenic factors, excessive fire of the liver and gallbladder, and lingering pannus due to latent pathogenic factors. Since the disease arises from the meridians of the liver and lung or from lung involving liver, treatment should focus on removing pathogenic heat from the lung and liver simultaneously. And, according to the severity of the two involved organs, treatment should mainly be put on removing pathogenic heat either from the liver or from the lung.

1. Syndrome of Initial Affection of Epidemic and Noxious Pathogenil Factors

Main Symptoms and Signs   At the beginning, photophobia and dacryorrhea with alternate itching and unsmooth sensations, obvious redness and slight swelling of the bulbar conjunctiva, sometimes visible star-like corneal pannus, fever and aversion to cold, and stuffy nose with discharge; thin whitish tongue coating and floating rapid pulse.

Therapeutic Methods   Dispelling wind and removing heat.

Recipe   The modified Yinqiaosan Decoction: Lianqiao (*Fructus Forsythiae*) 15 g, Jinyinhua (*Flos Lonicerae*) 15 g, Jiegeng (*Radix Platycodi*) 10 g, Niubangzi (*Fructus Arctii*) 10 g, Jingjiesui (*Spica Schizonepetae*) 6 g, Bohe (*Herba Menthae*, to be decocted later) 5 g, Dandouchi (*Semen Sojae Praeparatum*) 10 g, Lugen (*Rhizoma Phragmitis*) 10 g, Zhuye (*Folium Phyllostachydis Henonis*) 10 g, and Shenggancao (*Radix Glycyrrhizae*) 6 g.

Modification   In the cases of piles of star-like corneal pannus and serious photophobia and dacryorrhea, respective 6 g, 10 g, 20 g and 10 g of Chantui (*Periostra-*

泌物培养后分离出腺病毒。

【辨证论治】

本病临床主要分为初感疫毒证、肝胆实火证、邪退翳留证。病位在肝肺二经,由肺及肝,治当清肝泻肺并举,并根据二者轻重缓急,或以清肝为主,或以泻肺为主。

1. 初感疫毒证

主要证候 病势初起,羞明流泪,刺痒交作,白睛红赤明显,轻微浮肿,或可见黑睛星翳稀疏散在,发热恶寒,鼻塞流涕。舌苔薄白,脉浮数。

治 法 疏风清热。

方 药 银翘散加减。连翘15 g,金银花15 g,桔梗10 g,牛蒡子10 g,荆芥穗6 g,薄荷(后下)5 g,淡豆豉10 g,芦根10 g,竹叶10 g,生甘草6 g。

加 减 若黑睛星翳簇生,畏光流泪甚者,加蝉蜕6 g,白蒺藜10 g,石决明(先煎)

cum Cicadae）, Baijili (*Fructus Tribuli*), Shijueming (*Concha Haliotidis*, decocted first), and Qingxiangzi (*Semen Celosiae*) are added.

2. Syndrome of Excessive Fire of the Liver and Gallbladder

Main Symptoms and Signs　Serious photoporbia and dacryorrhea, conjunctival hyperemia and even ciliary hyperemia, dense gray-white starry pannus of the superficial cornea in a large spotty shape, bitter taste in the mouth and dry throat; red tongue with yellowish coating and thready, rapid and strong pulse.

Therapeutic Method　Removing pathogenic fire by purging the liver.

Recipe　The modified Longdan Xiegan Decoction: Longdancao (*Radix Gentianae*) 6 g, Huangqin (*Radix Scutellariae*) 10 g, Shanzhizi (*Fructus Gardeniae*) 10 g, Zexie (*Rhizoma Alismatis*) 10 g, Mutong (*Caulis Akebiae*) 10 g, Cheqianzi (*Semen Plantaginis*, bagged) 10 g, Shengdihuang (*Radix Rehmanniae*) 10 g, Danggui (*Radix Angelicae Sinensis*) 10 g, Chaihu (*Radix Bupleuri*) 6 g, and Gancao (*Radix Glycyrrhizae*) 3 g.

Modification　In the cases of serious hyperemia of bulbar conjunctiva, respective 10 g of Lianqiao (*Fructus Forsythiae*) and Sangbaipi (*Cortex Mori*) are added; in the cases of serious photophobia and dacryorrhea, 10 g of Manjingzi (*Fructus Viticis*), 6 g Juhua (*Flos Chrysanthemi*) and 10 g Baijili (*Fructus Tribuli*) are added.

3. Syndrome of Lingering Pannus due to Latent Pathogenic Factors

Main Symptoms and Signs　Symptomatic relief and disappearance of redness and pain of the affected eye, while starry corneal nebula in large spotty shape still being remained, accompanied sometimes by photophorbia, dacryorrhea and poor vision, bitter taste in the mouth and dry

20 g,青葙子10 g。

2. 肝胆实火证

主要证候　羞明流泪特甚,白睛红赤不甚而以抱轮红赤为主,黑睛浅层大点状灰白色星翳密集,口苦咽干。舌红苔黄,脉弦数有力。

治　法　清肝泻火。

方　药　龙胆泻肝汤加减。龙胆草6 g,黄芩10 g,山栀子10 g,泽泻10 g,木通10 g,车前子（包煎）10 g,生地黄10 g,当归10 g,柴胡6 g,甘草3 g。

加　减　白睛红赤甚者,加连翘10 g,桑白皮10 g;羞明流泪甚者,加蔓荆子10 g,菊花6 g,白蒺藜10 g。

3. 邪退翳留证

主要证候　患眼红赤疼痛诸症减退或消失,唯黑睛遗留大点状星翳不退,时有畏光流泪,视物欠清,口苦咽干。苔薄白或薄黄,脉弦。

throat; thin whitish tongue coating and thready pulse.

Therapeutic Methods Removing pathogenic heat by calming the liver, and improving visional acuity by relieving nebula.

Recipe The modified Shijuemingsan Decoction: Shijueming (*Concha Haliotidis*, to be decocted first) 30 g, Caojueming (*Semen Cassiae*) 15 g, Qingxiangzi (*Semen Celosiae*) 10 g, Muzeicao (*Herba Equiseti Hiemalis*) 10 g, Shanzhizi (*Fructus Gardeniae*) 10 g, Chishaoyao (*Radix Paeoniae Rubra*) 10 g, Jingjie (*Herba Schizonepetae*) 6 g, Qianghuo (*Rhizoma et Radix Notopterygii*) 6 g, Maimendong (*Radix Ophiopogonis*) 10 g, Gujingcao (*Flos Eriocauli*) 10 g, and Mimenghua (*Flos Buddlejae*) 10 g.

Modification In the cases of no pathogenic wind, Qianghuo and Jingjie are removed.

[**Other Treatments**]

1. Chinese Patent Drugs

(1) **Yinqiao Jiedu Tablet** 4 tablets each time, three times a day and applicable to the syndrome of initial affection of epidemic and noxious pathogenic factors.

(2) **Huanglian Shangqing Pill** 6 g each time, twice a day and applicable to the syndrome of excessive stagnation of toxic heat.

(3) **Shangqing Pill** 6 g each time, twice a day and applicable to the syndrome of excessive stagnation of toxic heat.

(4) **Niuhuang Shangqing Pill** 6 g each time, twice a day and applicable to the syndrome of excessive stagnation of toxic heat.

(5) **Longdan Xiegan Pill** 6 g each time, twice a day and applicable to the syndrome of excessive fire of the liver and ballgladder.

(6) **Qingre Jiedu Pill** 10 pills once, three times a

治　法　清热平肝,明目退翳。

方　药　石决明散加减。石决明(先煎)30 g,草决明15 g,青葙子10 g,木贼草10 g,山栀子10 g,赤芍药10 g,荆芥6 g,羌活6 g,麦门冬10 g,谷精草10 g,密蒙花10 g。

加　减　若无风证者,去羌活、荆芥。

【其他疗法】

1. 中成药

(1) 银翘解毒片　每服4片,每日 3 次。适用于初感疫毒证。

(2) 黄连上清丸　每服6 g,每日 2 次。适用于热毒壅盛证。

(3) 上清丸　每服6 g,每日2～3 次。适用于热毒壅盛证。

(4) 牛黄上清丸　每服6 g,每日2～3 次。适用于热毒壅盛证。

(5) 龙胆泻肝丸　每服6 g,每日 2 次。适用于肝胆实火证。

(6) 清热解毒丸　每服

day and applicable to the syndrome of excessive fire of the liver and ballgladder.

(7) Anti-virus Oral Drink　10 ml each time, three times a day and applicable to all syndromes of the disease.

2. Simple and Proved Recipes

(1) Mangxiao (*Natrii Sulphas*), Huangdan (*Minium*), Ruxiang (*Resina Olibani*), and Moyao (*Myrrha*), 6 g of each and 3 g of Xionghuang (*Realgar*), all the drugs are ground into powder which is applied for nasal insufflation for the mild cases of the disease.

(2) 120 g of fresh Pugongying (*Herba Taraxaci*) is decocted with water for oral application to treat the mild cases of the disease.

(3) Sangye (*Folium Mori*) 5 g, Juhua (*Flos Chrysanthemi*) 5 g, Bohe (*Herba Menthae*, to be decocted later) 3 g, Kuzhuye (*Folium Pleioblasti Amari Juvenile*) 30 g, all these herbs are washed cleanly, steeped with hot boiled water in a teapot for 10 minutes. The beverage is applicable to the mild cases of the disease.

(4) The ingredients of the porridge include Sangbaipi (*Cortex Mori*, honeyed) 50 g, Yiyiren (*Semen Coicis*) 20 g, and 100 g of rice fruit. After steeped with water, Sangbaipi is boiled twice. With the dregs being removed, Yiyiren and rice are put into the decoction which is then cooked well into porridge. The porridge is applicable to the disease in its later course or with the remaining pathogenic factors.

(5) Danggui (*Radix Angelicae Sinensis*), Huangbai (*Cortex Phellodendri*), Fangfeng (*Radix Ledebouriellae*), Xingren (*Semen Armeniacae Amarum*), each 3 g, and respective 6 g of Gancao (*Radix Glycyrrhizae*), Tonglü (*Arerugo*) and Danfan (*Chalcanthitum*), all are decocted for fumigating and washing the eye, which is ap-

10 粒,每日 3 次。适用于肝胆实火证。

（7）抗病毒口服液　每服 10 ml,每日 3 次。适用各类型。

2. 单验方

（1）芒硝、黄丹、乳香、没药各 6 g,雄黄 3 g。共研细末,含水吹鼻。适用于本病轻症。

（2）新鲜蒲公英 120 g,水煎饮之,适用于本病轻症。

（3）桑叶 5 g,菊花 5 g,薄荷(后下)3 g,苦竹叶 30 g。将上药洗净,放入茶壶内,用开水泡 10 分钟即可饮用。适用于本病轻症。

（4）蜜炙桑白皮 50 g,薏苡仁 20 g,粳米 100 g。桑白皮以水浸泡,熬煎 2 次,弃渣留汤,加入薏苡仁、粳米,煮之熟烂。适用于本病后期,余邪滞留证。

（5）当归、黄柏、防风、杏仁各 3 g,甘草、铜绿、胆矾各 6 g,煎汤薰洗眼睛。适用于本病各证。

plicable to all syndromes of the disease.

(6) Some fresh Biqi (*Cormus Eleocharitis Dulcis*) is cleaned by washing and, with its skin being removed, is pounded to pieces. The juice, which is taken with a piece of sterilized gauze, is mixed with a little salt for the washing of the affected eye. The method is applicable to the mild cases of the disease.

(7) The method consists of five slices of Huanglian (*Rhizoma Coptidis*) and 10 ml of human milk. The slices are soaked in the milk for 15 minutes, and then removed. The affected eye is dropped with the prepared milk three times a day. The method is applicable to epidemic keratoconjunctivitis in the mild cases.

3. External Therapies

(1) Eye Drops   a. Coptis-watermelon-frost Eye Drops   It is given 3 to 4 times a day, which is applicable to all types of the disease. b. Qianliguang Eye Drops: It is given 3 to 4 times a day, which is applicable to all syndromes of the disease. c. Danzhi Erlian Ointment: The eye is smeared before sleeping and the method is applicable to all syndromes of the disease.

(2) Fumigation-Washing   Method   20 g of fresh Yejuhua (*Flos Chrysanthemi Indici*), 30 g of Pugongying (*Herba Taraxaci*), 30 g of Cheqiancao (*Herba Plantaginis*), 30 g of Zihuadiding (*Herba Violae*), all are decocted with water for fumigating and washing the eye once or twice a day. The method is applicable to the severe cases.

2.3.3   Spring Conjunctivitis

[Introduction]

Spring conjunctivitis, also called spring catarrhal

（6）鲜荸荠洗净去皮，捣烂，以纱布绞汁，加食盐少许洗眼。适用于本病轻症。

（7）黄连（切片）5 片，人乳10 ml。黄连片浸入人乳内，等待 15 分钟后，去黄连。滴眼，每日 3 次。适用于流行性角膜结膜炎轻症。

3. 外治法

（1）点眼药   ① 黄连西瓜霜眼药水：每日点眼3～4次。适用于本病各证。② 千里光眼药水：每日点眼3～4次。适用于本病各证。③ 胆汁二连膏：每晚临睡前涂眼。适用于本病各证。

（2）薰洗法   新鲜野菊花20 g，蒲公英30 g，车前草30 g，紫花地丁30 g，煎水薰洗患眼。每日1～2 次。适用于本病重症。

第三节   春季
结膜炎

【概述】

春季结膜炎，又称春季卡

conjunctivitis, is a kind of allergic ophthalmopathy characterized by unusual ocular itching in clinic. As a seasonal
and periodical disease, it often starts in warm spring and
becomes worse in summer and relieves or disappears in
autumn and winter. In the coming spring, it relapses and
lasts several or dozens of years without recovery, but it
may gradually turn better and even recovered as the patients are aging. The case is common in children and
young people with the male more than the female, and
both eyes are usually affected in most cases.

It is often believed that the disease, though the real
cause is unknown, is a sort of immune trouble or an allergic conjunctivitis and pertains to allergic type I. The sen-
sitinogens of the disease may be different plant pollens,
microbial antigenic components, filthy dust, animal fur-
furs, feathers, changes of sunlight and temperature, and
so on.

Clinical manifestations of the disease show that the
case should pertain in traditional Chinese medicine to Shi-
fuzheng (seasonal and periodical ophthalmopathy), Mu-
yang (ocular itching) and Yangruo Chongxingzheng (insect-moving itching of eye). It is caused in most cases by
the fact that the invasion of pathogenic wind repeatedly
attacks between the lids and the connecting tissues, or
that, when internal accumulated dampness of the spleen
and stomach is frequently affected by pathogenic wind,
the combatting pathogenic wind, dampness and heat all
accumulates up to the eye and stagnates in the lid. It may
arise as a result of deficiency of the liver and blood, for
blood asthenia can raise endopathic wind which causes
itching.

[Main Diagnostic Points]

1. Clinical Manifestations

Usually, the disease attacks binocularly in spring and

他性结膜炎,是一种变态反应
性疾病,临床主要表现为眼部
奇痒。其发病季节性强,大多
于春暖时节发病,至盛夏加剧,
秋冬时症状减轻或消失,次年
春季来临时又复发,如此反复
不已,可延续数年或十余年之
久,随年龄增长而逐年减缓或
痊愈。本病好发于儿童和少
年,男性较多,多为双眼患病。

本病的真正病因尚不明
确,多数人认为本病为免疫性疾
病,为过敏反应性结膜炎,属变
态反应第Ⅰ型。其过敏原可能
为各类植物的花粉、各种微生物
的抗原成分、污尘、动物皮屑、羽
毛、阳光及温度的变化等。

根据本病的临床表现,当
属于中医学"时复症"、"目
痒"、"痒若虫行症"等范畴。
病因多因风邪侵袭,邪气往来
于睑眦腠理之间;或脾胃内蕴
湿热,复感风邪,风湿热邪相
搏,上壅于目,停留于睑内而
发;亦可因肝虚血少,血虚风
动而作痒。

【诊断要点】

1. 临床表现

常双眼发病,多于春夏季

summer and disappears naturally in autumn and winter, but recurs next spring and lasts years without recovery. Its typical symptom is unbearable ocular itching accompanied by photophobia, dacryorrhea, foreign body sensation and a little eye secretion.

Clinically, the disease is divided into three types according to the part of pathogenic changes.

(1) **Type of palpebral conjunctiva** It is the most common type with the lesion often localized in the upper palpebral conjunctiva. At the beginning of its occurrence, there is a small amount of adhensive and thready secretion, congestion of the conjunctiva, lots of flat cobble-like and light red papillae in the upper palpebra conjunctiva which are of various sizes and shapes with a layer of milk-like substance painted on, and the tarsal becomes hyperplastic and pachyntic.

(2) **Type of corneal limbus (*bulbar conjunctiva*)** The lesion starts in the corneal limbus and near the bulbar conjunctiva. One or many grayish yellow colloid projecting nodules appear at the corneal limbus, and the surrounding part of the bulbar conjunctiva congested, especially the palpebral fissure.

(3) **Mixed Type** Both of the above pathogenic changes exsist in the affected eye simultaneously.

2. Laboratory Examination

Acidocyte can be found on the secretion smear of conjunctival sac or by conjunctival scaling.

[**Syndrome Differentiation and Treatment**]

In clinic, the disease is mainly classified into the syndromes of invasion of pathogenic wind, ocular accumulation of pathogenic wind-heat, pathogenic damp-heat plus wind, and endopathic wind due to blood asthenia. The

起病,秋冬季自行消退,翌年春季又犯,反复多年不止。其最典型的症状是眼部奇痒,患者难以忍受,此外常伴有畏光流泪,灼热异物感,及少量分泌物。

临床上根据病变发生部位,分为三种类型。

(1)睑结膜型 是最常见的一种类型。病变多局限于上睑结膜,下睑较少发病。发病时,有少量黏丝状分泌物,结膜充血,上睑结膜有多数硬韧而扁平的乳头,大小不一,形状不规则,色淡红,似铺路的石子,上涂有薄层牛奶状,睑板可以增生肥厚。

(2)角膜缘型(球结膜型) 病变发生于角膜缘及其附近的球结膜。角膜缘部出现一个或多数灰黄胶状隆起结节,周围球结膜充血,睑裂部充血尤为常见。

(3)混合型 一眼中同时存在以上两型病变。

2. 实验室检查

结膜囊分泌物涂片或结膜刮片中可查见嗜酸性白细胞。

【辨证论治】

本病临床主要分为风邪侵袭证、风热壅目证、湿热挟风证、血虚生风证。治疗当内外兼施。内治以祛风止痒为

treatment, therefore, should include internal and external methods. The internal treatment principle, based on the discrimination of asthenia and sthenia, should focus on removing wind to relieve itching. In sthenia cases, the methods of removing wind, heat and dampness should be applied while, in asthenia cases, nourishing blood and dispelling wind to stop itching should be applied with the support of proper external treatment ways.

基本治法,分清虚实,实证当祛风清热除湿止痒,虚证当养血熄风以止痒,并适当配合外治方法。

1. Syndrome of Invasion of Pathogenic Wind

Main Symptions and Signs Uncomfortable sensation of eye, constant itching, normal eyesight, and light red eyelid with a few red granules; thin whitish tongue coating and floating pulse.

Therapeutic Method Removing pathogenic wind to stop itching.

Recipe The modified Qufeng Yizi Powder: Paochuanwu (*Radix Corniti*, prepared) 1.5 g, Chuanxiong (*Rhizoma Ligustici Chuanxiong*) 6 g, Jingjiesui (*Spica Schizonepetae*) 5 g, Qianghuo (*Rhizome seu Radix Notopterygii*) 5 g, and Bohe (*Herba Menthae*, to be decocted later) 5 g.

Modification In the cases of unbearable itchiness, 10 g of Gaoben (*Rhizoma et Radix Ligustici*) and 6 g of Wushaoshe (*Zaocys*) are added; in the cases of pathogenic heat, Huangqin (*Radix Scultellariae*), Shengdihuang (*Radix Rehmanniae*) and Kushen (*Radix Sophorae Flavescentis*), each 10 g, are added; in debility cases, 10 g of Dangshen (*Radix Codonopsis Pilosulae*) and 10 g of Huangqin (*Radix Scultellariae*) are added.

2. Syndrome of Ocular Accumulation of pathogenic Wind-heat

Main Symptoms and Signs Burning itching in the eye, repeated occurrence in spring, cobble-like reddish granules in eyelid tidily arranged, severe condition when

1. 风邪侵袭证

主要证候　眼部不适,时时作痒,视力正常,睑内微红,少许红色颗粒。舌苔薄白,脉浮。

治　法　祛风止痒。

方　药　驱风一字散加减。炮川乌1.5 g,川芎6 g,荆芥穗5 g,羌活5 g,薄荷(后下)5 g。

加　减　痒甚难忍者,加藁本10 g,乌梢蛇6 g;兼挟热邪者,加黄芩10 g,生地黄10 g,苦参10 g;若兼体虚者,加党参10 g,黄芪10 g。

2. 风热壅目证

主要证候　眼内灼痒,每于春暖季节发作,睑内红色颗粒,排列整齐,如铺路卵石样。

facing wind blow, sunshine or fire fumigation; thin yellowish tongue coating and floating rapid pulse.

Therapeutic Methods Removing wind and heat and activating blood circulation to stop itching.

Recipe The modified Jiajian Siwu Decoction: Shengdihuang (*Radix Rehmanniae*) 10 g, Kushen (*Radix Sophorae Flavescentis*) 10 g, Bohe (*Herba Menthae*, to be decocted later) 5 g, Chuanxiong (*Rhizoma Ligustici Chuanxiong*) 10 g, Niubangzi (*Fructus Arctii*) 10 g, Lianqiao (*Fructus Forsythiae*) 10 g, Tianhuafen (*Radix Trichosanthis*) 10 g, Fangfeng (*Radix Ledebouriellae*) 6 g, Chishaoyao (*Radix Paeoniae Rubra*) 10 g, Danggui (*Radix Angelicae Sinensis*) 10 g, and Jingjiesui (*Herba Schizonepetae*) 10 g.

Modification In the cases of severe heat, 10 g of Huangqin (*Radix Scutellariae*) and 10 g of Huangbai (*Cortex Phellodendri*) and 15 g of Huzhang (*Rhizoma Polygoni Cuspidati*) are added.

3. Syndrome of Pathogenic Damp-heat Plus Wind

Main Symptoms and Signs Peculiar and unbearable eye-itching, tears with mucopurulent secretion, thickness and heaviness of the palpebra, yellowish and turbid bulbar conjunctiva, and thickness of corneal boundaries; red tongue with yellowish greasy coating and smooth pulse.

Therapeutic Method Removing wind, heat and dampness to arrest itching.

Recipe The modified Chushi Decoction: Lianqiao (*Fructus Forsythiae*) 10 g, Huashi (*Talcum*) 10 g, Cheqianzi (*Semen Plantaginis*, bagged) 10 g, Zhike (*Fructus Aurantii*) 6 g, Huangqin (*Radix Scutellariae*) 10 g, Huanglian (*Rhizoma Coptidis*) 5 g, Mutong

遇风吹日晒或近火薰灼后,症情往往加重。舌苔薄黄,脉浮数。

治 法 祛风清热,活血止痒。

方 药 加减四物汤加减。生地黄10 g,苦参10 g,薄荷(后下)5 g,川芎10 g,牛蒡子10 g,连翘10 g,天花粉10 g,防风6 g,赤芍药10 g,当归10 g,荆芥穗10 g。

加 减 热盛者,加黄芩10 g,黄柏10 g,虎杖15 g。

3. 湿热挟风证

主要证候 眼内奇痒难忍,眵多胶粘,胞睑厚重,白睛黄浊,黑睛边缘增厚如厚胶。舌红苔黄腻,脉滑。

治 法 祛风清热,除湿止痒。

方 药 除湿汤加减。连翘10 g,滑石10 g,车前子(包煎)10 g,枳壳6 g,黄芩10 g,黄连5 g,木通5 g,陈皮5 g,荆芥10 g,茯苓10 g,防风

(*Caulis Akebiae*) 5 g, Chenpi (*Pericarpium Citri Reticulatae*) 5 g, Jingjie (*Herba Schizonepetae*) 10 g, Fuling (*poria*) 10 g, Fangfeng (*Radix Ledebouriellae*) 10 g, and Gancao (*Radix Glycyrrhizae*) 3 g.

Modification In the cases of severe pathogenic wind, 5 g of Wushaoshe (*Zaocys*), 10 g of Chuanxiong (*Rhizoma Ligustici Chuanxiong*), 6 g of Qianghuo (*Rhizoma seu Radix Notopterygii*), 5 g of Bohe (*Herba Menthae*, to be decocted later) and 5 g of Chantui (*Periostracum Cicadae*) are added; in the cases of serious itching, respective 10 g of Tufuling (*Rhizoma Smilacis Glabrae*), Baixianpi(*Crotex Dictamni Radicis*) and Difuzi (*Fructus Kochiae*) are added.

4. Syndrome of Endogenic Wind due to Blood Asthenia

Main Symptoms and Signs Mild itching of eye now and then, recurrence without recovery, accompanied by a dry and uncomfortable sensation in the eye, light red palpebral conjunctiva and a few scattering and soft granules; pale tongue with thin coating and thin pulse.

Therapeutic Method Nourishing blood to dispel wind.

Recipe The modified Siwu Decoction: Chuanxiong (*Rhizoma Ligustici Chuanxiong*) 10 g, Danggui (*Radix Angelicae Sinensis*) 10 g, Baishaoyao (*Radix Paeoniae Alba*) 10 g, Shudihuang (*Radix Rehmanniae Praeparata*) 10 g, Baijiangchan (*Bombyx Batryticatus*)10 g, Baijili (*Fructus Tribuli*) 10 g, Baizhi (*Radix Angelicae Dahuricae*) 10 g, Fangfeng (*Radix Ledebouriellae*) 6 g, and Jingjie (*Herba Schizonepetae*) 6 g.

[Other Treatments]

1. Chinese Patent Drugs

(1) **Yufeng Pill** 6 g each time, three times every day and applicable to the syndrome of invasion of pathogenic wind.

10 g,甘草3 g。

加 减 风邪较重,加乌梢蛇5 g,川芎10 g,羌活6 g,薄荷(后下)5 g,蝉蜕5 g;痒甚者,加土茯苓10 g,白鲜皮10 g,地肤子10 g。

4. 血虚生风证

主要证候 眼痒势轻,时作时止,反复难愈,兼有干涩不舒,睑内微红,颗粒稀少,形体不实。舌淡苔薄,脉细。

治 法 养血熄风。

方 药 四物汤加减。川芎10 g,当归10 g,白芍药10 g,熟地黄10 g,白僵蚕10 g,白蒺藜10 g,白芷10 g,防风6 g,荆芥6 g。

【其他疗法】

1. 中成药

(1)愈风丸 每服6 g,每日3次。适用于风邪侵袭证。

(2) Xiaofeng Granule   10 g each time, three times every day and applicable to the syndrome of ocular accumulation of pathogenic wind-heat.

2. Simple and Proved Recipes

The ingredients of ten Chinese dates and 100 g of barley are decocted with water for oral taking, twice or three times a day, which is applicable to the syndrome of endopathic wind due to blood asthenia.

3. External Therapies

(1) Eye Drops   a. Chunxue (*Spring-snow*) Ointment: It is given with the ointment twice a day, which is applicable to pathogenic damp-heat plus wind. b. Red Eye Ointment: It is given with the ointment three times a day, which is applicable to all syndromes of the disease. c. Qingliang (*Cooling*) Ointment: A small amount of the ointment is pasted on the canthus twice or three times a day, and it is applicable to all syndromes of the disease. d. Xiongdan Eye Drops: It is given four times a day, which is applicable to the cases with severe itching.

(2) Fumigation-Washing Method   10 g of Longdancao (*Radix Gentianae*) and of Fangfeng (*Radix Ledebouriellae*) and 3 g of Xixin (*Herba Asari*) and of Gancao (*Radix Glycyrrhizae*) are decocted with water, and the eye is fumigated and washed with the decoction twice a day. Or the dregs of oral decoctions are decocted with water for fumigating and washing the eye twice a day. The method is applicable to the syndrome of ocular accumulation of pathogenic wind-heat.

2.3.4   Phlyctenular Conjunctivitis

[Introduction]

Phlyctenular conjunctivitis is a kind of allergic con-

（2）消风冲剂　每服 10 g，每日 3 次。适用于风热壅目证。

2. 单验方

大枣 10 枚，大麦100 g。加水煎服，每日2～3 次。适用于血虚生风证。

3. 外治法

（1）点眼药　① 春雪膏：每日点眼 2 次。适用于湿热挟风证。② 红眼药：每日点眼 3 次。适用于本病各证。③ 清凉膏：用时少许贴眼角上，每日2～3 次。适用于本病各证。④ 熊胆眼药水：每日点眼 4 次。适用于本病痒甚者。

（2）薰洗法　龙胆草 10 g，防风10 g，细辛3 g，甘草 3 g。煎水，或以内服药渣煎水薰洗患眼，每日 2 次。适用于风热壅目证。

第四节　泡性结膜炎

【概述】

泡性结膜炎是一种变态

junctivitis which often starts in spring and summer. Clinically, it mainly manifests the symptoms of repeated nodular damage of the conjunctiva and local congestion of the nearby conjunctiva. In most cases, one eye is affected and sometimes both eyes are involved at the same time or one after the other. The disease is common in children of debility, malnutrition and bad living conditions or in those who prefer to sweet and starchy foods.

The case may occur only in the bulbar conjunctiva, or simultaneously in the cornea and conjunctiva, and sometimes in the cornea alone. If the lesion is in the bulbar conjunctiva, the case is refered to as phlyctenular conjunctivitis. If in the corneal margin, it is called phlyctenular keratoconjunctivitis, and it can be defined as phlyctenular keratitis if in the cornea. And phlyctennular ophthelmia is a general term of all.

Pathogenetically and etiologically, the disease is a kind of delayed hypersensitivity to the microorganic protein. The concerned microorganisms include tubercle bacillus, staphylococcus, Candida albicans, Conidiosporalis and Chlamydia trachomatis and so on.

From the clinical manifestations, the disease should pertain to "Jingan" or "Jinyang" (fallicular conjunctivitis) in traditional Chinese medicine. Pathogenic dryness-heat in the lung meridian, deficiency of lung yin or weakness of the spleen and stomach and incoordination of the lung and spleen, all these are the crucial factors to the occurrence of the disease. The pathogenic dryness-heat in the lung meridian makes the lung lose its dispelling-releasing function which gives rise to qi stagnancy and blood stasis, thus the bulbar conjunctiva being affected. If the deficiency of lung yin initiates hyperactivity of deficient fire, the bulbar vessels are affected and stagnated, and qi and blood are accumulated, causing malnutritional disorders of the eye.

反应性结膜炎,本病多发生在春夏季节,临床主要表现为结膜上反复出现结节状损害,附近结膜局限性充血。单眼发病为多,亦有双眼同时或先后发病者,本病多见于体弱、营养不良、环境卫生欠佳或喜食糖果、淀粉类食物的儿童。

本病可单独发生于球结膜,也可同时侵犯角膜结膜或单独侵犯角膜,病变位于球结膜者称为泡性结膜炎,位于角膜缘者称为泡性角膜结膜炎,位于角膜者称之为泡性角膜炎,可统称为泡性眼炎。

本病的病因病机是一种对微生物蛋白质的迟发过敏反应。相关的微生物有结核杆菌、葡萄球菌、白色念珠菌、球孢子菌属及沙眼衣原体等。

根据本病的临床表现,当属于中医学"金疳"、"金疡"范畴。肺经燥热,肺阴不足或脾胃虚弱,肺脾失调为导致本病发生的重要因素。肺经燥热,失其清肃宣发之功,则气机郁滞,气滞而致血瘀,故病发于白睛;若肺阴不足,火无水济,虚火上炎,白睛血络受迫,滞而不行,气血瘀滞,聚而成疳。另外,脾胃虚弱,运化无力,土不生金,肺失所养,气化不利,气血郁滞亦可发为本病。

Besides, the poor transforming function of the spleen due to deficiency of the spleen and stomach and the nourishing disfunction of the lung due to the failure of the spleen (earth) to generate the lung (gold) may cause the obstruction of qi activities, for stagnancy of qi and blood can also start the disease.

[Main Diagnostic Points]

(1) The affected eye suffers from the symptoms of slight pain, photophobia, dacryorrhea and an uncomfortable and foreign body sensation.

(2) In the bulbar conjunctiva occurs a local projecting nodule which is round, grayish red, 1 to 4mm in diameter and with local congestion around. When the tip of the nodule is necrotic and deciduous in 2 to 4 days, ulcer is formed, which often heals naturally in 8 to 10 days with no scar left.

(3) The lesion usually starts in the palpebral fissure with one nodule in most cases and two or more in a severe case.

[Syndrome Differentiation and Treatment]

Clinically, the case is mainly classified into the syndromes of pathogenic dryness-heat of lung meridian, deficiency of lung yin and asthenia of both the lung and spleen. The principle of treatment should focus on the lung because it is the crucial organ involved in this disease. At the beginning of the disease, the treatment method is to purge lung heat to promote the circulation of qi while, in the repeated and lingering cases without recovery, the treatment method is mainly to nourish the lung and spleen to reduce deficient fire and restore the normal function of the lung.

1. Syndrome of Pathogenic Dryness-heat of Lung Meridian

Main Symptoms and Signs   Astringing pain,

【诊断要点】

(1) 患眼轻度异物感,或有微痛畏光,流泪不适感。

(2) 球结膜出现局限性隆起结节,圆形,直径1～4 mm,灰红色,周围局限性充血。2～4日后,小结顶部坏死脱落,形成溃疡,常于8～10 日后自行愈合,结节消退后而不留瘢痕。

(3) 病变好发于睑裂部,通常发生一个结节,严重者可发生两个甚至两个以上的结节。

【辨证论治】

本病临床主要分为肺经燥热证、肺阴不足证、肺脾两虚证。主脏在肺,治疗总宜治肺为本。病初起,宜泻肺利气散结,使气血畅行;如病情反复发作或病势缠绵不愈,则应润肺健脾,使脾土健而肺金生,肺润而虚火平,复其宣发肃降之功。

1. 肺经燥热证

主要证候 涩痛畏光,流

photophobia, dacryorrhea with profuse secretion, protrusion of phlyctenular granules surrounded by congested capillaries on the bulbar conjunctiva, dryness in the mouth and throat, cough with scanty sputum, constipation and brownish urine; reddish tongue with thin yellowish coating and rapid pulse.

泪眵多,白睛表面小泡样颗粒隆起,周围赤丝环绕,口渴鼻干,咳嗽少痰,便秘溲赤。舌红苔薄黄,脉数等。

Therapeutic Methods　Removing lung heat and resolving mass.

治　法　清肺散结。

Recipe　The modified Qingfei Decoction: Sangbaipi (*Cortex Mori*) 10 g, Huangqin (*Radix Scutellariae*) 10 g, Digupi (*Cortex Lycii Radicis*) 10 g, Zhimu (*Rhizome Anemarrhenae*) 10 g, Maimendong (*Radix Ophiopogonis*) 10 g, Jiegeng (*Radix Platycodi*) 5 g, Fangfeng (*Radix Ledebouriellae*) 10 g, Chishaoyao (*Radix Paeoniae Rubra*) 10 g, and Lianqiao (*Fructus Forsythiae*) 10 g.

方　药　泻肺汤加减。桑白皮10 g,黄芩10 g,地骨皮10 g,知母10 g,麦门冬10 g,桔梗5 g,防风10 g,赤芍药10 g,连翘10 g。

2. Syndrome of Deficiency of Lung Yin

2. 肺阴不足证

Main Symptoms and Signs　Slight pain with a faint astringing sensation, a few tears and secretion, small granules of the bulbar conjunctiva with light red capillaries around, lingering and repeated history, dryness in the mouth and throat, dry cough, feverish sensation in chest, palms and soles; red tongue with thin coating and rapid pulse.

主要证候　隐涩微痛,眵泪不多,白睛颗粒小而不高,周围血丝淡红,且病程较久,反复难愈,口咽干燥,干咳无痰,五心潮热。舌红,苔薄,脉细数。

Therapeutic Methods　Nourishing yin, moistening the lung and dissipating stagnation.

治　法　滋阴润肺散结。

Recipe　The modified Yangyin Qingfei Decoction: Shengdihuang (*Radix Rehmanniae*) 12 g, Maimendong (*Radix Ophiopogonis*) 10 g, Baishaoyao (*Radix Paeoniae Alba*) 10 g, Xuanshen (*Radix Scrophulariae*) 10 g, Mudanpi (*Cortex Moutan Radicis*) 10 g, Bohe (*Herba Menthae*, to be decocted later) 5 g, Beimu (*Bulbus Fritillariae*) 6 g, Shenggancao (*Radix Glycyrrhizae*) 3 g, Xiakucao (*Spica Prunellae*) 10 g, and Lianqiao (*Fructus Forsythiae*) 10 g.

方　药　养阴清肺汤加减。生地黄12 g,麦门冬10 g,白芍药10 g,玄参10 g,牡丹皮10 g,薄荷(后下)5 g,贝母6 g,生甘草3 g,夏枯草10 g,连翘10 g。

3. Syndrome of Asthenia of Both Lung and Spleen

Main Symptoms and Signs Slight astringing and uncomfortable sensation in the eye, repeated occurrence of bulbar conjunctiva nodules surrounded by mild capillaries, mental tiredness and fatigue, shortness of breath and no desire to speak, anorexia, cough with sputum, abdominal distension, loose stool or constipation; whitish tongue with thin coating and weak-thready pulse.

Therapeutic Methods Nourishing the spleen and benefiting the lung.

Recipe The modified Liujunzi Decoction: Dangshen (*Radix Codonopsis Pilosulae*) 10 g, Baizhu (*Rhizoma Atractylodis Macrocephalae*) 10 g, Fuling (*Poria*) 10 g, Zhigancao (*Radix Glycyrrhizae Praeparata*) 5 g, Chenpi (*Pericarpium Citri Reticulatae*) 6 g, Banxia (*Rhizoma Pinelliae*) 10 g, Fangfeng (*Radix Ledebouriellae*) 10 g, Sangbaipi (*Cortex Mori*) 10 g, Chishaoyao (*Radix Paeoniae Rubra*) 10 g, Shengjiang (*Rhizoma Zingiberis Recens*) 2 slices, and Dazao (*Fructus Jujubae*) 4 pieces.

[Other Treatments]

1. Chinese Patent Drugs

Yangyin Qingfei Ointment 15 g each time, twice a day for oral taking and applicable to the syndrome of deficiency of lung yin.

2. External Therapies

(1) Coptidis – Watermelon-Frost Eye Drops It is given 4 times every day and applicable to the syndrome of pathogenic dryness-heat of lung meridian.

(2) Qianliguang Eye Drops It is given 4 times every day and applicable to the syndrome of pathogenic dryness-heat of lung meridian.

(3) Sanhuang Eye Drops It is given 4 times every

3. 肺脾两虚证

主要证候 微涩不适,白睛小泡反复难愈,周围赤丝轻微,神疲乏力,少气懒言,纳谷不佳,咳嗽有痰,腹胀不舒,便溏或便秘。舌淡苔薄,脉细无力。

治 法 补脾益肺。

方 药 六君子汤加减。党参10 g,白术10 g,茯苓10 g,炙甘草5 g,陈皮6 g,半夏10 g,防风10 g,桑白皮10 g,赤芍药10 g,生姜 2 片,大枣 4 枚。

【其他疗法】

1. 中成药

养阴清肺膏 每服15 g,每日 2 次。适用于肺阴不足证。

2. 外治法

(1) 黄连西瓜霜眼药水 每日点眼 4 次。适用于肺经燥热证。

(2) 千里光眼药水 每日点眼 4 次。适用于肺经燥热证。

(3) 三黄眼液 每日点

day and applicable to the syndrome of pathogenic dryness-heat of lung meridian.

(4) Xiongdan Eye Drops   It is given 4 times every day and applicable to the syndrome of pathogenic dryness-heat of lung meridian.

(5) Guangming Eye Ointment   Smear the eye every night before sleep and it is applicable to the syndrome of pathogenic dryness-heat of lung meridian.

2.3.5 Episcleritis

[**Introduction**]

Episcleritis, an inflammation of superficial tissues overlaying the sclera, is a sort of recurrent, transient, self-limited and often nonspecific ophthalmopathy. It is common among the middle-aged people, of whom women are more than men. In clinic, the disease mainly manifests the symptom of local or diffuse dark-red prominence of the outermost layer of the sclera. The pathogenic change of the disease usually appears in the part between the corneal limbus of the anterior equator and the attachment line of the ocular rectus. The case may start either monocularly or binocularly with a favorable prognosis.

The cause and pathogensis of the disease, as many researchers think, are related either with autoimmune desmosis, or with the general infection, or with the allergic reaction caused by local infection and endocrine factors. In addition, there might be some idiopathic causes.

Clinical manifestations show that the disease should pertain to "Huogan" or "Huoyang" (acute scleritis) in traditional Chinese medicine. In most cases, hyperactivity

眼 4 次。适用于肺经燥热证。

（4）熊胆眼液　每日点眼 4 次。适用于肺经燥热证。

（5）光明眼膏　每晚临睡前涂眼。适用于肺经燥热证。

第五节　浅层巩膜炎

【概述】

浅层巩膜炎是指浅层巩膜组织的炎症。临床主要表现为巩膜表层暗红色局限性或弥漫性隆起。本病多见于壮年人，女性多于男性。它是一种复发性、短暂性、自限性、并常为非特异性的眼病。病变多位于眼球赤道前部角膜缘与眼直肌附着线之间，可一眼或双眼发病，预后良好。

其病因和发病机理，多数学者认为与自身免疫性结缔组织疾病有关，或与多种全身感染性疾病有关，也可能与病灶感染引起的过敏反应以及内分泌因素有关，此外，还有一些原因不明引起者。

根据本病的临床表现，当属于中医学"火疳"、"火疡"范畴。病因多为肺热亢盛，气机

of lung heat and stagnancy of qi's activities accumulates up to the bulbar conjunctiva, thus giving rise to the disease. When the concerned meridian is obstructed by the interior retention of pathogenic damp-heat and attack of pathogenic wind, the lung qi fails to flow freely and pathogenic factors retain in the bulbar conjunctiva, eventually bringing about this disease. It may also be caused by deficient fire. For example, if the impairment of yin by lung heat results in deficiency of lung yin which causes fire hyperactivity and yin deficiency, the bulbar conjunctiva is harassed and episleritis may occur.

[**Main Diagnostic Points**]

(1) At the initial stage, the affected eye suffers from the symptoms of astringing pain, photophobia, dacryorrhea, which repeat and last a long time.

(2) In the pathogenic area, there is diffuse congestive edema on the outmost layer of the sclera, or local mild prominent scarlet nodules caused by infiltration in the round or elliptic shapes and of various sizes, the bulbar conjunctiva over the nodules being movable and tender to compression. The prominent nodules, which increase gradually in size, are seldom diabrotic and can be absorbed in several weeks.

(3) Usually, one eye is affected and both may be affected occasionally at the same time or one after another.

[**Syndrome Differentiation and Treatment**]

The disease is mainly classified in clinic into the syndromes of hyperactivity of lung heat, combinating stagnancy of wind, damp and heat, and hyperacitivity of fire due to yin deficiency. Since the lesion is in the white of eye or aerorbiculus, lung is the crucial organ that is involved in the case, and stagnant accumulation of lung heat is therefore the key cause of the disease. The treatment meth-

滞塞,郁于白睛而发;或湿热内蕴,兼感风邪,阻滞经络,肺气失宣,郁久白睛而发病;亦有因虚火所致者,如肺热伤阴,肺阴不足,阴虚火旺,上扰白睛而发病。

【诊断要点】

(1) 初起患眼涩痛,畏光流泪,病程长,易反复发作。

(2) 病变区巩膜表层弥漫性充血水肿,或有浸润而形成局限性微凸的结节,色鲜红,形状呈圆形或椭圆形,大小不等,结节上的球结膜可以推移,微痛拒按,隆起之结节可由小渐渐增大,一般很少破溃。病变持续数星期后,结节可吸收。

(3) 单眼发病者多,也有双眼同时或先后发病者。

【辨证论治】

本病临床主要分为肺热亢盛证、风湿热结证、阴虚火旺证。病发于白睛,属气轮,主脏在肺,以肺热蕴结为多。故治疗应以泻肺热为本,酌加活血散结之品。若反复发作者,应调理全身。

ods, in principle, should be to dispel lung heat with adjuvant drugs of activating blood circulation to remove stasis in some cases. For the recurrent cases, the treatment method for the general regulation should be considered and applied.

1. Syndrome of Hyperactivity of Lung Heat

Main Symptoms and Signs   Slow attack, photophobia, slight tearing, vague pain, local fire-red nodule prominence with tenderness, cough, sore throat and constipation; yellowish tongue coating and rapid pulse.

Therapeutic Methods   Reducing lung-heat to smooth qi and activating blood to dissipate stagnation.

Recipe   The modified Xiebaisan Decoction: Sangbaipi (*Cortex Mori*) 10 g, Digupi (*Cortex Lycii Radicis*) 10 g, Jingmi (*Fructus Oryzae Sativae*) 20 g, Tinglizi (*Semen Lepidii seu Descurainiae*) 10 g, Lianqiao (*Fructus Forsythiae*) 10 g, Zhebeimu (*Bulbus Fritillariae*) 10 g, Honghua (*Flos Carthomi*) 6 g, and Gancao (*Radix Glycyrrhizae*) 3 g.

2. Syndrome of Combinating Stagnancy of Wind, Damp and Heat

Main Symptoms and Signs   Scarlet-red nodule prominence of the bulbar conjunctiva with capillaries around, depressing and distending pain in the eyeball, photophobia, dacryorrhea, aching pain of joints, swollen limbs, repeating attacks and lingering course; red tongue with whitish coating and slippery rapid pulse.

Therapeutic Methods   Dispelling wind and damp and removing heat and stasis.

Recipe   The modified Sanfeng Chushi Huoxue Decoction: Qianghuo (*Rhizoma seu Radix Notopterygii*) 5 g, Duhuo (*Radix Angelicae Pubescentis*) 5 g, Fangfeng (*Radix Ledebouriellae*) 5 g, Danggui (*Radix Angelicae Sinensis*) 10 g, Chuanxiong (*Rhizoma Ligustici*

1. 肺热亢盛证

主要证候 发病稍缓,畏光流泪轻微,隐隐作痛,局部火红色结节隆起,压痛轻微,咳嗽咽痛,便秘。苔黄,脉数。

治 法 泻肺利气,活血散结。

方 药 泻白散加减。桑白皮10 g,地骨皮10 g,粳米20 g,葶苈子10 g,连翘10 g,浙贝母10 g,红花6 g,甘草3 g。

2. 风湿热结证

主要证候 白睛结节隆起,色较鲜红,周围有赤丝牵绊,眼珠闷胀而疼,羞明流泪,关节酸痛,肢节肿胀。反复发作,病程缠绵。舌红,苔白腻,脉滑数。

治 法 祛风化湿,清热散结。

方 药 散风除湿活血汤加减。羌活5 g,独活5 g,防风5 g,当归10 g,川芎6 g,赤芍药10 g,鸡血藤10 g,红花6 g,苍术10 g,白术10 g,金银花

Chuanxiong) 6 g, Chishaoyao (*Radix Paeoniae Rubra*) 10 g, Jixueteng (*Caulis Spatholobi*) 10 g, Honghua (*Flos Carthomi*) 6 g, Cangzhu (*Rhizoma Atratylodis*) 10 g, Baizhu (*Rhizoma Atractylodis Macrocephalae*) 10 g, and Jinyinhua (*Flos Lonicerae*) 10 g.

Modification   In the cases of severe swelling redness of bulbar conjunctiva and obvious pain, 10 g of Huangqin (*Radix Scutellariae*) and 10 g of Lianqiao (*Fructus Forsythiae*) and 15 g of Shengshigao (*Gypsum Fibrosum*, to be decocted first) are added.

3. Syndrome of Hyperactivity of Fire due to Yin Deficiency

Main Symptoms and Signs   Recurrent onset of the disease with the symptoms of red bulbar conjunctiva, nodules occurring now and then, dark purple capillaries with slight swelling around, very light tenderness, dry and unsmooth sensation of the eye, dryness in the mouth and throat, night sweat with low fever and constipation; red tongue lack of fluid and thready rapid pulse.

Therapeutic Method   Nourishing yin to remove heat and mass.

Recipe   The modified Yangyin Qingfei Decoction: Shengdihuang (*Radix Rehmanniae*) 10 g, Maimendong (*Radix Ophiopogonis*) 10 g, Xuanshen (*Radix Scrophulariae*) 10 g, Beimu (*Bulbus Fritill a riae*) 10 g, Mudanpi (*Cortex Moutan Radicis*) 10 g, Chaobaishaoyao (*Radix Paeoniae Alba*) 10 g, Bohe (*Herba Menthae*, to be decocted later) 6 g, and Shenggancao (*Radix Glycyrrhizae*) 3 g.

Modification   In the cases of obvious hyperactivity of fire, Bohe is removed and respective 10 g of Zhimu (*Rhizoma Anemarrhenae*), Shihu (*Herba Dendrobii*) and Digupi (*Cortex Lycii Radicis*) are added; in the cases of nodules in the bulbar conjunctiva for a long time,

10 g。

加　减　白睛红甚,疼痛明显者,加黄芩10 g,连翘10 g,生石膏(先煎)15 g。

3. 阴虚火旺证

主要证候　病情反复发作,白睛红赤,结节时隐时现,血丝色偏紫暗,四周有轻度肿胀,压痛不甚明显,眼干涩,口干咽燥,盗汗低热,便秘不畅。舌红少津,脉细数。

治　法　养阴清热,兼以散结。

方　药　养阴清肺汤加减。生地黄10 g,麦门冬10 g,玄参10 g,贝母10 g,牡丹皮10 g,炒白芍药10 g,薄荷(后下)6 g,生甘草3 g。

加　减　若火旺明显者,去薄荷,加知母10 g,石斛10 g,地骨皮10 g;若白睛结节日久,难以消退者,用赤芍药易白芍药,加丹参10 g,广郁金

Baishaoyao is replaced by Chishaoyao (*Radix Paeoniae Rubra*) and respective 10 g of Danshen (*Radix Salviae Miltiorrhizae*), Guangyujin (*Radix Curcumae*) and Haifushi (*Fumex*) and 15 g of Walengzi (*Concha Arcae*) are added.

[Other Treatments]

1. Chinese Patent Drugs

Yangyin Qingfei Ointment　15 g each time for oral taking, twice a day and applicable to the syndrome of hyperac-tivity of due to yin deficiency.

2. External Therapies

(1) Moist-hot Compress　The affected eye is compressed with the hot salt water or the hot liquid decocted from the dregs of the oral decoctions. This moist-hot compress is performed for 20 minutes once, three to four times every day, and is applicable to the cases with severe pain.

(2) Eye Drops　a. Xihuang Powder　It is given with the powder once or twice a day, which is applicable to all syndromes of the disease. b. Coptidis Eye Drops (10%)　It is given three times a day, which is applicable to all syndromes of the disease. c. Xiongdan Eye Drops It is given three times a day, which is applicable to all syndromes of the disease.

10 g,瓦楞子15 g,海浮石10 g。

【其他疗法】

1. 中成药

养阴清肺膏　每服15 g,每日 2 次。适用于阴虚火旺证。

2. 外治法

(1) 湿热敷　用盐水湿热敷,或内服药渣煎水作湿热敷,每日3～4 次,每次 20 分钟。适用于疼痛较甚者。

(2) 点眼药　① 犀黄散:每日点眼1～2 次。适用于本病各证。② 10%黄连眼药水:每日点眼 3 次。适用于本病各证。③ 熊胆眼药水:每日点眼 3 次。适用于本病各证。

2.4 Diseases of Cornea

2.4.1 Bacterial Corneal Ulcer

[Introduction]

Bacterial corneal ulcer is a kind of acute suppurative inflammation of the cornea caused by the bacterial infection. Clinically, it usually manifests the symptoms of cloudy infiltration focus in the cornea that quickly amplifies to form ulcer. Although every one may suffer from it in all seasons of a year, the disease often attacks in summer and autumn and old people of debility are easy to be affected. It usually starts suddenly, develops rapidly and changes greatly. If it is not treated instantly and properly, there may arise corneal perforation and iridoptosis, and adhesive leukoma, after recovery, may be formed that greatly affects vision or even causes blindness. Sometimes, it may give rise to endophthalmitis or panophthalmia and even destroy the whole eyeball.

The common pathogens of the disease are Diplococcus pneumoniae, Staphylococcus aureus, Staphylococcus opidermidis, Pseudomonas aerugmosa, Bacillus coli, Streptococci and so on.

The disease, from its clinical manifestations, should pertain to "Ningzhiyi" (purulent keratitis) in traditional Chinese medicine. It is often caused by the ocular abrasions due to the wheat or rice awns or due to twigs or

第四章 黑睛疾病

第一节 细菌性角膜溃疡

【概述】

细菌性角膜溃疡是指由细菌感染引起的角膜的急性化脓性炎症。临床主要表现为角膜上出现混浊浸润灶,并迅速扩大,形成溃疡。任何年龄、任何季节均可发病。但以夏秋收割季节多见,年老体弱者易发病。一般起病急,发展快,变化多。若治疗不及时或处理不当,可造成角膜穿孔,虹膜脱出,愈后形成粘连性角膜白斑,严重影响视力,甚至失明。少数情况,还可引起眼内炎或全眼球炎,甚至毁坏整个眼球。

本病的致病菌常见的有肺炎双球菌、金黄色葡萄球菌、表皮葡萄球菌、绿脓杆菌、大肠杆菌、链球菌等。

根据本病的临床表现,当属于中医学"凝脂翳"范畴。病因多为黑睛被谷芒、麦刺、树枝、树叶等擦伤,或角膜异

leaves or due to the removal of a foreign body on the cornea, for pathogenic factors, taking advantage of the injury, invade the eye and the disease arises. And those with a history of dacryocystitis may easily be its victims. When the pathogenic heat transformed from the invasion of pathogenic wind and heat or the pathogenic fire-heat accumulated from the long-time preference for pepper and frying foods causes excessive visceral heat and hyperactivity of pathogenic fire and heat, the eye is flamed and the disease occurs. Besides, the protracted course of keratomalicia, denditic keratitis and other disorders, when exacerbated by virulent factors, may also bring about the case.

[Main Diagnostic Points]

(1) Preliminarily, the eye suffers from the subjective symptoms of sandy-unsmooth feeling, twinge with a burning sensation, photophobia, dacryorrhea, blepharospasm and visual disturbance. In severe cases, there may be dramatic headache and ophthalmagra and serious photophobia.

(2) Ciliary or mixed congestion appears and in the cornea occurs the dense inflammatory infiltration, which is usually round and grayish-whitish or yellow with cloudiness protruding on the surface edged obscurely.

(3) If the condition is not treated in time, the lesion may spread around and in depth, and the inflammatory infiltration of the cornea may become the yellowish-white ulcer which often advances serpiginously towards the central part and simultaneously goes deeply, causing purulent ulceration of the corneal stroma. The iris shows the severe inflammatory reaction in the form of hypopyon.

(4) If the course continues with the necrotic tissues scaling, there may appear descemetocele and, further, corneal perforation. The final result is adhesive leukoma

物剔除术后,邪毒乘伤袭入所致。若素有漏睛者,更易罹患;或因风热外邪入里化热,或嗜食辛辣炙煿,日久酿成火热,致脏腑热盛,火热上炎,蒸灼而成,本病亦可由花翳白陷、聚星障等病情迁延,复加邪毒,恶化而来。

【诊断要点】

(1) 初起自觉眼内沙涩,灼热刺痛,畏光流泪,眼睑痉挛,视力障碍。重者头目剧痛,强烈羞明。

(2) 睫状充血或混合性充血,角膜出现致密的炎性浸润,一般呈圆形,色灰白或微黄,表面隆起污浊,边缘不清。

(3) 若治不及时,则病变向周围和深部发展。角膜炎性浸润变为黄白色溃疡,溃疡呈匍行性进展,多向中央部发展;同时,亦可向深部发展,出现角膜基质脓疡。虹膜出现严重的炎症反应,表现为前房积脓。

(4) 若病情继续进展,坏死组织不断脱落,可出现后弹力层突出,进而角膜穿孔,最

and serious visual disturbance. If bacteria invade the intraocular part through the perforation, endophthalmitis arises and the atrophy of the eyeball is caused in the end.

If corneal ulcer is caused by Pseudomonas aeruginosa, yellowish-green secretion is attached to the surface of the ulcer. The condition of the disease develops rapidly with drastic symptoms and the whole cornea and eyeball may be destroyed in 24 hours.

[Syndrome Differentiation and Treatment]

In clinic, the disease is mainly classified into the syndromes of excessive accumulation of wind and heat, flaming fire of the liver and gallbladder, excessive noxious heat, and deficiency of healthy qi and retention of pathogenic factors. The treatment, in principle, should be based on removing heat and virulent pathogens and, in long-standing cases with weak healthy qi, the method of dispelling pathogenic factors to strengthen healthy qi should be considered.

1. Syndrome of Excessive Accumulation of Wind and Heat

Main Symptoms and Signs   Photophobia, dacryorrhea, ophthalmalgia, headache, visual diminution, ciliary hyperemia, corneal opacity with obscure edge and filthy surface; reddish tongue with thin yellowish coating and floating rapid pulse.

Therapeutic Methods   Dispelling wind and removing heat.

Recipe   The modified Wind-Heat-Removing Decoction: Jingjie (*Herba Schizonepetae*) 10 g, Fangfeng (*Radix Ledebouriellae*) 10 g, Chaihu (*Radix Bupleuri*) 6 g, Manjingzi (*Fructus Viticis*) 10 g, Huanglian (*Rhizoma Coptidis*) 6 g, Huangqin (*Radix Scultellariae*) 10 g, Shanzhizi (*Fructus Gardeniae*) 10 g,   Jinyinhua

后形成粘连性角膜白斑,严重障碍视力。若细菌乘穿孔部进入眼内,可形成眼内炎,最终导致眼球萎缩。

绿脓杆菌引起的角膜溃疡,则溃疡表面附有黄绿色分泌物,症状剧烈,发展迅速,可于 24 小时内毁坏整个角膜或眼球。

【辨证论治】

本病临床主要分为风热壅盛证、肝胆火炽证、热毒炽盛证、正虚邪留证。治疗以清热解毒为原则,病久正虚者,应扶正祛邪。

1. 风热壅盛证

主要证候　畏光流泪,目痛头痛,视力下降,抱轮红赤,黑睛混浊,边缘不清,表面污浊,舌红苔薄黄,脉浮数。

治　法　祛风清热。

方　药　祛风清热方加减。荆芥10 g,防风10 g,柴胡6 g,蔓荆子10 g,黄连6 g,黄芩10 g,山栀子10 g,金银花12 g,千里光12 g,甘草3 g。

(*Flos Lonicerae*) 12 g, Qianliguang (*Herba Senecionis Scandentis*) 12 g, and Gancao (*Radix Glycyrrhizae*) 3 g.

Modification　In the cases of serious headache indicating severe wind, 10 g of Qianghuo (*Rhizoma seu Radix Notopterygii*) and 10 g of Baizhi (*Radix Angelicae Dahuricae*) are added; in the cases of corneal opacity indicating the severity of stomach fire, 10 g of Zhimu (*Rhizoma Anemarrhenae*) and 20 g of Shengshigao (*Gypsum Fibrosum*, to be decocted first) are added.

2. Syndrome of Flaming Fire of Liver and Gallbladder

Main Symptoms and Signs　Swelling of eyelid, photophobia and ophthalmalgia with hot tears, cloudy-reddish edema of bulbar conjunctiva, corneal ulcer with the middle part pitting deeply and spreading serpiginously towards the center, hypopyon, accompanied by a bitter taste in the mouth and yellowish urine; reddish tongue with yellowish coating and thready rapid pulse.

Therapeutic Method　Removing pathogenic heat of the liver.

Recipe　The modified Longdan Xiegan Decoction: Longdancao (*Radix Gentianae*) 10 g, Shanzhizi (*Fructus Gardeniae*) 10 g, Huangqin (*Radix Scultellariae*) 10 g, Chaihu (*Radix Bupleuri*) 10 g, Zexie (*Rhizoma Alismatis*) 10 g, Cheqianzi (*Semen Plantaginis*, bagged) 20 g, Shengdihuang (*Radix Rehmanniae*) 10 g, Danggui (*Radix Angelicae Sinensis*) 10 g, Mutong (*Caulis Akebiae*) 6 g, and Gancao (*Radix Glycyrrhizae*) 3 g.

Modification　In the cases of profuse dry eye secretion indicating serious pathogenic heat, 5 g of Huanglian (*Rhizoma Coptidis*) and 10 g of Zhuye (*Folium Phyllostachydis Henonis*) are added, and in the cases of hy-

加　减　头痛明显为风邪偏胜，加羌活 10 g，白芷 10 g；黑睛混浊位于下方者，为胃火偏胜，加知母 10 g，生石膏（先煎）20 g。

2. 肝胆火炽证

主要证候　胞睑红肿，羞明眼痛，热泪如汤，白睛混赤水肿，黑睛溃疡，中间凹陷深大，并呈匐行性向中央进展，黄液上冲，伴口苦溲黄，舌红苔黄，脉弦数。

治　法　清肝泻火。

方　药　龙胆泻肝汤加减。龙胆草 10 g，山栀子 10 g，黄芩 10 g，柴胡 10 g，泽泻 10 g，车前子（包煎）20 g，生地黄 10 g，当归 10 g，木通 6 g，甘草 3 g。

加　减　眵多干结为心火甚，加黄连 5 g，竹叶 10 g；胃火亢盛者，加寒水石 10 g，生石膏（先煎）15 g，大黄 6 g。

peractivity of stomach fire, 10 g of Hanshuishi (*Calcitum*), 15 g of Shengshigao (*Gypsum Fibrosum*, to be decocted first) and 6 g of Dahuang (*Radix et Rhizoma Rhei*) are added.

3. Syndrome of Excessive Noxious Heat

Main Symptoms and Signs   Swollen eyelid, severe headache and ophthalmalgia, redness and opacity of bulbar conjunctiva, a large yellowish-green corneal ulcer in the shape of purulent keratitis, hypopyon; red tongue with yellow coating and rapid pulse.

Therapeutic Method   Removing heat, virulent and fire.

Recipe   The modified Wuwei Xiaodu Decoction and Huang-lian Jiedu Decoction: Jinyinhua (*Flos Lonicerae*) 10 g, Pugongying (*Herba Taraxaci*) 20 g, Yejuhua (*Flos Chrysanthemi Indici*) 10 g, Zihuadiding (*Herba Violae*) 20 g, Zibeitiankuicao (*Herba Senecionis Nudicaulis*) 20 g, Huanglian (*Rhizoma Coptidis*) 3 g, Huangqin (*Radix Scultellariae*) 10 g, Huangbai (*Cortex Phellodendri*) 10 g, and Shanzhizi (*Fructus Gardeniae*) 10 g.

Modification   In preliminary cases, 10 g of Fangfeng (*Radix Ledebouriellae*) and 5 g of Bohe (*Herba Menthae*, to be decocted later) are added; in the cases of constipation, 6 g of Dahuang (*Radix et Rhizoma Rhei*) and 10 g of Mangxiao (*Natrii Sulphas*) are added; in the cases of severe pain, 10 g of Zhiruxiang (*Resina Olibani*, processed) and 10 g of Zhimoyao (*Myrrha*, processed) are added; in the cases of accumulated heat and blood stasis, the drugs of Chishaoyao (*Radix Paeoniae Rubra*), Mudanpi (*Cortex Moutan Radicis*) and Shengdi huang (*Radix Rehmanniae*), each 10 g, are added.

4. Syndrome of Deficiency of Healthy Qi and Retention of Pathogenic Factor

Main Symptoms and Signs   A long-standing course

3. 热毒炽盛证

主要证候　胞睑红肿,头目痛甚,白睛混赤,黑睛大片溃陷,色带黄绿,状如凝脂,黄液上冲,舌红苔黄,脉数。

治　法　清热解毒泻火。

方　药　五味消毒饮合黄连解毒汤加减。金银花10 g,蒲公英20 g,野菊花10 g,紫花地丁20 g,紫背天葵草20 g,黄连3 g,黄芩10 g,黄柏10 g,山栀子10 g。

加　减　病初起者,加防风10 g,薄荷(后下)5 g;大便秘结者,加大黄6 g,芒硝10 g;疼痛剧烈者,加制乳香10 g,制没药10 g;热壅血滞者,加赤芍药10 g,牡丹皮10 g,生地黄10 g。

4. 正虚邪留证

主要证候　病情日久,眼

with symptoms of mild ophthalmalgia, photophobia and ciliary hyperemia, corneal ulcer and pitting without any healing; whitish tongue and weak pulse.

Therapeutic Method   Invigorating qi to dispel pathogenic factors.

Recipe   The modified Tuoli Xiaodusan Decoction: Huangqi (*Radix Astragali seu Hedysari*) 15 g, Dangshen (*Radix Codonopsis Pilosulae*) 10 g, Baizhu (*Rhizoma Atractylodis Macrocephalae*) 10 g, Fuling (*Poria*) 10 g, Danggui (*Radix Angelicae Sinensis*) 10 g, Baishaoyao (*Radix Paeoniae Alba*) 10 g, Chuanxiong (*Rhizoma Ligustici Chuanxiong*) 10 g, Jinyinhua (*Flos Lonicerae*) 12 g, Baizhi (*Radix Angelicae Dahuricae*) 10 g, Juhua (*Flos Chrysanthemi*) 6 g, Cijili (*Herba Chenopodii Aristati*) 10 g, Chantui (*Periostracum Cicadae*) 6 g, and Gancao (*Radix Glycyrrhizae*) 3 g.

Modification   In the cases of capillaries in the cornea indicating stagnation of qi and blood, 10 g of Danshen (*Radix Salviae Miltiorrhizae*) is added; in the cases of reddish tongue and no coating indiciating deficiency of qi and yin, 10 g of Maimendong (*Radix Ophiopogonis*) and 6 g of Wuweizi (*Fructus Schisandrae*) are added.

[Other Treatments]

1. Chinese Patent Drugs

(1) Yinqiao Jiedu Tablet   4 tablets each time, three times a day and applicable to the syndrome of excessive accumulation of wind and heat.

(2) Fangfeng Tongsheng Pill   6 g each time, twice a day and applicable to the syndrome of excessive accumulation of wind and heat.

(3) Mingmu Shangqing Pill   6 g each time, twice a day and applicable to the syndrome of excessive accumulation of wind and heat.

痛羞明较轻,轻度抱轮红赤, 黑睛溃陷不敛,舌淡,脉弱。

治　法　补气祛邪。

方　药　托里消毒散加减。黄芪15 g,党参10 g,白术10 g,茯苓10 g,当归10 g,白芍药10 g,川芎10 g,金银花12 g,白芷6 g,菊花6 g,刺蒺藜10 g,蝉蜕6 g,甘草3 g。

加　减　黑睛有赤脉伸入,为气血瘀滞,加丹参10 g;舌红无苔,为气阴不足,加麦门冬10 g,五味子6 g。

【其他疗法】

1. 中成药

(1) 银翘解毒片　每服4片,每日3次。适用于风热壅盛证。

(2) 防风通圣丸　每服6 g,每日2次。适用于风热壅盛证。

(3) 明目上清丸　每服6 g,每日2次。适用于风热壅盛证。

(4) Niuhuang Shangqing Pill 6 g each time, twice or three times a day and applicable to the syndrome of excessive accumulation of wind and heat.

(5) Shangqing Pill 6 g each time, twice or three times a day and applicable to the syndrome of excessive accumulation of wind and heat.

(6) Huanglian Shangqing Pill 6 g each time, twice a day and applicable to the syndrome of excessive accumulation of wind and heat.

(7) Yiqing Capsule 2 capsules each time, three times a day and applicable to the syndrome of excessive noxious heat.

(8) Longdan Xiegan Pill 6 g each time, twice a day and applicable to the syndrome of flaming fire of the liver and gallbladder.

(9) Xiongdan Jiedu Pill 6 g each time, three times a day and applicable to the syndrome of flaming fire of the liver and gallbladder.

(10) Sanhuang Pill 6 g each time, three times a day and applicable to the syndrome of excessive accumulation of wind and heat.

(11) Qingning Pill 6 g each time, twice or three times a day and applicable to the syndrome of excessive noxious heat.

(12) Boyun Tuiyi Pill 3 g each time, three times a day and applicable to the disease at the late stage.

2. Simple Proved Recipe

The recipe consists of Xiakucao (*Spica Prunellae*) 12 g, Luxiancao (*Herba Pyrolae*) 15 g, Gujingcao (*Flos Eriocauli*) 15 g, Mimenghua (*Flos Buddlejae*) 12 g, Zidanshen (*Radix Salviae Milyiorrhizae*) 15 g, and Xiaohongshen (*Radix Rubiae Yunnanesis*) 12 g. All the drugs are decocted with water one dose a day and the de-

（4）牛黄上清丸　每服 6 g,每日 2～3 次。适用于风热壅盛证。

（5）上清丸　每服6 g,每日 2～3 次。适用于风热壅盛证。

（6）黄连上清丸　每服 6 g,每日 2 次。适用于风热壅盛证。

（7）一清胶囊　每服 2 片,每日 3 次。适用于热毒炽盛证。

（8）龙胆泻肝丸　每服 6 g,每日 2 次。适用于肝胆火炽证。

（9）熊胆解毒丸　每服 6 g,每日 3 次。适用于肝胆火炽证。

（10）三黄丸　每服6 g, 每 日 3 次。适 用 于 热 毒 炽盛证。

（11）清宁丸　每服6 g, 每日 2～3 次。适用于热毒炽盛证。

（12）拨云退翳丸　每服 3 g,每日 3 次。适用于本病后期。

2. 单验方

夏枯草12 g,鹿衔草15 g, 谷精草15 g,密蒙花12 g,紫丹参15 g,小红参12 g。水煎服, 每日 1 剂,分 3 次服,6 日为 1 个疗程。适用于阴虚有热、气滞血瘀证。

coction is orally taken in three times, with six days as one treatment course. The recipe can be applied to treat the cases of yin deficiency with heat remaining or with qi stagnation and blood stasis.

3. External Therapies

(1) Eye Drops   a. Qianliguang Eye Drops: Applied to drop the eye six times a day, it is applicable to all syndromes of the disease. b. Pugongying Eye-Dropping Liquid: The liquid is applicable to all syndromes of the disease and is applied to drop the eye six times a day. c. Yuxingcao Eye Drops: By dropping the eye six times a day, it is applicable to all syndromes of the disease. d. Teling Eye Powder: By dipping a small amount of the powder with a sterilized glass rod to drop the lower eyelid twice every day, the powder is applicable to all syndromes of the disease.

(2) Fumigation-Washing Method   The ingredients in the therapy are: Jinyinhua (*Flos Lonicerae*) 10 g, Lianqiao (*Fructus Forsythiae*) 10 g, Banlangen (*Radix Isatidis*) 15 g, Yejuhua (*Flos Chrysanthemi Indici*) 6 g, Daqingye (*Folium Isatidis*) 10 g, Pugongying (*Herba Taraxaci*) 15 g, Jingjie (*Herba Schizonepetae*) 10 g, Fangfeng (*Radix Ledebouriellae*) 10 g, Baihuasheshecao (*Herba Hedyotis Diffusae*) 10 g, and Yuxingcao (*Herba Houttuymiae*) 10 g. All the above drugs are decocted with water. The warm filtrated liquid is used to wash the eye or first fumigate and then wash the eye with combination of damp-heat dressing. The therapy can be applied to all syndromes of the disease.

If the case is of emergency, western medicines must be used as a supplementary therapy.

3. 外治法

（1）点眼药　① 千里光眼药水：每日点眼6次。适用于本病各证。② 蒲公英滴眼液：每日点眼6次。适用于本病各证。③ 鱼腥草眼药水：每日点眼6次。适用于本病各证。④ 特灵眼药：用消毒玻璃棒蘸少许药粉，点于下眼睑内，每日2次。适用于本病各证。

（2）薰洗法　用金银花10 g，连翘10 g，板蓝根15 g，野菊花6 g，大青叶10 g，蒲公英15 g，荆芥10 g，防风10 g，白花蛇舌草10 g，鱼腥草10 g。煎水澄清过滤，乘温洗眼，或先薰后洗，并结合作湿热敷。适用于本病各证。

若本病急重，须配合必要的西药。

2.4.2 Herpes Simplex Keratitis

[Introduction]

Herpes simplex keratitis is a kind of inflammatory affection of the cornea due to the infection of herpes simplex virus. Usually, the invading virus cannot give rise to the disease but may, only when the body's resistance is weak. One eye is often affected, and sometimes both simultaneously or one after another. In clinic, the disease manifests the main symptom of dendritic or geographic or discoid inflammatory focus of the cornea. With a repeated and protracted course, the case can greatly affect a patient's vision or even cause blindness if it is not treated immediately.

In most cases, the infection of herpes simplex virus type I is the cause of the disease.

From the clinical manifestations, the disease at the early stage should pertain in traditional Chinese medicine to "Juxingzhang" (dendritic keratitis). When the punctuate infiltration becomes confluent to form a dendritic or geographic ulcer, there develops the case of the TCM's "Huayi Baixian" (Keratomalacia). In the cases of cold, fever, emotional trouble, menstrual disorder or chronic diseases due to the imbalance of yin and yang, qi and blood, the pathogenic factor of wind-heat or wind-cold, by taking advantage of the body's deficiency, invades the eye resulting in the disease. It may be caused by the fact that the internal pathogenic heat transformed from the invading external pathogenic factors or the latent fire of liver meridian recurrently affected by pathogenic wind brings about the conjoint wind-fire invasion and hyperactivity of

第二节　单纯疱疹性角膜炎

【概述】

单纯疱疹性角膜炎是指由单纯疱疹病毒引起的角膜炎性病变。这种病毒侵入机体后,在一般情况下是不会致病的,只有在机体抵抗力下降的情况下才会发病。常为单眼患病,也可双眼同时或先后发生,临床主要表现为树枝状、地图状或圆盘状角膜炎性病灶,病程长,常反复迁延,治疗不及时可严重影响视力,甚至失明。

本病病因多由单纯疱疹病毒I型感染所引起。

根据本病的临床表现,在早期当属于中医"聚星障"范畴,点状浸润相互融合,形成树枝状或地图状溃疡者则属于中医"花翳白陷"范畴。本病大多在感冒、高热、情志不遂、月经失调或慢性疾病等阴阳气血失调的情况下,风热或风寒之邪乘虚袭眼而致;或由外邪入里化热,或肝经伏火,复受风邪,风火相搏,火热上炎引起;或素食煎炒五辛,酿成脾胃湿热,上薰黑睛而成;亦可因素体偏于阴虚,或热病后灼伤津液,以致阴津亏乏,

fire and heat. When dampness and heat of the spleen and stomach is bred by the habitual preference of the pepper and frying foods, the eye is fumigated and the disease occurs. Sometimes, it may be formed due to yin deficiency or burning damage of body fluids after febrile diseases, for either of factors may cause the consumption of yin fluids which, when affected by pathogenic wind, may give rise to the disease.

[Main Diagnostic Points]

(1) The affected eye suffers from pain, photophobia, dacryorrhea and visual disturbance.

(2) Ciliary or mixed congestion occurs in the eye, and pathogenic change of different forms starts in the cornea.

1) Type of Superficial Keratitis a. Dendritic keratitis At the early stage, many needle-point-like infiltrating opacities on the cornea appear and turn immediately to alveoli. When the alveoli rupture and become confluent with each other, streak ulcer is formed, which takes the typical dendritic appearance in the fluorescing sodium staining. The corneal sensation of the damaged area is reduced. b. Geographic keratitis Most of the cases develop from dendritic keratitis. The ulcer goes deeper and spreads more outwards, confluently to form a geographic shape. The corneal stroma beneath the ulcer becomes cloudy, and much rugosty appears on the posterior elastic layer. Complicated iridocyclitis may happen in the course of the pathogenic change.

2) Type of Deep Keratitis Disciform keratitis The corneal stroma becomes cloudy with discoid edema edged tidily (sometimes irregular in shape). The corneal surface is shaggy and the posterior elastic layer rugose. If the case is severe, the whole stroma of the cornea may be affected, showing the symptoms of diffuse filtrative opacity,

兼感风邪所致。

【诊断要点】

(1) 患眼疼痛,畏光流泪,视力障碍。

(2) 眼部睫状充血或混合性充血,角膜有不同形态的病损。

1) 浅层型 ① 树枝状角膜炎:早期角膜有多个如针尖大小的浸润混浊,很快形成小泡,小泡破溃后即相互融合形成条状溃疡,用荧光素钠染色后呈典型的树枝状形态。病损区角膜知觉减退。② 地图状角膜炎:多由树枝状角膜炎发展而来,即溃疡向深部与边缘发展扩大,相互融合呈地图状。溃疡底部之基质混浊,后弹力层皱褶多,病变过程中可并发虹膜睫状体炎。

2) 深层型 盘状角膜炎:角膜基质混浊水肿,边缘较整齐,形如圆盘状,但也有不规则形状者。角膜表面粗糙,后弹力层皱褶。严重者可侵犯整个角膜基质层,出现弥

obvious edema of the corneal epithelium and recurrent alveoli, or increasing rugosity of the posterior elastic layer, more deposit on the inner ocular walls, and even hypopyon or secondary glaucoma. In a long time, neonatal vessels extend deeper into the cornea. After recovery, a white patch or leukoplacia may remain in the cornea, which greatly influences the vision.

[**Syndrome Differentiation and Treatment**]

In clinic practice, the disease is usually classified into the syndromes of wind-cold invasion of eye, wind-heat invasion of eye, excessive flaming fire of the liver, stagnant fumigation of damp-heat, and yin deficiency and pathogenic factors retention. Therefore, the treatment, in principle, should be based on removing wind and heat, and the specific methods of expelling wind, dispelling cold, clearing away heat and eliminating dampness should be respectively applied according to the severity of pathogenic factors. In the case of yin deficiency due to a long course of the condition, the method of nourishing yin to dispel pathogenic factors should be applied.

1. Syndrome of Wind-cold Invasion of Eye

Main Symptoms and Signs Delacrimation of the affected eye at first, photophobia, obscure congestion, occurrence of punctate or dendritic cloudiness of the cornea, accompanied by running nose, fever and severe aversion to cold; light-reddish tongue with thin whitish coating and floating tense pulse.

Therapeutic Method Dispersing pathogenic wind and cold.

Recipe The modified Jingfang Baidu Powder: Qianghuo (*Rhizoma seu Radix Notopterygii*) 6 g, Fang-feng (*Radix Ledebouriellae*) 10 g, Duhuo (*Radix Angelicae Pubescentis*) 6 g, Jingjie (*Herba Schizonepetae*) 6 g, Chaihu (*Radix Bupleuri*) 6 g, Jiegeng (*Radix Platycodi*)

漫性浸润混浊,上皮明显水肿,反复发生小泡;后弹力层皱褶增多,内壁有较多的沉着物,甚至前房积脓,可继发青光眼。病程较长,角膜深层可有新生血管伸入。愈后形成致密的白斑,视力严重障碍。

【辨证论治】

本病临床主要分为风寒犯目证、风热犯目证、肝火炽盛证、湿热蕴蒸证、阴虚邪留证。治疗以祛风清热为基本方法,根据病邪的偏胜,分别采用祛风、散寒、清热、除湿,病久伤阴者,则应养阴祛邪。

1. 风寒犯目证

主要证候 病初起患眼泪多,畏光羞明,红赤不显,黑睛出现点状或树枝状混浊,伴鼻流清涕,恶寒发热,寒重热轻,舌质淡红,苔薄白,脉浮紧。

治 法 发散风寒。

方 药 荆防败毒散加减。羌活6 g,防风10 g,独活6 g,荆芥6 g,柴胡6 g,桔梗10 g,川芎10 g,茯苓10 g,薄荷(后下)6 g,甘草3 g。

10 g, Chuanxiong (*Rhizoma Ligustici Chuanxiong*) 10 g, Fuling (*Poria*) 10 g, Bohe (*Herba Menthae*, to be decocted later) 6 g, and Gancao (*Radix Glycyrrhizae*) 3 g.

Modification In the cases of fever and severe aversion to cold without sweat, 5 g of Mahuang (*Herba Ephedrae*), 10 g of Gaoben (*Rhizoma et Radix Ligustici*) and 3 g of Xixin (*Herba Asari*) are added.

2. Syndrome of Wind-heat Invasion of Eye

Main Symptoms and Signs Photophobia and dacyorrhea with faint unsmooth or uncomfortable sensation, ciliary hyperemia, punctate or dendritic opacity of the cornea, or even grayish-whitish discoid cloudiness, accompanied by the general symptoms of headache and stuffy nose; thin yellowish tongue coating and floating rapid pulse.

Therapeutic Method Removing pathogenic wind and heat.

Recipe The modified Qianghuo Shengfeng Decoction: Qianghuo (*Rhizoma et Radix Notopterygii*) 6 g, Jingjie (*Herba Schizonepetae*) 6 g, Fangfeng (*Radix Ledebouriellae*) 10 g, Baizhi (*Radix Angelicae Dahuricae*) 6 g, Chaihu (*Radix Bupleuri*) 6 g, Qinpi (*Cortex Fraxini*) 10 g, Bohe (*Herba Menthae*, to be decocted later) 6 g, Gancao (*Radix Glycyrrhizae*) 3 g, Huangqin (*Radix Scutellariae*) 10 g, Banlangen (*Radix Isatidis*) 15 g, and Chuanxiong (*Rhizoma Ligustici Chuanxiong*) 10 g.

Modification In the cases of a reddish tongue and yellowish urine, 10 g of Shanzhizi (*Fructus Gardeniae*) is added.

3. Syndrome of Excessive Flaming Fire of Liver

Main Syndromes and Signs Obvious ophthalmalgia, photophobia and dacryorrhea, ciliary hyperemia and

加　减　若发热恶寒,寒重热轻又无汗者,加麻黄5g,藁本10g,细辛3g。

2. 风热犯目证

主要证候　羞明流泪,隐涩不舒,抱轮红赤,黑睛出现点状或树枝状混浊,甚至出现圆盘状混浊,色灰白,全身伴头痛鼻塞,苔薄黄,脉浮数。

治　法　疏风散热。

方　药　羌活胜风汤加减。羌活6g,荆芥6g,防风10g,白芷6g,柴胡6g,秦皮10g,薄荷(后下)6g,甘草3g,黄芩10g,板蓝根15g,川芎10g。

加　减　若舌红溲黄者,加山栀子10g。

3. 肝火炽盛证

主要证候　眼痛明显,畏光流泪,抱轮红赤或白睛混

bulbar conjunctival cloudiness, amplified and deeper corneal opacity in the geographic or discoid form, accompanied by the symptoms of yellowish-scanty urine and bitter taste in the mouth; yellowish tongue coating and thready rapid pulse.

Therapeutic Method   Clearing the liver to reduce pathogenic fire.

Recipe   The modified Longdan Xiegan Decoction: Longdancao (*Radix Gentianae*) 6 g, Shanzhizi (*Fructus Gardeniae*) 10 g, Huangqin (*Radix Scultellariae*) 10 g, Chaihu (*Radix Bupleuri*) 10 g, Zexie (*Rhizoma Alismatis*) 10 g, Shengdihuang (*Radix Rehmanniae*) 10 g, Danggui (*Radix Angelicae Sinensis*) 10 g, Fangfeng (*Radix Ledebouriellae*) 6 g, Juhua (*Flos Chrysanthemi*) 6 g, Jinyinhua (*Flos Lonicerae*) 10 g, Pugongying (*Herba Taraxaci*) 15 g, Banlangen (*Radix Isatides*) 10 g, and Gancao (*Radix Glycyrrhizae*) 3 g.

Modification   In the cases of hypopyon, 20 g of Shigao (*Gypsum Fibrosum*, to be decocted first) and 10 g of Hanshuishi (*Calcitum*) are added; in the cases of constipation, 6 g of Dahuang (*Radix et Rhizoma Rhei*) is added.

4. Syndrome of Stagnant Fumigation of Dampness-heat

Main Symptoms and Signs   Protracted course with the condition mild and severe alternatively and no recovery, dendritic or geographic or discoid opacity of the cornea, accompanied by the symptoms of carebaria, chest distress, yellowish urine and loose stool; reddish tongue with yellowish-greasy coating, and soft and rapid pulse.

Therapeutic Method   Removing pathogenic dampness and heat.

Recipe   The modified Ganlu Xiaodudan Decoction: Huashi (*Talcum*) 12 g, Yinchen (*Herba Artemisiae*

赤,黑睛混浊扩大加深,形成地图状或圆盘状,伴小便黄短,口苦,苔黄,脉弦数。

治　法　清肝泻火。

方　药　龙胆泻肝汤加减。龙胆草6 g,山栀子10 g,黄芩10 g,柴胡10 g,泽泻10 g,生地黄10 g,当归10 g,防风6 g,菊花6 g,金银花10 g,蒲公英15 g,板蓝根10 g,甘草3 g。

加　减　若前房积脓者,加石膏(先煎)20 g,寒水石10 g;大便秘结者,加大黄6 g。

4. 湿热蕴蒸证

主要证候　病情迁延不愈,时轻时重,黑睛出现树枝状、地图状或圆盘状混浊,伴头重胸闷,溲黄便溏,舌红苔黄腻,脉濡数。

治　法　化湿清热。

方　药　甘露消毒丹加减。滑石12 g,茵陈10 g,黄芩

Capillaris) 10 g, Huangqin (*Radix Scultellariae*) 10 g, Mutong (*Caulis Akebiae*) 6 g, Huoxiang (*Herba Agastachis*) 10 g, Doukouren (*Semen Amomi Rotundus*) 10 g, Yiyiren (*Semen Coicis*) 15 g, Houpo (*Cortex Magnoliae Officinalis*) 6 g, Chenpi (*Pericarpium Citri Reticulatae*) 10 g, and Huzhang (*Rhizoma Polygoni Cuspidati*) 10 g.

Modification In the cases of whitish-smooth tongue coating indicating severe dampness, the drug Yinchen is removed and 10 g of Cangzhu (*Rhizoma Atractylodis*) is added.

5. Syndrome of Yin Deficiency and Pathogenic Factors Retention

Main Symptoms and Signs Prolonged course being recovered or onsetting alternatively, obvious dry and unsmooth sensation of the eye, mild ciliary hyperemia, or appearance of active lesion on the recovered scars; reddish tongue with little fluid and thready or thready-rapid pulse.

Therapeutic method Nourishing yin to dispel pathogenic factor.

Recipe The modified Jia Jian Dihuangwan Decoction: Shengdihuang (*Radix Rehmanniae*) 12 g, Shudihuang (*Radix Rehmanniae Praeparata*) 12 g, Niuxi (*Radix Achyranthis Bidentatae*) 6 g, Dangguishen (*Radix Angelicae Sinensis*) 10 g, Qianghuo (*Rhizona seu Notopterygii*) 10 g, Fangfeng (*Radix Ledebouriellae*) 10 g, Xuanshen (*Radix Scrophulariae*) 10 g, Zhimu (*Rhizoma Anemarrhenae*) 10 g, Juhua (*Flos Chrysanthemi*) 6 g, and Chantui (*Periostracum Cicadae*) 6 g.

Modification In the cases of fever at a late stage indicating deficiency of yin and qi, 10 g of Dangshen (*Radix Codonopsis Pilosulae*) and of Maimendong (*Radix*

10 g,木通6 g,藿香10 g,豆蔻仁10 g,薏苡仁15 g,厚朴6 g,陈皮10 g,虎杖10 g。

　加　减　若舌苔白滑者,为湿重,去茵陈加苍术10 g。

5. 阴虚邪留证

　主要证候　病情日久,时愈时发,眼内干涩明显,轻度抱轮红赤;或于痊愈的瘢痕上又出现活动性病灶,舌红少津,脉细或细数。

　治　法　滋阴祛邪。

　方　药　加减地黄丸。生地黄12 g,熟地黄12 g,牛膝6 g,当归身10 g,羌活10 g,防风10 g,玄参10 g,知母10 g,菊花6 g,蝉蜕6 g。

　加　减　若见于高热后期,多为气阴不足,加党参10 g,麦门冬10 g,五味子6 g。

Ophiopogonis) and 6 g of Wuweizi (*Fructus Schisandrae*) are added.

[Other Treatments]

1. Chinese Patent Drugs

(1) **Yinqiao Jiedu Tablet**   4 tablets each time, three times a day and applicable to the syndrome of wind-heat invasion of eye.

(2) **Fangfeng Tongsheng Bolus**   6 g each time, twice a day and applicable to the syndrome of wind-heat invasion of eye.

(3) **Mingmu Shangqing Bolus**   6 g each time, twice a day and applicable to the syndrome of wind-heat invasion of eye.

(4) **Shangqing Bolus**   6 g each time, twice or three times a day and applicable to the syndrome of wind-heat invasion of eye.

(5) **Jingfang Baidu Pill**   6 g each time, twice or three times a day and applicable to the syndrome of wind-cold invasion of eye.

(6) **Longdan Xiegan Pill**   6 g each time, twice a day and applicable to the syndrome of excessive flaming fire of the liver.

(7) **Xiongdan Jiedu Pill**   6 g each time, three times a day and applicable to the syndrome of excessive flaming fire of the liver.

(8) **Yiqing Capsule**   two capsules each time, three times a day and applicable to the syndrome of excessive virulent heat.

(9) **Anti-virus Oral Liquid**   10 ml each time, three times a day and applicable to all syndromes of the disease.

2. Simple and Proved Recipes

(1) 10 to 15 g of Chaojuemingzi (*Semen Cassiae*, fried), 100 g of rice fruit and small amount of crystal sugar

【其他疗法】

1. 中成药

（1）银翘解毒片　每服 4 片，每日 3 次。适用于风热犯目证。

（2）防风通圣丸　每服 6 g，每日 2 次。适用于风热犯目证。

（3）明目上清丸　每服 6 g，每日 2 次。适用于风热犯目证。

（4）上清丸　每服 6 g，每日 2～3 次。适用于风热犯目证。

（5）荆防败毒丸　每服 6 g，每日 2～3 次。适用于风寒犯目证。

（6）龙胆泻肝丸　每服 6 g，每日 2 次。适用于肝火炽盛证。

（7）熊胆解毒丸　每服 6 g，每日 3 次。适用于肝火炽盛证。

（8）一清胶囊　每服 2 片，每日 3 次。适用于热毒炽盛证。

（9）抗病毒口服液　每服 10 ml，每日 3 次。适用于本病各证。

2. 单验方

（1）炒决明子 10～15 g，粳米 100 g，冰糖少许（或白菊

(or 10 g of white chrysanthemum flower), all the ingredients are cooked into porridge for the patient to take. The porridge is applicable to cases at late course with pathogenic heat and corneal opacity remained.

(2) Qianghuo (*Rhizoma seu Radix Notopterygii*), Yejuhua (*Flos Chrysanthemi Indici*), Jinyinhua (*Flos Lonicerae*), Shanzhizi (*Fructus Gardeniae*), Banlangen (*Radix Isatidis*), Huangqin (*Radix Scultellariae*), Lianqiao (*Fructus Forsythiae*) and Juemingzi (*Semen Cassiae*), each 9 g, and Jingjie (*Herba Schizonepetae*), Fangfeng (*Radix Ledebouriellae*), Daqingye (*Folium Isatidis*), each 6 g, all these drugs are decocted with water one dose a day. The decoction is orally taken in three times every day and it is applicable to the syndrome of wind-heat invasion of eye.

(3) The ingredients of 2 ml goat bile and 2 g honey are completely mixed. The mixture is used to drop the eye four times every day with three days as a treatment course. The method is applicable to the syndrome of yin deficiency and pathogenic factors retention.

3. External Therapies

(1) The affected eye is dropped three or four times a day with drugs which can remove virulent heat, such as Yuxingcao Eye Drops, Qianliguang Eye Drops, Zicao Eye Drops, Huangqin Eye Drops. Or the eye is smeared, before sleep, with the drugs of Chuanxinlian Eye Ointment or Danzhi Erlian Ointment.

(2) Subcutaneous conjunctival injection is performed with 1 ml of Yinhuang Injection once a day or once every other day. Or combined with the intramuscular injection, the eye is dropped with the drug which is twice diluted.

(3) With 5 ml balneo-soaking drug of Daqingye (*Folium Isatidis*) or compound Daqingye (*Isatidis*), the

花10 g)。适用于本病后期,余热未尽,黑睛仍留翳障者。

(2)羌活、野菊花、金银花、山栀子、板蓝根、黄芩、连翘、决明子各9 g,荆芥、防风、大青叶各6 g,每日1剂,水煎服,日服3次。适用于风热犯目证。

(3)羊胆汁2 ml,蜂蜜2 g。调匀点眼。每日4次,3日为1疗程。适用于阴虚邪留证。

3. 外治法

(1)选用清热解毒类中药制剂滴眼,如鱼腥草眼药水,千里光眼药水,紫草眼药水,黄芩眼药水等,每日滴眼3～4次。睡前涂穿心莲眼膏或胆汁二连膏。

(2)用银黄注射液作球结膜下注射,每次1 ml,每日或隔日1次;并可结合肌肉注射,还可以用此稀释1倍滴眼。

(3)用大青叶或复方大青叶眼浴剂浴眼,每次用5 ml,每

cornea is soaked for 15 to 20 minutes once every day, and then antibiotics eye-ointment is applied to the eye.

（4）Jinyinhua（*Flos Lonicerae*）10 g, Lianqiao（*Fructus Forsythiae*）10 g, Chaihu（*Radix Bupleuri*）8 g, Jingjie（*Herba Schizonepetae*）6 g, Fangfeng（*Radix Ledebouriellae*）6 g, Shanzhizi（*Fructus Gardeniae*）10 g, Pugongying（*Herba Taraxaci*）15 g, all the drugs are decocted with water. The decoction is used first to fumigate and then wash the eye.

次浸泡角膜 15～20 分，浸后上抗生素眼膏，每日 1 次，可连续进行。

（4）用金银花10 g，连翘10 g，柴胡8 g，荆芥6 g，防风6 g，山栀子10 g，蒲公英15 g，煎水先熏后洗。

2.5 Diseases of Pupil

2.5.1 Iridocyclitis

[Introduction]

Iridocyclitis, also called anterior uveitis, is a kind of uveitic inflammatory reaction caused by various pathogenic factors. Clinically, it is mainly characterized by the symptoms of ocular pain, photophobia, diminution of vision, ciliary or mixed congestion of the bulbar conjunctiva, deposit at the posterior cornea, aqueous opacity, iris edema, mitosis and so on. As a common ophthalmic disorder, it is frequently found in the young and middle-aged people with both eyes often affected repeatedly. The case is one of the common diseases leading to blindness.

Although its etiology is quite complex, the pathogenic cause of most iridocyclitis cases is endogenous besides some external factors like trauma, operation, infection and so on. It is reported that, in recent years, the morbidity of HLA – B27 in the acute cases of iridocyclitis has reached 60%.

From the clinical manifestations, the disease should pertain in traditional Chinese medicine to "Tongshen Jinxiao" (stenocoriasis) or to "Tongshen Ganque" (miosis). The exopathic cause of the disease is due to the invasion of pathogenic wind, heat and dampness, and the endopathic cause is concerned with constitutional yang excess and yin deficiency of the liver and kidney. The pathogenesis is

第五章 瞳神疾病

第一节 虹膜睫状体炎

【概述】

虹膜睫状体炎,又称前葡萄膜炎,是一种由多种原因引起的葡萄膜炎症反应疾病。临床上主要表现为患眼疼痛、畏光、视力下降、球结膜睫状充血或混合充血、角膜后沉着物、房水混浊及虹膜水肿、瞳孔缩小等。本病为常见的眼科疾病,多发生于青壮年,常累及双眼,易反复发作,也是常见的致盲眼病之一。

本病的病因较为复杂,其发病原因除外伤、手术、感染等因素外,绝大多数属内源性。近年来发现,HLA – B27在急性虹膜睫状体炎中的出现率高达60%。

根据本病的临床表现,当属于中医学"瞳神紧小"、"瞳神干缺"范畴。其外因为风、热、湿等外邪的侵入,内因与素体阳盛、肝肾阴亏有关。主要病机为邪热灼伤黄仁,以致黄仁展而不缩、瞳神紧小。病

mainly related with the fact that the pupil is fumigatedly injured by pathogenic heat, causing the expansion of iris without contraction and the contracted pupil. If the case is protracted for a long time, the condition of excessive heart fire and failure of the kidney will appear, indicating the intermingled syndrome of asthenia and sthenia.

[Main Diagnostic Points]

(1) The ocular symptoms indude: ophthalmagia, photophobia, dacryorrhea and visual diminution.

(2) There is tenderness in the ciliary area, ciliary or mixed congestion in the bulbar conjunctiva and deposit at the posterior cornea. The aqueous humor is of opacity, the iris becomes swollen, and the pupil is contracted.

(3) In the iris, posterior synechia of the pupil often occurs and, if it is not dilated in time, the occlusion of pupil or the seclusion of pupil may arise.

[Syndrome Differentiation and Treatment]

The sthenia syndrome and the intermingled syndrome of asthenia and sthenia are the common ones of the disease in clinic. The cause of sthenia syndrome is, in most cases, because of either exogenous wind, dampness and heat or stagnated heat of the liver and gallbladder, and the reason for the intermingled syndrome of asthenia and sthenia is often due to yin deficiency of the liver and kidney. In the sthenia cases, the treatment should include the methods of dispelling wind, removing dampness, clearing away heat, detoxicating, cooling blood and dissipating blood stasis while, in the intermingled cases of deficient yin causing hyperactivity of fire, the treatment method should be to nourish yin to lessen fire.

1. Syndrome of Pathogenic Wind-heat of Liver Meridian

Main Symptoms and Signs Acute attack with the ocular symptoms of dragging pain of the eyeball, photo-

久可致火盛水衰,表现为虚实夹杂之证。

【诊断要点】

(1) 眼部症状有疼痛、畏光、流泪、视力减退。

(2) 睫状区有压痛,球结膜睫状充血或混合充血,角膜后沉着物,房水混浊,虹膜肿胀,瞳孔缩小。

(3) 虹膜常发生瞳孔后粘连,如散瞳不及时常造成瞳孔膜闭或闭锁。

【辨证论治】

本病临床以实证及虚实夹杂证为常见。实证多因外感风、湿、热邪或肝胆郁热,虚实夹杂证常为肝肾阴亏。在治疗方面,实证用祛风、除湿、清热、解毒、凉血、散瘀等法;虚实夹杂的阴虚火旺证,则予以滋阴降火法。

1. 肝经风热证

主要证候　起病较急,眼珠坠痛,畏光流泪,视物模糊,

phobia, lacrimation, blurred vision, ciliary hyperemia, contracted pupil, opacity of aqueous humor dark and gloomy iris with obscure line, often accompanied by headache, fever and dry mouth; reddish tongue with thin yellowish or whitish coating and floating rapid pulse.

Therapeutic Methods　Removing wind and clearing away heat.

Recipe　The Modified New Chailian Decoction: Chaihu (*Radix Bupleuri*) 6 g, Huanglian (*Rhizoma Coptidis*) 6 g, Shanzhizi (*Fructus Gardeniae*) 10 g, Maijingzi (*Fructus Viticis*) 10 g, Chishaoyao (*Radix Paeoniae Rubra*) 10 g, Fangfeng (*Radix Ledebouriellae*) 6 g, and Gancao (*Radix Glycyrrhizae*) 3 g.

Modification　In the cases of severe redness and pain of the eye, Shengdihuang (*Radix Rehmanniae*), Mudanpi (*Cortex Moutan Radicis*), Danshen (*Radix Salviae Miltiorrhizae*) and Chongweizi (*Semen Leonuri*), each 10 g, are added.

2. Syndrome of Excessive Fire of the Liver and Gallbladder

Main Symptoms and Signs　Besides the same ocular symptoms of the above syndrome, there often occurs blood coagulation between the black of eye and the iris, or hypopyon will be seen, usually accompanied by dry mouth with bitter taste and susceptibility to losing temper; reddish tongue with yellowish coating and thread rapid pulse.

Therapeutic Method　Purging pathogenic fire of the liver and gallblader.

Recipe　The modified Longdan Xiegan Decoction: Longdancao (*Radix Gentianae*) 6 g, Shanzhizi (*Fructus Gardeniae*) 10 g, Huangqin (*Radix Scutellariae*) 10 g, Chaihu (*Radix Bupleuri*) 6 g, Shengdihuang (*Radix Rehmanniae*) 10 g, Mutong (*Caulis Akebiae*) 6 g, Zexie (*Rhizoma Alismatis*) 10 g, and Chishaoyao (*Radix*

抱轮红赤,瞳神紧小,神水混浊,黄仁晦暗,纹理不清。常伴有头痛发热,口干舌红,舌苔薄白或薄黄,脉浮数。

治　法　祛风清热。

方　药　新制柴连汤加减。柴胡6 g,黄连6 g,山栀子10 g,蔓荆子10 g,赤芍药10 g,防风6 g,甘草3 g。

加　减　目赤痛较甚者,加生地黄10 g,牡丹皮10 g,丹参10 g,茺蔚子10 g。

2. 肝胆实火证

主要证候　眼部见症同前。还可见黑睛与黄仁之间血液沉着,或黄液上冲。常伴有口干且苦,暴躁易怒,舌红苔黄,脉弦数。

治　法　清泻肝胆。

方　药　龙胆泻肝汤加减。龙胆草6 g,山栀子10 g,黄芩10 g,柴胡6 g,生地黄10 g,木通6 g,泽泻10 g,赤芍药10 g。

Paeoniae Rubra) 10 g.

Modification In the cases of severe ophthalmalgia or hyphema, 10 g of Mudanpi (*Cortex Moutan Radicis*) and 10 g of Puhuang (*Pollen Typhae*) and 15 g of Baimaogen (*Rhizoma Imperatae*) are added, and in the cases of thirsty sensation, constipation and hypopyon, 15 g of Shengshigao (*Gypsum Fibrosum*, to be decocted first), 10 g of Zhimu (*Rhizome Anemarrhenae*) and 6 g of Shengdahuang (*Radix et Rhizoma Rhei*) are added.

3. Syndrome of Pathogenic Wind-dampness plus Heat

Main Symptoms and Signs Urgent or slow onset with the same symptoms of above syndromes, or sometimes dim eyesight with the subjective feeling of dark objects moving about, often accompanied by headache, chest distress and arthrodynia of extremities; reddish tongue with yellowish greasy coating and thready rapid or soft rapid pulse.

Therapeutic Methods Dispersing wind and removing heat and dampness.

Recipe The modified Yiyang Jiuliansan Decoction: Duhuo (*Radix Angelicae Pubescentis*) 10 g, Qianghuo (*Rhizome seu Radix Notopterygii*) 6 g, Fangji (*Radix Stephaniae Tetrandrae*) 6 g, Baizhi (*Radix Angelicae Dahuricae*) 6 g, Manjingzi (*Fructus Viticis*) 10 g, Huanglian (*Rhizoma Coptidis*) 6 g, Huangqin (*Radix Scutellariae*) 10 g, Shanzhizi (*Fructus Gardeniae*) 10 g, Huangbai (*Cortex Phellodendri*) 10 g, Shengdihuang (*Radix Rehmanniae*) 10 g, and Gancao (*Radix Glycyrrhizae*) 3 g.

Modification In the cases of severe pathogenic wind-heat and serious pain and swelling, 10 g of Chongweizi (*Semen Leonuri*) and 10 g of Chishaoyao (*Radix Paeoniae Rubra*) are added with Duhuo and Baizhi being

加 减 眼痛较甚或前房积血者,加牡丹皮10 g,蒲黄10 g,白茅根15 g;口渴便秘,黄液上冲者,加生石膏(先煎)15 g,知母10 g,生大黄6 g。

3. 风湿挟热证

主要证候 发病或急或缓,眼部见证同前。或自觉眼前黑花飞舞。多伴有头痛胸闷,肢节酸痛,舌红苔黄腻,脉弦数或濡数。

治 法 祛风清热除湿。

方 药 抑阳酒连散加减。独活10 g,羌活6 g,防己6 g,白芷6 g,蔓荆子10 g,黄连6 g,黄芩10 g,山栀子10 g,黄柏10 g,生地黄10 g,甘草3 g。

加 减 风热偏盛,赤痛较甚者,去独活,羌活,白芷,加茺蔚子10 g,赤芍药10 g;风湿偏重,去黄柏,加厚朴10 g,

removed, and in the cases of severe wind-dampness, Huangbai is removed and respective 10 g of Houpo (*Cortex Magnoliae Officinalis*), Fuling (*Poria*) and Yiyiren (*Semen Coicis*) are added.

4. Syndrome of Hyperactivity of Fire due to Yin Deficiency

Main Symptoms and Signs The late or remission period of the disease with a dry and unsmooth sensation in the eye, repeated pain and swelling sometimes severe and sometimes mild, irregular posterior synechia of the pupil and dim eyesight, often accompanied by headache, sleepless, feverish sensation in the chest, palms and soles, dry mouth and throat; reddish tongue with a little coating and thready rapid pulse.

Therapeutic Method Nourishing yin to remove fire.

Recipe The modified Zhibai Dihuangwan Decoction: Zhimu (*Rhizome Anemarrhenae*) 10 g, Huangbai (*Cortex Phellodendri*) 10 g, Shengdihuang (*Radix Rehmanniae*) 10 g, Shanzhuyu (*Fructus Corni*) 10 g, Shanyao (*Rhizoma Dioscoreae*) 10 g, Fuling (*Poria*) 10 g, Zexie (*Rhizoma Alismatis*) 10 g, and Mudanpi (*Cortex Moutan Radicis*) 10 g.

5. Syndrome of Liver and Kidney Deficiency

Main Symptoms and Signs The late stage of the disease with dryness and uncomfortable sensation in the eye, dim vision with the subjective feeling of dark objects moving about, contracted pupil and even opacity of the lens, often accompanied by headache, tinnitus, sleepless with dreams and aching weakness in waist and legs; whitish tongue and thready pulse.

Therapeutic Method Nourishing the liver and kidney.

Recipe The modified Qiju Dihuangwan Decoction:

茯苓10 g,薏苡仁10 g。

4. 阴虚火旺证

主要证候 病至后期,或病势较缓,眼干涩不适,赤痛时轻时重,反复发作,瞳神后粘连不圆,视物昏花。常伴有头痛寐差,五心烦热,口干咽燥,舌红少苔,脉细数。

治 法 滋阴降火。

方 药 知柏地黄丸加减。知母10 g,黄柏10 g,生地黄10 g,山茱萸10 g,山药10 g,茯苓10 g,泽泻10 g,牡丹皮10 g。

5. 肝肾不足证

主要证候 病至后期,眼干不适,视物昏朦或自见黑花,瞳神干缺,甚至晶珠混浊。常伴有头晕耳鸣,少寐多梦,腰膝酸软,舌淡脉细。

治 法 滋补肝肾。

方 药 杞菊地黄丸加

Gouqizi (*Fructus Lycii*) 10 g, Juhua (*Flos Chrysanthemi*) 6 g, Shengdihuang (*Radix Rehmanniae*) 10 g, Zexie (*Rhizoma Alismatis*) 10 g, Fuling (*Poria*) 10 g, Nüzhenzi (*Fructus Ligustri Lucidi*) 10 g, Heshouwu (*Radix Polygoni Multiflori*) 10 g, Shanyao (*Rhizoma Dioscoreae*) 10 g, Mudanpi (*Cortex Moutan Radicis*) 10 g, and Shanyurou (*Fructus Corni*) 10 g.

[Other Treatments]

1. Chinese Patent Drugs

(1) Londan Xiegan Pill 5 g each time, twice a day and applicable to the syndrome of excessive fire of the liver and gallbladder.

(2) Zhibai Dihuang Pill 8 pills each time, twice a day and applicable to the syndrome of hyperactivity of fire due to yin deficiency.

(3) Qiju Dihuang Pill 8 pills each time, twice a day and applicable to the syndrome of liver and kidney deficiency.

2. Simple and Proved Recipes

(1) Compound Leigongteng Decoction The prescription consists of the herbal drugs of Leigongteng (*Radix Folium seu Flos Tripterygii Wilfordii*), Chongweizi (*Semen Leonuri*), Tusizi (*Semen Cuscutae*), and Hanliancao (*Herba Ecliptae*), each 10 g, and all the ingredients are simmered for an hour, one dose a day with the decoction being orally taken in the morning and evening. The recipe is applicable to the disease due to the deficiency of kidney qi and latent pathogenic factors.

(2) Xiakucao (*Spica Prunellae*) 60 g, Xiangfu (*Rhizoma Cyperi*) 60 g and Gancao (*Radix Glycyrrhizae*) 12 g, all are pounded into powder which is orally taken with green tea, 9 g each time, twice a day and it is applicable to the syndrome of stagnant heat of liver meridian.

减。枸杞子10 g,菊花6 g,生地黄10 g,泽泻10 g,茯苓10 g,女贞子10 g,何首乌10 g,山药10 g,牡丹皮10 g,山萸肉10 g。

【其他疗法】

1. 中成药

（1）龙胆泻肝丸　每服5 g,每日2次。适用于肝胆火炽证。

（2）知柏地黄丸　每服8粒,每日2次。适用于阴虚火旺证。

（3）杞菊地黄丸　每服8粒,每日2次。适用于肝肾不足证。

2. 单验方

（1）复方雷公藤汤　雷公藤10 g,茺蔚子10 g,菟丝子10 g,旱莲草10 g。文火煎1小时,每日1剂,分2次服。适用于本病肾气虚,余邪留恋者。

（2）夏枯草60 g,香附60 g,甘草12 g。共研细末,每日2次,每次9 g,清茶送服。适用于本病肝经郁热证。

(3) The Recipe of Uveitis No. I   The drugs used in the recipe are: Baimaogen (*Rhizoma Imperatae*) 10 g, Mudanpi (*Cortex Moutan Radicis*) 10 g, Huanglian (*Rhizoma Coptidis*) 6 g, Huangbai (*Cortex Phellodendri*) 10 g, Longdancao (*Radix Gentianae*) 6 g, Dahuang (*Radix et Rhizoma Rhei*) 6 g, Shigao (*Gypsum Fibrosum*, to be decocted first) 15 g, Mutong (*Caulis Akebiae*) 6 g and Niuxi (*Radix Achyranthis Bidentatae*) 10 g. All these drugs are decocted with water, one dose a day for oral taking. The decoction is applicable to the syndrome of excessive heat.

(4) The Recipe of Uveitis No. II   The drugs used in the recipe are: Zhimu (*Rhizoma Anemarrhenae*) 10 g, Huangbai (*Cortex Phellodendri*) 10 g, Mutong (*Caulis Akebiae*) 6 g, Mudanpi (*Cortex Moutan Radicis*) 10 g, Xuanshen (*Semen Plantaginis*) 10 g, Shihu (*Herba Dendrobii*) 10 g, Fuling (*Poria*) 10 g, Cheqianzi (*Semen Plantaginis*, bagged) 10 g, Zicao (*Radix Arnebiae seu Lithospermi*) 15 g, Niuxi (*Radix Achyranthis Bidentatae*) 10 g, and Baijili (*Fructus Tribuli*) 10 g, all are decocted with water for oral taking, one dose a day and the decoction is applicable to the syndrome of deficient heat.

(5) The modified Danggui Shaoyao Decoction   The ingredients of the decoction include Danggui (*Radix Angelicae Sinensis*) 10 g, Chishaoyao (*Radix Paeoniae Rubra*) 10 g, Chuanxiong (*Rhizoma Ligustici Chuanxiong*) 10 g, Fuling (*Poria*) 12 g, Zexie (*Rhizoma Alismatis*) 12 g, Baizhu (*Rhizoma Atractylodis Macrocephalae*) 10 g, Danshen (*Radix Salviae Miltiorrhizae*) 12 g, and Mimenghua (*Flos Buddlejae*) 12 g, all of which are decocted with water, one dose a day with the liquid being taken in the morning and evening. The decoction is applicable to the syndrome of the deficiency of both qi and blood attac-

（3）色素膜炎 I 号方
白茅根10 g,牡丹皮10 g,黄连6 g,黄柏10 g,龙胆草6 g,大黄6 g,石膏(先煎)15 g,木通6 g,牛膝10 g。水煎服,每日 1 剂。适用于实热证。

（4）色素膜炎 II 号方
知母10 g,黄柏10 g,木通6 g,牡丹皮10 g,玄参10 g,石斛10 g,茯苓10 g,车前子10 g,紫草15 g,牛膝10 g,白蒺藜10 g。水煎服,每日 1 剂,适用于虚热证。

（5）加味当归芍药汤
当归10 g,赤芍药10 g,川芎10 g,茯苓12 g,泽泻12 g,白术10 g,丹参12 g,密蒙花12 g。每日 1 剂,水煎服,每日 2 次。适用于本病气血虚弱,反复发作者。

king repeatedly.

(6) A proper amount of Huanglian (*Rhizoma Coptidis*) powder is made, by mixing with water, into a kind of paste which is applied externally to the foot soles to purge heat downwards.

3. External Therapies

(1) Eye Drops   a. Local Mydriatic Application The drug commonly used is 1% of atropine or the eye ointment, which is applied to drop the eye once or twice every day (after the dropping of atropine, the inner canthus is pressed for 3 to 5 minutes). b. Application of eye drops for removing heat and virulent pathogenic factors The drug often used is either 1% of Baicalein Eye Drops or 10% to 50% of Qianliguang Eye Drops, which is used to the eye several times a day.

(2) Wet-hot Dressing   The affected eye is compressed with the hot water or hot liquid by decocting the oral drugs with water. The wet-compressing method, which is performed three times a day and ten minutes for each time, can improve the circulation of qi and blood so as to relieve swelling and pain.

(3) Hormones or Antibiotics   In the very severe cases, the eye is dropped with some hormones or antibiotics, or subconjunctival injection may be needed.

2.5.2 Acute Angle-closure Glaucoma

[**Introduction**]

Acute angle-closure glaucoma is a kind of ophthalmopathy characterized by the rapid rise of intraocular pressure accompanied by the corresponding symptoms and tissue changes of the anterior chamber of the eye. Clinically, it often manifests the symptoms of the increasing

（6）黄连末外敷　黄连适量,研成细末,用水调成糊状,外敷足心,引热下行。

3. 外治法

（1）点眼药　① 局部点扩瞳剂:常用药为 1% 阿托品液或眼膏,每日点眼 1～2 次(每次点阿托品液后,应压迫内眦部 3～5 分钟)。② 点清热解毒眼液:常用 1% 黄芩素眼液或 10%～50% 千里光眼液,每日点眼数次。

（2）湿热敷　患眼用热水或内服药渣煎水作湿热敷,每日 3 次,每次 10 分钟。湿热敷可促进气血流通,以退赤止痛。

（3）激素、抗生素　病情严重者,可用激素或抗生素类药物滴眼或结膜下注射。

第二节　急性闭角型青光眼

【概述】

急性闭角型青光眼是一种以眼压急剧升高并伴有相应症状和眼前段组织改变为特征的眼病。临床主要表现为眼压升高,瞳孔散大,视力

intraocular pressure, platycoria and serious visual diminution. A common disease in China with a morbidity of 0.21% to 1.64%, it is the fourth disease to cause blindness. Persons over fifty years old are easy to develop the disease and most of them are women. Usually, both eyes are affected one after the other or simutaneously.

The cause of the disease, though unclear at present, is generally believed to be concerned with the blockage of trabecular network by the peripheral iris or with the permanent adhension of the trabecular network, causing the aqueous outflow to be obstructed, and the increase in the intraocular pressure occurs.

The disease, from its clinical manifestations, should pertain to "Lüfeng Neizhang" (green glaucoma) in traditional Chinese medicine. Usually, it arises from the invasion of eye by pathogenic wind-fire and phlegm. The upward invasion of eye by pathogenic factors, disorder of qi and blood, obstruction of meridian and vessel, closure of sweat pore, stagnation of qi and blood as well as accumulation of aqueous humor, all these form the pathogenesis of the disease.

[Main Diagnostic Points]

1. Clinical Symptoms

Severe headache, distending pain of eye, iridization and visual deterioration or only light sensation remaining in severe cases.

2. Clinical Physical Signs

(1) The increase of the intraocular pressure Often above 6.65 kPa (50 mmHg) or over 13.3 kPa (100 mmHg) in some serious cases.

(2) Platycoria Moderate in degree and veridical or oval in shape, disappearance of photoreaction and visible dark-green reflection in the pupillary zone. It is for this

严重减退。本病在中国为常见病,占致盲眼病的第四位,人群中发病率约为 0.21%～1.64%。发病以 50 岁以上的老年人为多,女性更常见。常两眼先后或同时发病。

本病的病因尚不十分清楚。一般认为是由于周边虹膜堵塞小梁网,或与小梁网产生永久性粘连,以致房水外流受阻,引起眼压升高。

根据本病的临床表现,当属于中医学"绿风内障"范畴。其病因为风、火、痰上犯目窍。主要病机为邪气上犯目窍,气血失和,经脉不利,玄府闭塞,气滞血郁,神水瘀积所致。

【诊断要点】

1. 临床症状

剧烈头痛,眼胀痛,虹视,视力减退,严重者视力降至仅留光感。

2. 临床体征

(1) 眼压升高 一般在 6.65 kPa(50 mmHg)以上,个别严重病例可达 13.3 kPa(100 mmHg)以上。

(2) 瞳孔散大 瞳孔常中等度散大,多呈垂直椭圆形,光反应消失,瞳孔区可见

reason that the case is called "Lüfeng Neizhang " (green glaucoma) in traditional Chinese medicine.

(3) Ocular hyperemia   Mixed congestion of conjunctiva accompanied sometimes by chemosis and palpebral edema in some serious cases.

(4) Corneal edema   Edema of corneal epithelium in the fog-like or ground-glass-like form.

(5) Obstruction in the anterior chamber and the angle   The anterior chamber becomes shallow and the angle is blocked.

(6) Opacity of the aqueous humor   The aqueous humor is cloudy even with the flocculent exudate.

(7) Iris Lesion   The iris is of segmental strophy and posterior synechia, and fine dust-like pigmentation is often found behind the cornea and in front of the iris.

[**Syndrome Differentiation and Treatment**]

Clinically, the disease is usually classified into the syndromes of excessive fire of the liver and gallbladder, phlegm-fire with wind disturbance, stagnation of live qi, yin deficiency and yang hyperactivity, and asthenia cold of the liver and stomach. The treatment of the disease, on one hand, should be to remove the pathogenic factors and cure the principal symptoms and, on the other hand, special attention must be paid to the improving of blood circulation, opening sweat pore, dispersing of obstruction and stagnation, contracting of the pupil so that the symptoms can be immediately relieved and the eyesight protected.

1. Syndrome of Excessive Fire of the Liver and Gallbladder

Main Symptoms and Signs   Acute onset, headache, ocular swelling involving orbit, rapid deterioration of vision or even blindness, ciliary or bulbar conjunctival hyperemia, fog-like pancorneal opacity, platycoria, light-

青绿色反光,故中医学称"绿风内障"。

（3）眼部充血　结膜呈混合性充血或伴球结膜水肿,严重者可出现眼睑水肿。

（4）角膜水肿　角膜上皮水肿,呈雾状或毛玻璃状混浊。

（5）前房、房角闭塞　前房变浅甚至房角闭塞。

（6）房水混浊　房水混浊,甚至出现絮状渗出物。

（7）虹膜病变　虹膜节段状萎缩及后粘连,角膜后面及虹膜前面常见到微细的尘状色素沉着。

【辨证论治】

本病临床主要分为肝胆火炽证、痰火动风证、肝郁气滞证、阴虚阳亢证、肝胃虚寒证,治疗除应消除病因,治其根本外,同时要注意通血脉,开玄府,宣壅滞,缩瞳神,尽快改善症状,以保存视力。

1. 肝胆火炽证

主要证候　发病急剧,头痛目胀,连及目眶,视力急降,甚至失明,抱轮红赤或白睛混赤,黑睛混浊呈雾状,瞳神散

green pupil, hard eyeball or even stonily swollen, and accompanied by nausea, vomiting, or fever with aversion to cold, yellowish urine and constipation; reddish tongue with yellowish coating and thready rapid pulse.

Therapeutic Methods　Removing heat and fire and calming endopathic wind by cooling the liver.

Recipe　The modified Lüfeng Lingyang Beverage or Longdan Xiegan Decoction: Longdancao (*Radix Gentianae*) 6 g, Chaoshanzhizi (*Fructus Gardeniae*, fried) 10 g, Huangqin (*Radix Scutellariae*) 10 g, Gouteng (*Ramulus Uncariae cum Uncis*) 10 g, Cheqianzi (*Semen Plantaginis*, bagged) 10 g, Shengdihuang (*Radix Rehmanniae*) 10 g, Baishaoyao (*Radix Paeoniae Alba*) 10 g, Dahuang (*Radix et Rhizoma Rhei*) 10 g, and Niuxi (*Radix Achyranthis Bidentatae*) 10 g.

Modification　In the cases of serious vomiting, Zhuru (*Caulis Bambusae in Taeniam*), Banxia (*Rhizoma Pinelliae*) and Tianzhuhuang (*Concretio Silicea Bambusae*), each 10 g, are added; in the cases of severe ciliary hyperemia, Chishaoyao (*Radix Paeoniae Rubra*), Taoren (*Semen Persicae*) and Zelan (*Herba Lycopi*), each 10 g, are added.

2. Syndrome of Phlegm-fire with Wind Disturbance

Main Symptons and Signs　Acute onset, distending eyes and head, ophthalmalgia, platycoria, light green pupil, turgid eyeball, full and oppressed sensation in the chest and stomach, nausea, vomiting, frequent vertigo, yellowish urine and constipation; reddish tongue with yellowish greasy coating and thready-slippery-rapid pulse.

Therapeutic Methods　Removing phlegm-fire and calming endopathic wind from the Liver.

Recipe　The modified Jiangjun Dingtongwan or Wendan Decoction: Dahuang (*Radix et Rhizoma Rhei*)

大,瞳色淡绿,眼珠变硬,甚至胀硬如石。可伴有恶心呕吐或恶寒发热,尿黄便结,舌红苔黄,脉弦数等。

治　法　清热泻火,凉肝熄风。

方　药　绿风羚羊饮或龙胆泻肝汤加减。龙胆草6 g,炒山栀子10 g,黄芩10 g,钩藤10 g,车前子(包煎)10 g,生地黄10 g,白芍药10 g,大黄10 g,牛膝10 g。

加　减　呕吐甚者,加竹茹10 g,半夏10 g,天竺黄10 g;抱轮红赤甚者,加赤芍药10 g,桃仁10 g,泽兰10 g。

2. 痰火动风证

主要证候　起病急骤,头胀眼痛,瞳神散大,瞳色淡绿,眼珠胀硬,胸脘满闷,恶心呕吐,动辄眩晕,尿黄便结,舌红苔黄腻,脉弦滑数。

治　法　降火逐痰,平肝熄风。

方　药　将军定痛丸或温胆汤加减。大黄10 g,黄芩

10 g, Huangqin (*Radix Scutellariae*) 10 g, Baijiangcan (*Bombyx Batryticatus*) 6 g, Chenpi (*Pericarpium Citri Reticulate*) 10 g, Banxia (*Rhizoma Pinelliae*) 10 g, Fuling (*Poria*) 12 g, Zhishi (*Fructus Aurantii Immaturus*) 10 g, Cheqianzi (*Semen Plantaginis*, bagged) 10 g, and Mutong (*Caulis Akebiae*) 6 g.

Modification In the cases of serious vertigo, 10 g of Tianma (*Rhizoma Gastrodiae*) is added; in the cases of severe fullness in the chest and stomach, Zexie (*Rhizoma Alismatis*), Laifuzi (*Semen Raphani*) and Baijiezi (*Semen Sinapis Albae*), each 10 g, are added.

3. Syndrome of Stagnation of Liver Qi

Main Symptoms and Signs Serious frontal headache on the sick side, unbearable distending pain of eye, platycoria, vision diminishment, hard eyeball, accompanied by emotional disturbance, oppressed chest, eructation, loss of appetite, nausea, vomiting and bitter taste in the mouth; reddish tongue with yellowish coating and thready rapid pulse.

Therapeutic Methods Dispersing stagnated liver by removing heat and lowering adverse qi to regulate stomach.

Recipe The modified Danzhi Xiaoyaosan Decoction: Chaihu (*Radix Bupleuri*) 10 g, Danggui (*Radix Angelicae Sinensis*) 10 g, Baishaoyao (*Radix Paeoniae Alba*) 10 g, Fuling (*Poria*) 10 g, Baizhu (*Rhizoma Atractylodis Macrocephalae*) 10 g, Mudanpi (*Cortex Moutan Radicis*) 10 g, Shanzhizi (*Fructus Gardeniae*) 10 g, Huanglian (*Rhizoma Coptidis*) 6 g, and Wuzhuyu (*Fructus Evodiae*) 3 g.

Modification In the cases of serious vomiting, 10 g of Xuanfuhua (*Flos Inulae*) and 10 g of Daizheshi (*Ochrae Haematitum*) are added; in the cases of severe ophthalmalgia, 15 g of Shijueming (*Concha Haliotidis*, to be decocted first), 10 g of Caojueming (*Herba Cassiae*)

10 g,白僵蚕6 g,陈皮10 g,半夏10 g,茯苓12 g,枳实10 g,车前子(包煎)10 g,木通6 g。

加 减 头昏甚者,加天麻10 g;胸脘满甚者,加泽泻10 g,莱菔子10 g,白芥子10 g。

3. 肝郁气滞证

主要证候 患侧头额痛甚,目赤胀痛难忍,瞳神散大,视力下降,眼珠变硬。常伴有情志不舒,胸闷嗳气,食少纳呆,呕吐泛恶,口苦,舌红苔黄,脉弦数等。

治 法 疏肝清热,降逆和胃。

方 药 丹栀逍遥散加减。柴胡10 g,当归10 g,白芍药10 g,茯苓10 g,白术10 g,牡丹皮10 g,山栀子10 g,黄连6 g,吴茱萸3 g。

加 减 呕逆甚者,加旋覆花10 g,代赭石10 g;目赤痛较甚者,加石决明(先煎)15 g,草决明10 g,夏枯草10 g;胸闷甚者,加郁金10 g。

and 10 g of Xiakucao (*Spica Prunellae*) are added; in the cases of serious oppressed sensation in the chest, 10 g of Yujin (*Radix Curcumae*) is added.

4. Syndrome of Yin Deficiency and Yang Hyperactivity

Main Symptoms and Signs Distending pain of head and eye, platycoria, dim eyesight, hard eyeball, restlessness and sleeplessness, dry mouth and throat, vertigo and tinnitus; reddish tongue with little coating and thready rapid pulse.

Therapeutic Methods Nourishing yin to remove fire and calming endopathic wind from the liver.

Recipe The modified Zhibai Dihuangwan Decoction: Zhimu (*Rhizoma Anemarrhenae*) 10 g, Huangbai (*Cortex Phellodendri*) 10 g, Shengdihuang (*Radix Rehmanniae*) 10 g, Zexie (*Rhizoma Alismatis*) 10 g, Shijueming (*Concha Haliotidis*, to be decocted first) 15 g, Gouteng (*Ramulus Uncariae cum Uncis*) 10 g, and Baishaoyao (*Radix Paeoniae Alba*) 10 g.

Modification In the cases of constipation, 10 g of Juemingzi (*Semen Cassiae*) is added; in the cases of serious dry mouth, 10 g of Tianhuafen (*Radix Trichosanthis*) is added.

5. Syndrome of Asthenia Cold of Liver and Stomach

Main Symptoms and Signs In addition to the ocular symptoms, acute attack with symptoms of severe headache and ophthalmalgia involving vertex, retching with saliva, poor appetite, tiredness and cold limbs; pale tongue with whitish coating and thready pulse.

Therapeutic Method Warming the liver and stomach to lower adverse qi and arrest pain.

Recipe The modified Wuzhuyu Decoction: Wuzhuyu (*Fructus Evodiae*) 5 g, Shengjiang (*Rhizoma Zingib-*

4. 阴虚阳亢证

主要证候　头眼胀痛,瞳神散大,视物昏朦,眼珠变硬,心烦失眠,口干咽燥,眩晕耳鸣,舌红少苔,脉弦细而数。

治　法　滋阴降火,平肝熄风。

方　药　知柏地黄丸加减。知母10 g,黄柏10 g,生地黄10 g,泽泻10 g,石决明(先煎)15 g,钩藤10 g,白芍药10 g。

加　减　大便干结者,加决明子10 g;口干甚者,加天花粉10 g。

5. 肝胃虚寒者

主要证候　急性发作,除眼部症状外,尚有头目剧痛,头痛上及巅顶,干呕吐涎,食少神疲,四肢不温,舌淡苔白,脉细。

治　法　温肝暖胃,降逆止痛。

方　药　吴茱萸汤加减。吴茱萸5 g,生姜10 g,陈皮

eris Recens) 10 g, Chenpi (*Pericarpium Citri Reticulatae*) 10 g, Fuling (*Poria*) 12 g, Baizhi (*Radix Angelicae Dahuricae*) 10 g, Chuanxiong (*Rhizoma Ligustici Chuanxiong*) 6 g, and Gancao (*Radix Glycyrrhizae*) 3 g.

Modification   In the cases of severe headache, 3 g of Xixin (*Herba Asari*) is added; in the cases of limbs aversing to cold, 6 g of Guizhi (*Ramulus Cinnamomi*) is added; in the cases of oppressed chest and poor appetite, 10 g of Baizhu (*Rhizoma Atractylodis Macrocephalae*) and 10 g of Baikouren (*Semen Amomi Rotundus*) are added.

[Other Treatments]

1. Chinese Patent Drugs

(1) **Longdan Xiegan Pill**   5 g each time, twice a day and applicable to the syndrome of excessive fire of the liver and gallbladder.

(2) **Danzhi Xiaoyao Pill**   5 g each time, twice a day and applicable to the syndrome of pathogenic fire due to stagnated liver.

(3) **Zhibai Dihuang Pill**   8 pills each time, twice a day and applicable to the syndrome of fire hyperactivity due to yin deficiency.

(4) **Jiangjun Dingtong Pill**   6 pills each time, twice a day and applicable to the syndrome of phlegm-fire with wind disturbance.

2. Simple and Proved Recipes

(1) **Anti-glaucoma No. Ⅱ Decoction**   The herbs used in the recipe are: Shijueming (*Concha Haliotidis*, to be decocted first) 18 g, Caojueming (*Herba Cassiae*) 12 g, Shengdihuang (*Radix Rehmanniae*) 15 g, Shengshigao (*Gypsum Fibrosum*, to be decocted first) 24 g, Huanglian (*Rhizoma Coptidis*) 1.5 g, Huangqin (*Radix Scutellariae*) 9 g, Danggui (*Radix Angelicae Sinensis*) 10 g, Chishaoyao (*Radix Paeoniae Rubra*) 12 g, Qianghuo (*Rhizoma seu Radix Notopterygii*) 3 g, Juhua

10 g,茯苓12 g,白芷10 g,川芎6 g,甘草3 g。

加 减 头痛甚者,加细辛3 g;四肢逆冷者,加桂枝6 g;胸闷纳差者,加白术10 g,白蔻仁10 g。

【其他疗法】

1. 中成药

(1)龙胆泻肝丸 每服5 g,每日 2 次。适用于肝胆火炽证。

(2)丹栀逍遥丸 每服5 g,每日 2 次。适用于肝郁化火证。

3)知柏地黄丸 每服8粒,每日 2 次。适用于阴虚火旺证。

(4)将军定痛丸 每服6 g,每日 2 次。适用于痰火动风证。

2. 单验方

(1)抗青光眼Ⅱ号方石决明(先煎)18 g,草决明12 g,生地黄15 g,生石膏(先煎)24 g,黄连1.5 g,黄芩9 g,当归10 g,赤芍药12 g,羌活3 g,菊花6 g,防风3 g,蔓荆子9 g。水煎服,每日 1 剂。适用于其他方法降眼压效果不显著者。

(*Flos Chrysanthemi*) 6 g, Fangfeng (*Radix Ledebouriellae*) 3 g, and Manjingzi (*Fructus Viticis*) 9 g. All the drugs are decocted with water for oral taking one dose a day. The recipe can be applied when other methods of decreasing the intraocular pressure is not very effective.

(2) Sanzi Yicaoling Decoction The ingredients of the recipe are：Nüzhenzi (*Fructus Ligustri Lucidi*) 10 g, Chongweizi (*Semen Leonuri*) 10 g, Wuweizi (*Fructus Schisandrae*) 6 g, Xiakucao (*Spica Prunellae*) 10 g, and Fuling (*Poria*) 12 g. All the herbs are decocted with water one dose a day. The recipe is applicable to glaucoma at all stages or the high intraocular pressure after operation.

3. External Therapies

(1) Eye Drops a. Arecoline Eye-Dropping Liquid (1%)：Drop the eye with the liquid once every 15 to 30 minutes when the case is severe, and 3 to 5 times every day when the pupil is contracted. b. Arecoline Medicated Film：Place the film in the interior conjunctival fornix until it dissolves itself. In 15 minutes, the pupil begins to contract, lasting 6 to 8 hours. The method can be applied twice or three times a day. c. Anti-glaucoma Ointment：Drop the eye with the ointment twice a day and the pupil begins to contract in 15 minutes and becomes contracted in 45 minutes.

(2) Operation Peripheral iridectomy or laser iridectomy may be performed. If extensive adhension exists at the corner of the camera, the trabecular removal should be chosen.

2.5.3 Primary Open-angle Glaucoma

[**Introduction**]

Primary open-angle glaucoma is a kind of ophthamop-

（2）三子一草苓汤　女贞子10 g，茺蔚子10 g，五味子6 g，夏枯草10 g，茯苓12 g。水煎服，每日 1 剂。适用于各期青光眼或术后眼压不降者。

3. 外治法

（1）点眼药　①1%槟榔碱滴眼液：重症每15～30 分钟滴眼 1 次，瞳神缩小后每日滴 3～5 次。② 槟榔碱药膜：将药膜置于下睑穹窿部，待其自行溶化。每日 2～3 次，用药后 15 分钟瞳神开始缩小，可维持6～8 小时。③ 抗青膏：每日滴眼 2 次，点 15 分钟开始缩瞳，45 分钟瞳神缩小。

（2）手术　可作周边虹膜切除术或激光虹膜切开术。如房角已有广泛性粘连，应选用小梁切除术。

第三节　原发性开角型青光眼

【概述】

原发性开角型青光眼，又

athy also termed as chronic simple glaucoma. Its onset is because the chronic progressive obstruction of the aqueous humor leads to the increase of intraocular pressure or nervous lesion of the anterior segment. The clinical manifestations of the diseases include opened and widened anterior angle, enlargement of ophthalmic cup, opic astrophy and visual field detect. The disease, often with obvious familial tendency, is usually found among people at the age of 20 to 60 and men patients are more than women ones.

It is generally thought, though unclear at present, that the disease is caused by polygene or multiple factors.

From its clinic manifestations, the disease should pertain to "Qingfeng Neizhang" (bluish glaucoma) in traditional Chinese medicine. Its occurrence is much concerned with the factors of qi stagnation, phlegm-fire, injury from overstrain, yin deficiency and so on. The main pathogensis of the case is due to the fact that the invasion of eye by pathogenic factor causes the circulation disorder of qi and blood and obstruction in vessel and meridian so that accumulation of the aqueous humor arises. And those who often show wind syndrome of head, phlegm-fire and deficiency of yin and blood may easily develop the disease.

[Main Diagnostic Points]

1. Clinical Manifestations

Usually, there is not any subjective symptom at the beginning but only some mild symptoms such as distending pain of eye, headache and dim eyesight. In the middle and late stages, it is difficult for the patient to get about because of contraction of visual field.

2. Intraocular Pressure

At first, the intraocular pressure is unstable and

称慢性单纯性青光眼。此型青光眼为慢性进行性房水排出受阻,而导致眼压增高或前段视神经病变。临床主要表现为高眼压状态下房角宽而开放,视杯扩大,视神经萎缩,视野缺损。本病发病年龄在20～60岁,男性患者略多于女性,有明显的家族倾向。

本病的病因尚不完全明了,普遍认为本病为多基因或多因素疾病。

根据本病的临床表现,当属于中医学"青风内障"范畴。其发生主要与气郁、痰火、劳伤、阴亏等有关。主要病机为邪气上犯目窍,气血失和,脉络不利,神水瘀滞。素有头风、痰火及阴虚血少之人,尤易罹患。

【诊断要点】

1. 临床表现

早期往往无任何自觉症状,仅少数偶有轻微眼胀、头痛、视朦等。中晚期因视野缩小而行动不便。

2. 眼压

早期眼压不稳定,多间歇

often increases intermittently. If the pressure is examined within 24 hours, the climax tilter can be easily found out. The average reading of the pressure is a little higher than usual in most cases.

3. Fundus Examination

The enlargement of ophthalmic cup is one of the common signs, with the ratio frequently over 0.6 or the difference of two eyes over 0.2.

4. Visual Field

Characteristic changes of the visual field is one of the important bases to diagnose chronic simple glaucoma. The early field defect shows paracentral scotoma or paranasal stepladder-like scotoma and so on. There may be, in the middle stage, circular scotoma, paranasal visual field defect and concentric visual field contraction while, in the late stage, tubular visual field and temporal visual island occurs.

The diagnosis of the disease can be determined if two of the three indications — increase of intraocular pressure, damage of optic disc and visual field defect — are positive and the anterior chamber examination shows the opened angle.

[Syndrome Differentiation and Treatment]

In clinic practice, the disease is mainly classified into the syndromes of pathogenic fire due to qi stagnation, ocular invasion of phlegm-fire, fire hyperactivity due to yin deficiency, and asthenia of the liver and kidney. In treatment, the specific methods should include removing pathogenic fire, calming the liver and tranquilizing endogenous wind and, in long-standing cases, the method of nourishing the liver and kidney may be applied.

1. Syndrome of Pathogenic Fire due to Qi Stagnation

Main Symptoms and Signs　Distending pain of head

性增高,测量 24 小时眼压易发现眼压高峰值。总的眼压水平,多较正常值略微偏高。

3. 眼底

视杯增大是常见体征之一。杯盘比值常超过 0.6 或两眼之差超过 0.2。

4. 视野

特征性视野改变是诊断慢性单纯性青光眼的重要依据之一。早期视野缺损表现为旁中心暗点或鼻侧阶梯状暗点等。中期改变可有环状暗点、鼻侧视野缺损及向心性视野缩小等。晚期主要有管状视野和颞侧视岛。

眼压增高,视乳头损害,视野缺损三大指征中,如两项为阳性,另外检查房角属开角,即可诊断为开角型青光眼。

【辨证论治】

本病临床主要分为气郁化火证、痰火上扰证、阴虚动风证、肝肾两亏证。治疗分别采用泻火、平肝、熄风等法;病久者则应补益肝肾。

1. 气郁化火证

主要证候　头目胀痛,情

and eye, discomfort in emotion, fullness in chest and hypochondrium, vexation with a bitter taste in the mouth, poor appetite and mental tiredness; reddish tongue with yellowish coating and thready pulse.

Therapeutic Methods Removing pathogenic heat and dispersing stagnated liver.

Recipe The modified Danzhi Xiaoyaosan Decoction: Mudanpi (*Cortex Moutan Radicis*) 10 g, Shanzhizi (*Fructus Gardeniae*) 10 g, Chaihu (*Radix Bupleuri*) 6 g, Baishaoyao (*Radix Paeoniae Alba*) 10 g, Shengdihuang (*Radix Rehmanniae*) 10 g, Danggui (*Radix Angelicae Sinensis*) 10 g, Zexie (*Rhizoma Alismatis*) 10 g, Yujin (*Radix Curcumae*) 10 g, and Fuling (*Poria*) 10 g.

Modification In the cases of stagnated liver and yin deficiency, Shudihuang (*Radix Rehmanniae Praeparata*), Nüzhenzi (*Fructus Ligustri Lucidi*) and Sangshenzi (*Fructus Mori*), each 10 g, are added, and in the cases of pathogenic fire and wind due to stagnated liver, 10 g of Xiakucao (*Spica Prunellae*), 6 g of Juhua (*Flos Chrysanthemi*) and 10 g of Gouteng (*Ramulus Uncariae cum Uncis*) are added.

2. Syndrome of Ocular Invasion of Phlegm-fire

Main Symptoms and Signs Vertigo, ophthalmalgia, fullness of head, poor appetite, chest distress and much sputum, nausea, and a bitter taste in the mouth; reddish tongue with yellowish greasy coating and thready smooth pulse.

Therapeutic Methods Removing heat and sputum and regulating the stomach to lower adverse qi.

Recipe The modified Huanglian Wendan Decoction: Chenpi (*Pericarpium Citri Reticulatae*) 6 g, Banxia (*Rhizoma Pinelliae*) 10 g, Fuling (*Poria*) 10 g, Zhuru (*Caulis Bambusae in Taeniam*) 10 g, Zhishi (*Fructus Aurantii Immaturus*) 6 g, Huanglian (*Rhizoma Copti-*

志不舒,胸胁胀满,心烦口苦,食少神疲,舌红苔黄,脉弦细。

治 法 清热疏肝。

方 药 丹栀逍遥散加减。牡丹皮10 g,山栀子10 g,柴胡6 g,白芍药10 g,生地黄10 g,当归10 g,泽泻10 g,郁金10 g,茯苓10 g。

加 减 肝郁而阴虚者,加熟地黄10 g,女贞子10 g,桑椹子10 g;肝郁化火生风者,加夏枯草10 g,菊花6 g,钩藤10 g。

2. 痰火上扰证

主要证候 头眩目痛脑胀,食少痰多,胸闷恶心,口苦舌红,苔黄而腻,脉弦滑。

治 法 清热祛痰,和胃降逆。

方 药 黄连温胆汤加减。陈皮6 g,半夏10 g,茯苓10 g,竹茹10 g,枳实6 g,黄连6 g,黄芩6 g,甘草3 g。

dis) 6 g, Huangqin (*Radix Scutellariae*) 6 g, and Gancao (*Radix Glycyrrhizae*) 3 g.

3. Syndrome of Wind Stirring due to Yin Deficiency

Main Symptoms and Signs　Vertigo, distending pain of eye, dim eyesight, sleeplessness, tinnitus, dysphoria and feverish sensation in the five centers (chest, palms and soles), dryness in the mouth and throat, and slight platycoria; a reddish tongue with a little coating and a thready rapid pulse.

Therapeutic Methods　Nourishing yin and blood and regulating liver to calm endopathic wind.

Recipe　The modified Qiju Dihuangwan Decoction: Gouqizi (*Fructus Lycii*) 12 g, Juhua (*Flos Chrysanthemi*) 6 g, Shengdihuang (*Radix Rehmanniae*) 10 g, Shanyao (*Rhizoma Dioscoreae*) 10 g, Zexie (*Rhizoma Alismatis*) 10 g, Heshouwu (*Radix Polygoni Multiflori*) 10 g, Tusizi (*Semen Cuscutae*) 10 g, Wuweizi (*Fructus Schisandrae*) 6 g, Danggui (*Radix Angelicae Sinensis*) 10 g, and Baishaoyao (*Radix Paeoniae Alba*) 10 g.

Modification　In the cases of qi and blood asthenia, 10 g of Dangshen (*Radix Codonopsis Pilosulae*) and 10 g of Huangqi (*Radix Astragali seu Hedysari*) and 6 g of Chuanxiong (*Rhizoma Ligustici Chuanxiong*) are added; in the cases of deficiency of kidney yang, 6 g of Fuzi (*Radix Aconiti Praeparata*) and 6 g of Rougui (*Cortex Cinnamoni*) are added.

[Other Treatments]

1. Chinese Patent Drugs

(1) Danzhi Xiaoyao Pill　5 g each time, twice a day and applicable to the syndrome of pathogenic fire due to stagnated qi.

(2) Zhibai Dihuang Pill　8 pills each time, twice a day and applicable to the syndrome of fire hyperactivity

3. 阴虚动风证

主要证候　头眩眼胀,视物昏朦,失眠耳鸣,五心烦热,口燥咽干,瞳神略散大,舌红少苔,脉细数。

治　法　滋阴养血,柔肝熄风。

方　药　杞菊地黄丸加减。枸杞子12 g,菊花6 g,生地黄10 g,山药10 g,泽泻10 g,何首乌10 g,菟丝子10 g,五味子6 g,当归10 g,白芍药10 g。

加　减　气血不足者,加党参10 g,黄芪10 g,川芎6 g;肾阳偏虚者,加附子6 g,肉桂6 g。

【其他疗法】

1. 中成药

(1) 丹栀逍遥丸　每服5 g,每日 2 次。适用于气郁化火证。

(2) 知柏地黄丸　每服8粒,每日 2 次。适用于阴虚火

due to yin asthenia.

(3) Qiju Dihuang Pill 8 pills each time, twice a day and applicable to the syndrome of yin deficiency of the liver and kidney.

(4) Shihu Yeguang Pill 5 g each time, twice a day and applicable to the syndrome of yin deficiency of the liver and kidney.

(5) Lüfengan Capsule Luhui (*Aloe*), Dingxiang (*Flos Caryophylli*), and Heichou (*Semen Pharbitidis*), each for 50 g, and 100 g of Cishi (*Magnetitum*), all the ingredients are ground into powder which, after being mixed completely, is capsulized and orally taken an hour after meals, 3 to 5 capsules each time, twice a day. The method is applicable to all syndromes of glaucoma.

2. Simple and Proved Recipes

(1) Cheqianzi Decoction The recipe consists of only 60 g of Cheqianzi (*Semen Plantaginis*, bagged) which is decocted with 30 ml water for oral taking. It is applicable to the syndrome of excessive phlegm-fire.

(2) Recipe for Chronic Glaucoma The herbs used in the recipe are: Fangfeng (*Radix Ledebouriellae*) 5 g, Qianghuo (*Rhizoma seu Radix Notopterygii*) 5 g, Xixin (*Herba Asari*) 3 g, Chantui (*Periostracum Cicadae*) 3 g, Shijueming (*Concha Haliotidis*, to be decocted first) 24 g, Juhua (*Flos Chrysanthemi*) 5 g, Mimenghua (*Flos Buddlejae*) 9 g, Shengdihuang (*Radix Rehmanniae*) 15 g, Chuanxiong (*Rhizoma Ligustici Chuanxiong*) 5 g, Shihu (*Herba Dendrobii*) 5 g, and Baijiangcan (*Bombyx Batryticatus*) 6 g. All are decocted with water for oral taking, one dose a day. The recipe is applicable to all syndromes of the disease.

(3) Pinggan Xifeng Jiangya Decoction The herbs in the decoction include Shengdihuang (*Radix Rehmanniae*) 15 g, Heshouwu (*Radix Polygoni Multiflori*)

（3）杞菊地黄丸　每服8粒,每日2次。适用于肝肾不足证。

（4）石斛夜光丸　每服5 g,每日2次。适用于肝肾不足证。

（5）绿风安胶囊　芦荟50 g,丁香50 g,黑丑50 g,磁石100 g,共研细末,混合均匀,装入空心胶囊内,每服3～5粒,每日2次,饭后1小时服。适用于各类青光眼。

2. 单验方

（1）车前子煎服　车前子60 g,加水30 ml,1次煮服。适用于痰火炽盛证。

（2）慢性青光眼方　防风5 g,羌活5 g,细辛3 g,蝉蜕3 g,石决明(先煎)24 g,菊花5 g,密蒙花9 g,生地黄15 g,川芎5 g,石斛9 g,白僵蚕6 g。每日1剂,水煎服。适用于本病各证。

（3）平肝熄风降压方　生地黄15 g,何首乌15 g,女贞子9 g,天麻5 g,钩藤5 g,白僵

15 g, Nüzhenzi (*Fructus Ligustri Lucidi*) 9 g, Tianma (*Rhizoma Gastrodiae*) 5 g, Gouteng (*Ramulus Uncariae cum Uncis*) 5 g, Baijiangcan (*Bombyx Batryticatus*) 6 g, Tongjili (*Semen Astragali Complanati*) 10 g, Manjingzi (*Fructus Viticis*) 10 g, Dongchongxiacao (*Cordyceps*) 6 g, Juemingzi (*Semen Cassiae*) 12 g, Chuanxiong (*Rhizoma Ligustici Chuanxiong*) 5 g, and Shenqu (*Massa Fermentata Medicinalis*) 12 g. They are decocted with water for oral taking, one dose a day. The decoction is applicable to the syndromees of yang hyperactivity due to yin deficiency.

3. External Therapies

(1) Eye Drops　a. Arecoline Eye Drops (1%): The eye is dropped 3 to 4 times every day. Or the arecoline film, twice every day, is placed in the sac of lower palpebral conjunctiva until it dissolves itself. Or the dropping method can be applied during the day and the film application in the night. b. Dinggongteng (*Caulis Erycibes*) Eye Drops: The liquid is used to drop the eye 3 to 4 times a day.

(2) Operation　If the condition of the disease can not be controlled after the above methods, operation is needed.

2.5.4　Senile Cataract

[Introduction]

Senile cataract, a type of common cataract, is one of the major causes of blindness worldwide at present. It is clinically defined as an opacity of the lens of the eye with progressive deterioration of vision. The prevalence of the disease is often seen in the aged above 50 and its incidence usually increases with age. The onsetting age of 60% to 70% patients of the disease is over 50 to 60 and that of

蚕 6 g,潼蒺藜 10 g,蔓荆子 10 g,冬虫夏草 6 g,决明子 12 g,川芎 5 g,神曲 12 g。水煎服,每日 1 剂。适用于阴虚阳亢证。

3. 外治法

(1) 点眼药　① 1%槟榔碱滴眼液:每日滴眼 3～4 次。亦可用槟榔碱药膜,每日 2 次,置患眼下睑结膜囊内,待其自溶。还可白天滴眼液,晚上用药膜。② 1%丁公藤滴眼液:每日滴眼 3～4 次。

(2) 手术　经治疗病情不能得到有效控制,可以手术。

第四节　老年性白内障

【概述】

老年性白内障是常见的白内障。临床主要表现为晶状体混浊,视力渐进性减退。本病是目前世界上主要致盲眼病之一。多见于 50 岁以上的老年人,其发病率随年龄的增长而增加。60% ～70% 患

80% patients over 70.

The pathogensis of the disease, which is not totally known now, is generally believed to be related to ultraviolet ray and holopathy such as diabetes, hypertension, arteriosclerosis, genetic factor, lens nutrition and metabolic condition.

From the clinical manifestations, the disease should pertain to "Yuanyi Neizhang" (cataract) in traditional Chinese medicine. Usually, it occurs as the result of aging, debility, deficiency of liver and kidney yin and asthenia of essence and blood, or ocular malnutrition caused by digestive disorder due to spleen asthenia. In addition, when the eye is affected by the stagnated heat of liver meridian or by yin deficiency with damp-heat, the disease may also arise.

[Main Diagnostic Points]

1. Cortical Cataract

It can be classified, in relation to the stages, into incipient, oncotic, mature and hypermature stages.

(1) Incipient stage When the pupil is dilated for many times, the lens opacity can be found with the vision almost normal.

(2) Oncotic stage This is a further stage of lens opacification which is gray-white with water fissure and visual deterioration. Since the crystal cortex is swollen because of water accumulation, the iris bombé appears and the anterior chamber becomes shallow.

(3) Mature stage The vision deteriorates only to sense hand movement or light perception, and the lens is cloudy in uniform gray-white colour. The iris bombé disappears gradually and the depth of the anterior chamber returns to normal.

者的发病年龄在 50～60 岁,80％ 患者的发病在 70 岁以上。

本病的发病机理尚不完全了解,一般认为与紫外线、全身疾病如糖尿病、高血压、动脉硬化、遗传因素及晶状体营养和代谢状况等有关。

根据本病的临床表现,当属于中医学"圆翳内障"范畴。本病多因年老体弱,肝肾两亏,精血不足,或脾虚失运,精气不能上荣于目,晶珠失养所致。此外,肝经郁热或阴虚夹湿热上攻于目,也能引起本病。

【诊断要点】

1. 皮质性白内障

一般分为初发期、肿胀期、成熟期和过熟期。

(1) 初发期 视力可正常,多散瞳才能发现晶体混浊。

(2) 肿胀期 视力可逐渐减退,晶体混浊程度加重,呈灰白色仍可见水裂。由于晶体皮质吸收水分肿胀,可使虹膜膨隆前房变浅。

(3) 成熟期 视力降至眼前手动或光感,晶体呈灰白色均匀混浊。晶体膨胀现象逐渐消退,前房深浅恢复正常。

(4) Hypermature stage　This is an overdue state of the mature stage in which the lenticular water keeps on losing, the lens has shrunk, the capsule is wrinkled, the anterior chamber is deepened and the iris vibrates.

2. Nuclear cataract

The case is not as common as that of cortical cataract and develops slowly. At the initial stage, the opacity starts from the embryonic nucleus or from the adult nucleus with the former to be more often found. Then it spreads gradually to the adult nucleus. The colour of the opacity turns slowly from grayish yellow at the beginning to yellowish brown, then to dark brown or brownish black finally. The vision is greatly reduced and the ocular fundus cannot be found at this stage.

3. Capsule cataract

The opacity occurs beneath the anterior or posterior capsule, and the cataract beneath the anterior capsule may gradually develop to a cortical opacity until a complete cataract is formed.

[Syndrome Differentiation and Treatment]

Medicinal treatment of the disease is only applicable to cases at the early stage. If the lens becomes a gray-white opaque with the vision interfered, operation should be applied in treatment. In clinic, the disease is mainly classified into the syndromes of deficiency of liver and kidney yin, asthenia of spleen qi, invasion of liver heat and yin deficiency with damp-heat.

1. Syndrome of Deficiency of Liver and Kidney Yin

Main Symptoms and Signs　Opacity of lens, dim eyesight, dizziness and tinnitus, lassitude in loin and legs; a pale tongue and thready pulse; or cold limbs with aversion to cold, clear and profuse urine and heavy thready pulse.

（4）过熟期　成熟期持续时间过长,晶状体内水分继续丢失,晶状体体积缩小,囊膜皱缩,前房加深,虹膜有震颤。

2. 核性白内障

较皮质性白内障少见,发展较为缓慢,混浊开始于胚胎核或成人核,前者较多见,以后逐渐发展到成人核。核的混浊开始是灰黄色,以后逐渐加重而成黄褐色、棕色或棕黑色。此时视力极度减退,眼底窥不见。

3. 囊性白内障

混浊发生在前囊下或后囊下。囊膜下白内障逐渐会发展为皮质性混浊直至发展为完全性白内障。

【辨证论治】

本病药物治疗适用于早期。若晶珠灰白混浊,视力明显障碍,则需手术治疗。本病临床上主要分为肝肾两亏证、脾虚气弱证、肝热上扰证、阴虚夹湿热证。

1. 肝肾两亏证

主要证候　晶珠混浊,视物模糊,头晕耳鸣,腰膝酸软,舌淡脉细,或肢冷畏寒,小便清长,脉沉细。

Therapeutic Method Nourishing the liver and kidney to improve eyesight.

Recipe The modified Qiju Dihuangwan or Yougui Pill Decoction: Gouqizi (*Fructus Lycii*) 10 g, Juhua (*Flos Chrysanthemi*) 5 g, Shudihuang (*Radix Rehmanniae Praeparata*) 12 g, Shanyurou (*Fructus Corni*) 10 g, Zexie (*Rhizoma Alismatis*) 10 g, Fuling (*Poria*) 10 g, Tusizi (*Semen Cuscutae*) 10 g, Shanyao (*Rhizoma Dioscoreae*) 10 g, Baishaoyao (*Radix Paeoniae Alba*) 10 g, and Chushizi (*Fructus Broussonetiae*) 10 g.

Modification In the cases of asthenia of kidney yang, 6 g of Fuzi (*Radix Aconiti Praeparata*) and 6 g of Rougui (*Cortex Cinnamomi*) are added. In the cases of severe lassitude in loin and legs, 10 g of Duzhong (*Cortex Eucommiae*) and 10 g of Sangjisheng (*Ramulus Loranthi*) are added.

2. Syndrome of Spleen Asthenia and Qi Deficiency

Main Symptoms and Signs Opacity of lens, dim vision, listlessness, poor appetite, mental tiredness, sallow complexion and hypodynamic limbs; pale tongue with thin coating and thready weak pulse.

Therapeutic Methods Invigorating spleen and replenishing qi.

Recipe The modified Buzhong Yiqi Decoction: Huangqi (*Radix Astragali seu Hedysari*) 15 g, Dangshen (*Radix Codonopsis Pilosulae*) 10 g, Baizhu (*Rhizoma Atractylodis Macrocephalae*) 10 g, Chenpi (*Pericarpium Citri Reticulatae*) 6 g, Danggui (*Radix Angelicae Sinensis*) 10 g, Shengma (*Rhizoma Cimicifugae*) 6 g, Gouqizi (*Fructus Lycii*) 10 g, Fuling (*Poria*) 12 g, and Gancao (*Radix Glycyrrhizae*) 3 g.

Modification In the cases of spleen asthenia with damp retention and loose stool, the drug Danggui is re-

治　法　补益肝肾明目。

方　药　杞菊地黄丸或右归丸加减。枸杞子10 g,菊花 5 g,熟地黄12 g,山萸肉10 g,泽泻10 g,茯苓10 g,菟丝子10 g,山药10 g,白芍药10 g,楮实子10 g。

加　减　肾阳不足者,加附子 6 g,肉桂 6 g;腰膝酸软甚者,加杜仲10 g,桑寄生10 g。

2. 脾虚气弱证

主要证候　晶珠混浊,视物昏花,精神倦怠,食少神疲,面色萎黄,肢体乏力,舌淡苔薄,脉细弱。

治　法　补脾益气。

方　药　补中益气汤加减。黄芪15 g,党参10 g,白术10 g,陈皮 6 g,当归10 g,升麻6 g,枸杞子10 g,茯苓12 g,甘草 3 g。

加　减　脾虚湿停,大便溏泻者,去当归,加扁豆10 g,

moved and 10 g of Biandou (*Semen Dolichoris*) and 10 g of Yiyiren (*Semen Coicis*) are added.

薏苡仁10 g。

3. Syndrome of Ocular Invasion by Liver Heat

3. 肝热上扰证

Main Symptoms and Signs Opacity of lens, dim eyesight, headache, dryness of eye, bitter taste in the mouth and dry throat; thin yellowish tongue coating and thready rapid pulse.

主要证候 晶珠混浊,视物模糊,头痛目涩,口苦咽干,舌苔薄黄,脉弦而数。

Therapeutic Methods Removing heat and calming liver.

治 法 清热平肝。

Recipe The modified Shijuemingsan Decoction: Shijueming (*Concha Haliotidis*, to be decocted first) 15 g, Caojueming (*Semen Cassiae*) 12 g, Shanzhizi (*Fructus Gardeniae*) 6 g, Dahuang (*Radix et Rhizoma Rhei*) 6 g, Chishaoyao (*Radix Paeoniae Rubra*) 10 g, Muzei (Herba Equiseti Hiemalis) 10 g, Qianghuo (*Rhizoma seu Radix Notopterygii*) 6 g, Jingjie (*Herba Schizonepetae*) 6 g, and Qingxiangzi (*Semen Celosiae*) 10 g.

方 药 石决明散加减。石决明(先煎)15 g,草决明12 g,山栀子6 g,大黄6 g,赤芍药10 g,木贼10 g,羌活6 g,荆芥6 g,青葙子10 g。

Modification In the cases without excessive liver fire, Dahuang and Shanzhizi are removed; in the cases without exopathogens, Jingjie and Qianghuo are removed; in the cases of irritability, 6 g of Chaihu (*Radix Bupleuri*) and 6 g of Xiangfu (*Rhizoma Cyperi*) are added; in the cases of serious dim vision, 10 g of Gouqizi (*Fructus Lycii*) and 6 g of Juhua (*Flos Chrysanthemi*) are added.

加 减 肝火不盛者,去大黄、山栀子;无外邪者,去荆芥,羌活;急躁易怒者,加柴胡6 g,香附6 g;视物模糊甚者,加枸杞子10 g,菊花6 g。

4. Syndrome of Yin Deficiency with Damp-heat

4. 阴虚夹湿热证

Main Symptoms and Signs Opacity of lens, dim vision, dryness sensation in the eye, ozostomia, and dyschesia, reddish tongue with greasy coating in the root part and thready or thready rapid pulse.

主要证候 晶珠混浊,视物昏花,目涩口臭,大便不畅,舌红苔根腻,脉弦细或细数。

Therapeutic Methods Nourishing yin to removing heat and relieving epigastric distension to dispel pathogenic damp.

治 法 滋阴清热,宽中利湿。

Recipe The modified Ganluyin Decoction: Shengdi-

方 药 甘露饮加减。

huang (*Radix Rehmanniae*) 10 g, Maimendong (*Radix Ophiopogonis*) 10 g, Shihu (*Herba Dendrobii*) 10 g, Huangqin (*Radix Scutellariae*) 10 g, Yinchen (*Herba Artemisiae Scopariae*) 10 g, Pipaye (Folium Eriobotryae) 10 g, and Gancao (*Radix Glycyrrhizae*) 3 g.

Modification In the cases of more dampness than heat, 10 g of Huoxiang (*Herba Agastachis*) and 10 g of Cangzhu (*Rhizoma Atractylodis*) are added; in the cases of more heat than dampness, 10 g of Lianqiao (*Fructus Forsythiae*) is added; in the cases of dampness and heat both severe, Shengdihuang is removed and 12 g of Fuling (*Poria*), 6 g of Houpo (*Cortex Magnoliae officinalis*) and 6 g of Huanglian (*Rhizoma Coptidis*) are added; in the cases of yin deficient severely, 10 g of Gouqizi (*Fructus Lycii*) and 10 g of Nüzhenzi (*Fructus Ligustri Lucidi*) are added.

[Other Treatments]

1. Chinese Patent Drugs

(1) Shihu Yeguang Pill 5 g each time, twice a day and applicable to the syndrome of deficiency of the liver and kidney plus wind stirring due to yang hyperactivity.

(2) Qiju Dihuang Pill 8 pills each time, twice a day and applicable to the syndrome of deficiency of the liver and kidney.

(3) Zhangyanming (Cataract) Tablet 4 tablets each time, three times a day and applicable to the syndrome of asthenia of the liver and kidney and to deficiency of spleen qi.

(4) Fuming (Vision-recovery) Tablet 5 tablets at a time, three times a day and applicable to the syndrome of yin asthenia.

2. Simple and Proved Recipes

Mingmu Zhizhang (Vision-brightening and Cataract-treating) Syrup The recipe consists of Gouqizi

生地黄10 g,麦门冬10 g,石斛10 g,黄芩10 g,茵陈10 g,枇杷叶10 g,甘草3 g。

加　减　湿重于热者,加藿香10 g,苍术10 g;热重于湿者,加连翘10 g;湿热重者,去生地黄,加茯苓12 g,厚朴6 g,黄连6 g;阴虚重者,加枸杞子10 g,女贞子10 g。

【其他疗法】

1. 中成药

（1）石斛夜光丸　每服5 g,每日2次,适用于肝肾两亏,兼阳亢动风证。

（2）杞菊地黄丸　每服8粒,每日2次,适用于肝肾两亏证。

（3）障眼明片　每服4片,每日3次,适用于肝肾不足,脾虚气弱证。

（4）复明片　每服5片,每日3次,适用于阴虚证。

2. 单验方

明目治障糖浆　由枸杞子、桑椹子、五味子、谷精草、

(*Fructus Lycii*), Sangshenzi (*Fructus Mori*), Wuweizi (*Fructus Schisandrae*), Gujingcao (*Flos Eriocauli*), and Cijili (*Fructus Tribuli*). All these ingredients are made into syrup which is bottled with 500 ml as a unit. The syrup is orally taken with a dose of 50 ml each time, three times a day.

3. Extermal Therapies

(1) Eye Drops a. Shezhu Mingmu Eye Drops: The eye is dropped with the liquid three times a day. b. Zhangyi (Cataract) Powder: The eye is dropped with the agent three times a day. c. Zhenzhu Mingmu Eye Drops: The eye is dropped with the liquid three times a day. d. Xiaomeng (Dim-removing) Eye Ointment The eye is dropped with the ointment twice every day.

(2) Surgical Treatment If the cataract is mature, the pupil is normal and light location and color sense in a good condition, the surgical treatment by using metal needle to pluck the cataract should be considered, especially for those patients with senile debility.

Cataract-plucking Operation with Metal Needle

The method of plucking cataract by using metal needle, an ocular operation in which the opaque lens is removed into the vitreous body so that the vision is recovered again, is applicable to the mature senile cataract or cataract that is almost mature.

Simple and convenient in instruments and procedures, it does not cause much pain to the patients who do not need to stay in bed after the operation. According to the specific procedure, the surgery can be classified into the method of using flat needle and that of using round needle.

Preoperative preparation In a few days before the surgery, anti-inflammatory eye drops is applied to the patient's affected eye and the lacrimal passage is irrigated. Two hours prior to the surgery, 1% atropine solu-

刺蒺藜等组成，制成每瓶500 ml，每次50 ml，每日3次。

3. 外治法

（1）点眼药　①麝珠明目液：点眼，每日3次。②障翳散：点眼，每日3次。③珍珠明目液：点眼，每日3次。④消朦眼膏：点眼，每日2次。

（2）手术治疗　若圆翳内障成熟，瞳神如常，光定位及色觉良好者，宜行白内障针拨术，特别是对年老体弱多病者，效果尤佳。

白内障针拨术

通过手术将混浊的晶状体移位到玻璃体腔内，使患者复明。适应证为老年性白内障成熟期或近成熟期。

本手术具有患者痛苦少，术后不需卧床和器械简单，方法简便等优点。年老多病患者尤宜这种手术方法。具体操作又有扁针法和圆针法两种。

术前准备：术前数天患眼点消炎眼药水，冲洗泪道。术前2h滴1%阿托品液或1%～2.5%新福林液散瞳，直至瞳

tion or 1% to 25% neosynephrine solution is applied to the eye so as to have the pupil fully dilated (over 8 mm). Then routine sterilization must be done to the conjunctival sac and the palpebral skin, and the eye pad is placed onto the eye. When the patient is in the operation room, the sterilization of the conjunctival sac and palpebral skin should be performed again, and then surface anesthesia is carried out.

Surgical instruments　The instruments for both surgical procedures are needle-holder, mosquito forceps, fixation forceps, smooth conjunctival forceps, double-edged razor blade (turned to a triangular form in use with the long edge about 7 - 8 mm and the bottom side about 4 - 5 mm in width). In the surgery with the flat needle, the extra instruments include flat-headed cataract needle, dilating needle, eye-lid hook, eye scissors, suturing needle and thread while, in that with the round needle, added are the instruments of round-headed cataract needle and eye speculum.

Operative Procedure：

Operative procedure of the flat needle　Take the left eye as an example. The patient should take a semidecubitus position or a sitting position on the chair for eye-ear-nose-throat examination, with the head slightly leaning backward. Then the operative towel is spread and subcutaneous anesthesia or anesthesia by needling is done at the postbulbar or the 1/3 part of the lateral lower palpebral margin. The assistant uses the eyelid hook to pull up the upper palpebra and the suturing thread to tract the lower palpebra. The operator holds the fixation forceps with his left hand to grip the bulbar conjunctiva of the corneal margin at the 6 o'clock part to have the eyeball fixed and tracked towards the upper part of the nose and, meanwhile, takes the hemostatic forceps with the right hand to grip tightly the

孔充分放大（8 mm以上）。术眼结膜囊及术区皮肤按常规消毒，眼垫包封。进手术室后再冲洗结膜囊及消毒皮肤，做表面麻醉。

手术器械：持针器、小蚊式止血钳、固定镊、无齿结膜镊、双面刮胡须刀片（用时掰成三角形，刀锋长约 7 ～ 8 mm，底边宽约 4～5 mm）。扁针法加扁针头拨障针、扩张针、眼睑拉钩、眼科剪、针及线。圆针法加圆头拨障针、开睑器。

手术方法：

扁针操作法　以左眼为例，患者取半卧位，或用五官科检查椅取坐位，头微后仰，铺手术巾，左球后及下睑缘外侧 1/3 处皮下浸润麻醉或用针麻。助手用眼睑拉钩拉起上睑，下睑缝线牵引，术者左手用固定镊子挟持角膜缘 6 点钟处的球结膜以固定眼球，并牵拉眼球转向鼻上方，右手持止血钳夹紧掰成三角形的刀片，在角膜缘 4～5 点钟外 4 mm处，刀尖与巩膜垂直，作一平行于角膜缘，穿通眼球壁

ready-prepared triangular blade and then cut, at the part 4 mm away from the 4 to 5 o'clock surface of the corneal margin, a 3 mm long incision with the point of the knife vertical to the sclera, which is paralled to the corneal margin and passes through the full thickness of the eyeball wall.

The operater makes a change to take hold of the cataract needle with his right hand, the curved surface of the needle facing downwards and the point of the needle vertical to the sclera. After the flate part of the cataract needle is completely inserted into the cut, the head of the needle, slightly withdrawn, is kept 3 mm deep in the cut, the manubrium of the needle inclining towards the face, the front part of the needle toward the 1 to 12 o'clock part of the pupil, and then the front part of the needle being softly swayed between the ciliary body and the lens, so that the needle can be made to move forward. When it passes the posterior surface of the iris to reach the pupillary center, the concavity of the front part of the needle, which is pressed close to the lens, is moved downwards to steer clear of the 6 o'clock surface of the equatoral part and then it is turned to the posterior lens to cut directly off the ligment at the 4 to 6 o'clock surface. Next, the needle, laid flatly with its front resting at the retrolental 7 to 8 o'clock surface of the equatorial part, is horizontally swayed to the 4 to 5 o'clock surface to make the first laceration (scarification) of the vitreous prozonal membrane. At this moment, the curved surface of the needle has turned upward, so it is necessary to rotate the needle outward so as to get its curved surface downwards. Then the need is withdrawn a little and inserted again into the anterior surface of the lens, successively to press the 1 to 4 and 9 to 12 o'clock surfaces of the lens margin so as to have the lens incline backward and downwards, and, at the same time, the ligaments of the corresponding parts

全层的切口，切口长约3 mm。

右手换取拨障针，针头部的弯曲面朝下，针尖与巩膜垂直，将拨障针的扁平部全部插入切口，然后略退针，针头留在切口内约3 mm时，针柄倾向面部，保持针头朝向1～12点钟处，并在睫状体与晶状体之间轻轻摆动前进，经过虹膜后面，到达瞳孔中心部，然后将针头凹面贴住晶状体向下绕过晶状体赤道部6点钟处，转向晶状体后上，直接拨断4～6点钟处韧带，接着把针放平到针头在晶状体后7～8点钟赤道部处，向4～5点钟作水平摆动，做第一次划破玻璃体前界膜的动作。此时，针头的凹面已朝上，要注意针柄向外旋转，使针的凹面仍然朝下。然后退针，重新进入晶状体前，再依次压晶状体边缘的1～4点、9～12点，使晶状体向后下倾倒，相应处的韧带亦同时折断。此时，用拨障针由左向右第二次水平划破瞳孔区下1/3的玻璃体前界膜（划时将拨障针头超过晶状体赤道部）。最后将针头部移到8点钟处的晶状体边缘，将晶状体拨至眼

should be cut off. Now the needle is moved horizontally from the left to the right to make the second laceration (scarification) of the vitreous prozonal membrane at the lower 1/3 of the papillary zone (the head of the needle, when lacerating, should exceed the equatorial part of the lens). Finally, the needle head is moved to the lens margin at the 8 o'clock surface to pluck the lens to the intraocular subtemporal zigzag margin of the retina (cautiously not to make the lens backward). With the exception of leaving a few ligaments at the 6 o'clock surface, the others at the 6 : 30 to 9 : 30 o'clock surface should all be broken. The lens is pressed for a few minutes till it no longer floats up and the needle is withdrawn.

If the laceration of the vitreous prozonal membrane is not sure enough, the dilating needle, after the cataract needle is withdrawn, is inserted into the incision (it must direct to the centre of the eyeball), and is slowly being twirled at the angle of 90 to dilate the incision until a tightened and unsmooth sensation is felt in the operator's hand. Before withdrawing the dilating needle, let go the fixation forceps in the left hand for the change of the conjunctival forceps and then, with the dilating needle being withdrawn, transpose the conjunctival incision and the sclera incision so that the scleral incision get covered by the conjunctiva. When the operation is finished, 1% atropine eye ointment and antibiotic eye ointment are applied to the operated eye which is covered with an eye pad and wrapped up with bandage.

Operative procedure of the round needle   Take the right eye as an example. The patient should take a recumbent or horizontal position. A piece of operation towel is spread, postbulbar anesthesia is performed, and the eye speculum is placed with its cecum towards the nose. The operator takes hold of the fixation forceps with his right

球内颞下的视网膜锯齿缘附近（注意不可使晶状体靠后）。除 6 点钟处保留几根韧带外，务使 6 点半到 9 点半处韧带全部折断。稍压数分钟，起针后晶状体不再浮起，即可退针。

如对划破玻璃体前界膜没有把握，可在取出拨障针后，换用扩张针伸向切口（必须朝向球心），缓慢来回捻转扩张切口。捻转角度 90 度左右即可，使手上有紧涩感才能达到充分扩张的目的。去扩张针之前，左手松开固定镊，换取结膜镊去扩张针，使结膜切口与巩膜切口错位，达到用结膜遮盖巩膜切口的目的。术毕点 1% 阿托品眼膏加抗生素眼膏，术眼盖眼垫包封。

圆针操作方法   以右眼为例，患者取平卧或半卧位，铺手术巾，作球后麻醉，放置开睑器（盲端在鼻测）。术者右手持固定镊夹持角膜缘 6 点处的球结膜，并牵拉眼球转

hand to grip the bulbar conjunctiva of the corneal margin at the 6 o'clock part to have the eyeball fixed and tracked towards the upper part of the nose and, meanwhile, with the hemostatic forceps in his left hand grips tightly the ready-prepared triangular blade to cut, with the cutting edge of the knife outward, a 3 mm-long incision at the part 4 mm away from the 8 to 9 o'clock surface of the corneal margin. The incision should be vertical to the sclera and pass through the full thickness of the eyeball wall.

The cataract needle is vertically inserted 3 mm deep into the incision and the needle body is turned till it is almost paralled to the eyeball wall, and then is slowly moved from the part between the ciliary body and the lens to the pupillary zone so that it reaches the front part of the lens. The legaments at the corresponding parts of the lens are directly cut off with the cataract needle in the order of outward-down, outward-up, inward-up and inward-down directions. Then it is slightly pressed backwards. Next, the curved part of the needle, holding the equatoral part (at the 4 o'clock in the right eye and 8 o'clock in the left eye) of the opposite side of the lens, is drawn and pressed downwards to the subtemporal part so that the equatoral part is sticked to the internal wall of the eyeball between the ciliary flat part and the intraocular subtemporal zigzag margin. After a while, the needle is slowly raised to the pupillary zone. When the lens no longer floats up, the needle is withdrawn. The incision is softly pressed with a cotton stick so as to transpose the conjunctival incision and the scleral incision to have the scleral incision covered by the conjunctiva. When the operation is finished, antibiotic eye ointment and mydriatic mixture are applied to the operated eye, which is then covered with an eye pad and wrapped up with bandage.

Postsurgical care of cataract needle operation After

向鼻上方,左手持止血钳夹紧瓣成三角形的刀片,在角膜缘8～9点钟的外侧4mm处,与巩膜垂直,刀锋向外,作一垂直于角膜缘、穿通眼球壁全层的切口,切口长约3mm。

用拨障针从切口垂直穿入球内3mm深,再将针体转至与眼球壁接近平行,缓慢将针由睫状体与晶状体之间向瞳孔区推进,使针达晶状体前面。然后用拨障针按外下、外上、内上、内下等方向的顺序,将晶状体相应部位的韧带直接拉断,并向后方轻压。继而以拨障针头弯曲部抱着晶状体对侧赤道部(右眼4点,左眼8点钟处)拉压向颞下方,使之紧贴与睫状体扁平部和锯齿缘之间的球壁内侧。稍候片刻,徐徐起针至瞳孔区。如晶状体不再浮起,方可抽出拨障针。用小棉签轻轻揉按出针口,使结膜切口与巩膜切口错位,达到用结膜遮盖巩膜的目的。术毕涂抗生素眼药膏及散瞳剂,术眼盖眼垫包封。

白内障针拨术后处理:术

the operation, the patient should lie on his back with the head slightly high or take, on the first day or first two days, the semi-recumbent position of 30 to 40 degrees. He can have an ordinary diet and take care of himself in shit and urination and other daily matters. Dressing should be changed once a day, and the eye pad may be taken off in four or five days after the surgery. Before the pupil contracts to normal, the patient should not bend with the head hanging down in case the vitreous herniate into the anterior chamber. Optometry can be carried out two months after the operation.

2.5.5 Obstruction of Retinal Artery

[Introduction]

Obstruction of retinal artery is an acute and severe eye trouble which involves the obstruction of the central artery of retina and obstruction of the branched artery of retina. In clinic, the case mainly manifests the symptoms of sudden visual diminishment and even blindness. Although its incidence is not high, the consequence by the disease is very severe. If it can not be treated instantly, blindness may occur in the end. The elderly people are the common victims of the disease, with a proportion of two male patients to one female. There is no difference whether the left or the right eye is affected but, in most cases, the disease attacks one eye.

The disease occurs as the result of pachynsis, constricture and thrombosis caused by sclerosis of the vascular wall of retinal artery, and it may be caused by vasospasm and exfoliated emboli as well.

The clinical manifestations of the disease show that the case should pertain to "Baomang" (sudden blindness)

后取头部稍高位平卧,或于第一二日取 30～40 度之半卧位。普食。大小便等日常生活均可自理。每日换药 1 次,4～5 日后解除眼垫。瞳孔在未缩小到正常以前,不宜低头,以免玻璃体疝嵌入前房。术后两个月可验光配镜。

第五节　视网膜动脉阻塞

【概述】

视网膜动脉阻塞包括视网膜中央动脉和分支动脉阻塞。临床上主要表现为视力骤降,甚至失明。本病发病率较低,但其后果极为严重,如果不能及时抢救,终将失明。本病多发于老年人,男女比例为 2：1,左右眼无差异,多为单眼发病。

本病的发病原因是视网膜动脉因血管壁硬化导致管壁增厚、狭窄、血栓形成或血管痉挛,栓子脱落所致。

根据本病的临床表现,当属于中医学"暴盲"范畴。多

in traditional Chinese medicine. Emotional depression causes qi stagnancy and blood stasis; liver damage from violent anger leads to disorder of qi activity and blood stagnation; overeating fat and sweet foods gives rise to dysfunction of the spleen and further to meridian obstruction by turbid phlegm; or yin deficiency and yang hyperactivity brings about endogenous wind of the liver which affects upwards the seven orifices in the head. All these can cause qi and blood to be stagnated and ocular vessels obstructed, thus initiating the disease.

[**Main Diagnostic Points**]

1. Clinical Manifestations

The patient's vision diminishes abruptly, even with light sensation left and light reflex retardant or disappearing, and mydriasis occurs.

2. Fundus Examination

(1) The retinal arteries become as thin as lines with interrupted thrombus in segments, and the retinal veins also become thin.

(2) The retina being anemic, the posterior pole of the retina turns to cream white opacity with edema and typical "cherry-red" points occur in the macula.

(3) The boundary of the optic disc is cloudy and a little pale, and then turns to total paleness as the course of the disease advances.

(4) For those with obstruction only in the branched arteries, the above lesions occur only in the concerned parts and the symptoms of visual disturbance and cherry-red points in the macula are not obvious.

3. Fluorescein Fudus Angiography

The examination shows that the filling time of the retinal arteries is deferred and there is not any phenomena of fluorescence and perfusion to be seen in the front peak

因七情郁结,气滞血瘀;或暴怒伤肝,气机逆乱,气逆血壅;或过食肥甘,脾失健运,痰浊阻络;或阴虚阳亢,肝风内动,上扰清窍等,以致气血瘀阻,眼内脉道阻塞而发病。

【诊断要点】

1. 临床表现

视力骤降,甚至只有光感,瞳孔散大,直接对光反应迟钝或消失。

2. 眼底检查

(1) 视网膜动脉纤细如线,血栓常间断呈节段状,视网膜静脉变细;

(2) 视网膜呈贫血状态,后极部视网膜呈乳白色混浊,水肿,黄斑区呈典型的"樱桃红点";

(3) 视乳头边界模糊,颜色偏淡,随着病程的进展而渐趋苍白;

(4) 动脉分支阻塞者仅在相应区域出现上述病变,视力障碍,黄斑区樱桃红点不显著。

3. 眼底荧光血管造影

可见视网膜动脉充盈时间延缓,并可见荧光素充盈的前锋以及阻塞的血管无荧光

of fluorescein filling and in the obstructed vessels.

[Syndrome Differentiation and Treatment]

Clinically the disease is classified into the syndromes of stagnation of qi and blood, turbid-phlegm attack of eye and endogenous wind of the liver. In an emergent case, the treatment should be put on the subordinate symptoms, or on subordinate and principal symptoms simultaneously. The therapeutic methods should include in clinic activating blood circulation, removing blood stasis and calming endogenous wind.

1. Syndrome of Qi and Blood Stagnation

Main Symptoms and Signs Abrupt onset after a period of bad mood or a violent rage, sudden diminishment of vision, boundary cloudiness of the optic disc, gray-whitish opacity of the posterior pole of retina with retinal ateries becoming obviously slender, cherry-red points in macula and accompanied by the general symptoms of dizziness, bitter taste in the mouth and distending pain in the chest; thready or unsmooth pulse.

Therapeutic Methods Promoting blood circulation and unblocking orifices.

Recipe The modified Tongqiao Huoxue Decoction: Taoren (*Semen Persicae*) 10 g, Honghua (*Flos Carthomi*) 6 g, Chishaoyao (*Radix Paeoniae Rubra*) 10 g, Chuanxiong (*Rhizoma Ligustici Chuanxiong*) 10 g, Danshen (*Radix Salviae Miltiorrhizae*) 15 g, Yimucao (*Herba Leonuri*) 15 g, Yujin (*Radix Curcumae*) 10 g, and Qingpi (*Pericarpium Citri Reticulatate Viride*) 10 g.

2. Syndrome of Turbid-phlegm Attack on Eye

Main Symptoms and Signs Besides the same ocular symptoms as the above, the accompanied symptoms and signs include dizziness with carebaria, fat stature, chest distress, poor appetite and nausea; greasy tongue coating and thready slippery pulse.

与灌注等现象。

【辨证论治】

本病临床上主要分为气血瘀阻证、痰浊上扰证、肝风内动证。治疗应急则治标，或标本兼治。临证以活血、祛瘀、熄风为主。

1. 气血瘀阻证

主要证候 其人情志不舒，或暴怒之后突然发病，视力骤降，视乳头边界模糊，后极部网膜灰白混浊，视网膜动脉显著变细，黄斑区呈樱桃红点。全身可伴有头晕，口苦，胸胁胀痛，脉弦或涩。

治 法 活血通窍。

方 药 通窍活血汤加减。桃仁10 g，红花6 g，赤芍药10 g，川芎10 g，丹参15 g，益母草15 g，郁金10 g，青皮10 g。

2. 痰浊上扰证

主要证候 眼症同前。伴头晕而重，形体肥胖，胸闷，食少恶心，舌苔腻，脉弦滑。

Therapeutic Mothod　Removing phlegm by activating meridian and blood circulation.

Recipe　The modified Ditan (phlegm-removing) Decoction: Banxia (*Rhizoma Pinelliae*) 10 g, Chendanxing (*Arisaem cum Bile*) 9 g, Zhuru (*Caulis Bambusae in Taeniam*) 10 g, Zhishi (*Fructus Aurantii Immaturus*) 10 g, Fuling (*Poria*) 12 g, Shichangpu (*Rhizoma Acori Graminei*) 10 g, Danshen (*Radix Salviae Miltiorrhizae*) 15 g, Chuanxiong (*Rhizoma Ligustici Chuanxiong*) 10 g, Dilong (*Lumbricus*) 12 g, Baijiangcan (*Bombyx Batrticatus*) 6 g, and Gancao (*Radix Glycyrrhizae*) 3 g.

Modification　In the cases of severe heat pathogen, 10 g of Huangqin (*Radix Scutellariae*) and 6 g of Huanglian (*Rhizoma Coptidis*) are added.

3. Syndrome of Endogenous Wind of Liver

Main Symptoms and Signs　Easy attack of hypetension patients with the same ocular symptoms as the above, accompanied by the general symptoms and signs of dizziness, headache, flushed face, tinnitus, being choleric and irritable and bitter taste in the mouth; reddish tongue with thin yellowish coating.

Therapeutic Mothods　Extinguishing endogenous wind of the liver and activating blood circulation to remove stasis.

Recipe　The modified Tianma Goutengyin Decoction: Tianma (*Rhizoma Gastrodiae*) 15 g, Gouteng (*Ramulus Uncariae cum Uncis*) 15 g, Shijueming (*Concha Haliotidis*, to be decocted first) 15 g, Shanzhizi (*Fructus Gardeniae*) 10 g, Niuxi (*Radix Achyranthis Bidentatae*) 10 g, Yimucao (*Herba Leonuri*) 15 g, Danshen (*Radix Salviae Miltiorrhizae*) 15 g, Taoren (*Semen Persicae*) 10 g, Honghua (*Flos Carthomi*) 6 g, Dilong (*Lumbricus*) 10 g, and Quanxie (*Scorpio*) 6 g.

Modification　In the cases of palpitation and sleep-

治　法　涤痰通络,活血开窍。

方　药　涤痰汤加减。半夏10 g,陈胆星9 g,竹茹10 g,枳实10 g,茯苓12 g,石菖蒲10 g,丹参15 g,川芎10 g,地龙12 g,白僵蚕6 g,甘草3 g。

加　减　热邪较甚者,加黄芩10 g,黄连6 g。

3. 肝风内动证

主要证候　眼症同前。多见于素有高血压病患者,全身症见头晕头痛,面红耳鸣,急躁易怒,口苦舌红,苔薄黄。

治　法　平肝熄风,破瘀行血。

方　药　天麻钩藤饮加减。天麻15 g,钩藤15 g,石决明(先煎)15 g,山栀子10 g,牛膝10 g,益母草15 g,丹参15 g,桃仁10 g,红花6 g,地龙10 g,全蝎6 g。

加　减　心悸失眠者,加

lessness, 10 g of Yuanzhi (*Radix Polygalae*) and 10 g of Suanzaoren (*Semen Ziziphi Spinosae*) are added; in the cases of chest distress and qi stagnation, 10 g of Zisuzi (*Fructus Perillae*) and 15 g of Gualou (*Fructus Fricho-santhis*) are added.

[Other Treatments]

1. Chinese Patent Drugs

(1) Compound Danshendi Pill   10 pills each time, three times a day, applicable to all the syndromes of the disease.

(2) Xuefu Zhuyu Oral Liquid   10 ml each time, three times a day, applicable to all the syndromes of the diesase.

2. Simple and Proved Recipe

The recipe consists of 12 g of Wulingzhi (*Faeces Trogopterorum*) and 15 g of Xiangfuzi (*Semen Cyperi*), which, fried with vinegar, are ground into powder and orally taken 5 g with two spoonful of wine once and twice a day.

When the case is emergent and severe, it is impor-tant first to save the patient's vision with some necessary western drugs.

2.5.6 Retinal Vein Obstruction

[Introduction]

Retinal vein obstruction, a quite common disease of the eyeground, is classified into the obstruction of the central vein of the retina and that of branched veins of the retina according to the part being obstructed. Clinically, it is characterized by the sudden diminution of vision. Common in the middle-aged and the elder, the case usual-ly occurs unilaterally, seldom bilaterally, with no sexual difference.

远志10 g,酸枣仁10 g;胸闷气结者,加紫苏子10 g,瓜蒌15 g。

【其他治疗】

1. 中成药

（1）复方丹参滴丸　每服10粒,每日3次。适用于临床各证。

（2）血府逐瘀口服液每服10 ml,每日3次。适用于临床各证。

2. 单验方

五灵脂12 g,香附子15 g,醋炒为散,兑入甜酒2匙服。每次服5 g,每日2次。

本病急重,为及时抢救视力,宜配合使用必要的西药。

第六节　视网膜静脉阻塞

【概述】

视网膜静脉阻塞是一种较为常见的眼底疾病。依据其阻塞部位不同,而分为视网膜中央静脉和分支静脉阻塞两种类型。其临床表现为视力急剧下降。本病多发于中老年人,男女无差异,常单眼发病,双眼发病较少。

The cause of the disease, which is complicated, is often related with multiple factors and closely associated with hypertension, arteriosclerosis, hyperlipernia, blood viscosity and hemodynamics.

The clinical manifestations of the disease indicate that the case should pertain to "Baomang" (sudden blindness) in traditional Chinese medicine. The seven emotions, diet, overworking and phlegm-fire are often the causes of the case. Its main pathogenesis is that hyperactivity of liver yang causes upward invasion of liver qi, or that stagnation of liver qi leads to blood stasis, or that endogenous phlegm-heat accumulates in the eye, or that excessive fire due to yin deficiency affects upwards the eye, and all the factors may obstruct the ocular channel (or veins), causing the occurrence of the disease.

[Main Diagnostic Points]

1. Clinical Symptom

The patient's vision diminishes abruptly.

2. Fundus Examination

(1) The retinal veins are coarsely large, tortuous, ectatic, obstructed and dark red, and the retinal artery becomes thin and thready.

(2) The retina is of hemorrhage, edema and exudation, and the massive hemorrhage is radiant, flaming-like, patchy and circle-pointed and spreads with the opatic disc as the center.

(3) The optic papilla is congested with edema and the surface is covered with hemorrhage.

3. Fluorescein fundus angiography

At the beginning, the fluorescein reflux of the retinal vein is slow, the filling time deferred, and the obstructed part is displayed in the branched veins. Later on, fluorescein effusion is clearly seen in the capillary with the

本病的病因比较复杂,常由多种因素造成,与高血压、动脉硬化、高血脂、血液黏滞度以及血液动力学均有密切关系。

根据本病的临床表现,当属于中医学"暴盲"范畴。其病因多与七情、饮食、劳累、痰火有关。主要病机为肝阳上亢,肝气上逆;或肝郁气滞,血行瘀滞;或痰热内生,上壅目窍;或阴虚火旺,上扰清窍,致眼络阻塞发为本病。

【诊断要点】

1. 临床症状

视力急剧下降。

2. 眼底检查

(1) 视网膜静脉粗大、纤曲、扩张、断流,血管呈黯红色,视网膜动脉细;

(2) 视网膜出血,水肿,渗出,大量出血呈放射状、火焰状、片状或圆点状,并以视乳头为中心分布;

(3) 视乳头充血、水肿,表面也被出血遮盖。

3. 眼底荧光血管造影

早期可见视网膜静脉荧光素回流缓慢,充盈时间延长,分支静脉阻塞可以显示阻塞的部位。造影后期可见毛

venous wall stained and the retina full of strong fluorescent light or covered with macular cystoid edema.

[Syndrome Differentiation and Treatment]

The disease is the obstruction of the retinal veins as a result of various causes with the fundus hemorrhage or blood stasis as the main change. In clinic, it is often classified into the syndromes of hyperactivity of liver yang, stagnation of qi and blood stasis, upward accumulation of phlegm-heat and excessive fire due to yin deficiency. The treatment methods, therefore, should include, whatever syndrome a case belongs to, activating blood circulation, removing blood stasis and dredging meridians in addition to the treatment aimed at its pathogensis. In the cases of the neonatal vessel and organic matter in the eye, the treatment method to soften hard lumps should also be applied.

1. Syndrome of Hyperactivity of Liver Yang

Main Symptoms and Signs   Sudden diminishment of vision, optic disc congestion and edema with obscure boundary, tortuosity and ectasia of the retinal vein in sausage shape, massive retinal hemorrhage distributing with the optic disc as the center, accompanied by the general symptoms of dizziness, headache, irritability, vexation, insomnia, tinnitus and hypochondiac pain; reddish tongue and thready pulse.

Therapeutic Methods   Calming the liver and suppressing yang hyperactivity.

Recipe   The modified Juhua Goutengyin Decoction: Gouteng (*Ramulus Uncariae cum Uncis*) 10 g, Juhua (*Flos Chrysanthemi*) 10 g, Zhenzhumu (*Concha Margaritifera Usta*, to be decocted first) 15 g, Chuanxiong (*Rhizoma Ligustici Chuanxiong*) 6 g, Danshen (*Radix Salviae Miltiorrhizae*) 15 g, Danggui (*Radix Angelicae*

细血管有明显的荧光素渗漏，静脉管壁染色，视网膜呈一片强荧光或有黄斑囊样水肿。

【辨证论治】

本病为各种原因引起的眼络阻塞，眼底以出血瘀血为主要改变。本病临床上主要分为肝阳上亢证、气滞血瘀证、痰热上壅证、阴虚火旺证。治疗时，无论何种证型，除针对病机治疗外，均应配合活血化瘀通络法。对眼内有新生血管、机化物者，当佐以软坚散结法。

1. 肝阳上亢证

主要证候   视力骤降，视乳头充血、水肿，边界模糊，视网膜静脉纤曲、扩张，呈腊肠状，视网膜有大量出血，以视乳头为中心呈放射状分布。全身伴有头晕头痛，急躁易怒，心烦失眠，耳鸣胁痛，舌红脉弦。

治   法   平肝潜阳。

方   药   菊花钩藤饮加减。钩藤10 g，菊花10 g，珍珠母（先煎）15 g，川芎6 g，丹参15 g，当归12 g，地龙10 g，蒲黄12 g，泽泻10 g，黄芩10 g，枳壳6 g。

Sinensis) 12 g, Dilong (*Lumbricus*) 10 g, Puhuang
(*Pollen Typhae*) 12 g, Zexie (*Rhizoma Alismatis*)
10 g, Huangqin (*Radix Scutellariae*) 10 g, and Zhike
(*Fructus Aurantii*) 6 g.

2. Syndrome of Qi Stagnation and Blood Stasis

Main Symptoms and Signs   The same ocular symptoms as the above, accompanied by depressed emotion,
distending pain in chest and hypochondrium, depressed
sensation in stomach and poor appetite; a dull purple
tongue and unsmooth pulse.

Therapeutic Method   Activating qi and blood circulation.

Recipe   The modified Xuefu Zhuyu Decoction:
Taoren (*Semen Persicae*) 12 g, Honghua (*Flos Cartho-
mi*) 10 g, Danggui (*Radix Angelicae Sinensis*) 12 g,
Shengdihuang (*Radix Rehmanniae*) 10 g, Chishaoyao
(*Radix Paeoniae Rubra*) 10 g, Chuanxiong (*Rhizoma
Ligustici Chuanxiong*) 10 g, Niuxi (*Radix Achyranthis
Bidentatae*) 10 g, Danshen (*Radix Salviae Miltiorrhi-
zae*) 15 g, Cebaiye (*Cacumen Biotae*) 10 g, and Zhike
(*Fructus Aurantii*) 10 g.

Modification   In the cases of severe stagnation of
liver qi, 10 g of Yujin (*Radix Curcumae*) and 10 g of
Qingpi (*Pericarpium Citri Rteiculatae*) are added; in
the cases of serious edema of retina, 3 g of amber powder
(*Succinum*, to be swallowed separately), 12 g of Zelan
(*Herba Lycopi*) and 15 g of Yimucao (*Herba leonuri*)
are added; in the cases of severe fundus hemorrhage, 10 g
of Puhuang (*Pallen Typhea*) and of Qiancao (*Radix Rubiae*) and 3 g of Sanqi (*Radix Notoginseng*, to be swallowed separately) powder are added.

3. Syndrome of Upward Accumulation of Phlegm-heat

Main Symptoms and Signs   The same ocular symp-

2. 气滞血瘀证

主要证候 眼症同前。
伴情志抑郁,胸胁胀痛,脘闷
食少,舌暗紫,脉涩。

治 法 行气活血。

方 药 血府逐瘀汤加
减。桃仁12 g,红花10 g,当归
12 g,生地黄10 g,赤芍药10 g,
川芎10 g,牛膝10 g,丹参15 g,
侧柏叶10 g,枳壳10 g。

加 减 肝郁气滞甚者,
加郁金10 g,青皮10 g;视网膜
水肿甚者,加琥珀粉(另吞)
3 g,泽兰12 g,益母草15 g;眼
底出血甚者,加蒲黄10 g,茜草
10 g,三七粉(另吞)3 g。

3. 痰热上壅证

主要证候 眼 症 同 前。

toms as the above, accompanied by dizziness and heavy sensation, nausea and vomiting, thick sputum with a bitter taste, and fat stature; a yellowish greasy tongue coating and thready pulse.

Therapeutic Methods   Removing phlegm-heat and activating blood circulation to improve vision.

Recipe   The modified Wendan Decoction: Bianxia (*Rhizoma Pinelliae*) 10 g, Fuling (*Poria*) 12 g, Zhike (*Fructus Aurantii*) 10 g, Zhuru (*Caulis Bambusae in Taeniam*) 10 g, Danxing (*Arisaema cum Bile*) 10 g, Shichangpu (*Rhizoma Acori Graminei*) 10 g, Danshen (*Radix Salviae Miltiorrhizae*) 15 g, Baimaogen (*Rhizoma Imperatae*) 15 g, Taoren (*Semen Persicae*) 10 g, Honghua (*Flos Carthomi*) 10 g, Baijiangcan (*Bombyx Batryticatus*) 10 g, and Puhuang (*Pollen Typhae*) 10 g.

4. Syndrome of Fire Hyperactivity due to Yin Deficiency

Main Symptoms and Signs   The same ocular symptoms as the above, accompanied by dizziness, tidal fever, night sweat, feverish sensation in chest, palms and soles; a reddish tongue with little coating and a thready pulse.

Therapeutic Methods   Nourishing yin and removing pathogenic fire.

Recipe   The modified Zhibai Dihuangwan Decoction: Shengdihuang (*Radix Rehmanniae*) 12 g, Shanzhuyu (*Fructus Corni*) 10 g, Fuling (*Poria*) 12 g, Zexie (*Rhizoma Alismatis*) 10 g, Mudanpi (*Cortex Moutan Radicis*) 10 g, Zhimu (*Rhizoma Anemarrhenae*) 10 g, Huangbai (*Cortex Phellodendri*) 10 g, Danggui (*Radix Angelicae Sinensis*) 10 g, Danshen (*Radix Salviae Miltiorrhizae*) 15 g, Yujin (*Radix Curcumae*) 10 g, Jixueteng (*Caulis Spatholobi*) 12 g, Cebaiye (*Cacumen Platycladi*) 10 g, and Zhike (*Fructus Aurantii*) 6 g.

伴头眩而重,恶心欲吐,痰稠而苦,形体肥胖,舌苔黄腻,脉弦。

治　法　清热祛痰,活血明目。

方　药　温胆汤加减。半夏10 g,茯苓12 g,枳壳10 g,竹茹10 g,胆星10 g,石菖蒲10 g,丹参15 g,白茅根15 g,桃仁10 g,红花10 g,白僵蚕10 g,蒲黄10 g。

4. 阴虚火旺证

主要证候　眼症同前。伴头晕目眩,潮热盗汗,五心烦热,舌红少苔,脉细数。

治　法　滋阴降火。

方　药　知柏地黄丸加减。生地黄12 g,山茱萸10 g,茯苓12 g,泽泻10 g,牡丹皮10 g,知母10 g,黄柏10 g,当归10 g,丹参15 g,郁金10 g,鸡血藤12 g,侧柏叶10 g,枳壳6 g。

[Other Treatments]

1. Chinese Patent Drugs

(1) **Sanqi Zongdai Tablet**   3 tablets each time, three times a day, applicable to all the syndromes of the disease.

(2) **Compound Danshendi Pill**   10 pills each time, three times a day, applicable to the syndrome of qi and blood stagnation.

(3) **Xuefu Zhuyu Oral Liquid**   10 ml each time, three times a day, applicable to the syndrome of qi and blood stagnation.

(4) **Zhibai Dihuang Pill**   8 pills each time, twice a day, applicable to the syndrome of hyperactivity due to yin deficiency.

2. Simple and Proved Recipes

(1) The recipe consists of the following herbs: Lianqiao (*Fructus Forsythiae*) 15 g, Puhuang (*Pollen Typhae*) 20 g, Cebaiye (*Cacumen Platycladi*) 10 g, Oujie (*Nodus Nelumbinis Rhizomatis*) 10 g, Chishaoyao (*Radix Paeoniae Rubra*) 10 g, Mudanpi (*Cortex Moutan Radicis*) 10 g, Danggui (*Radix Angelicae Sinensis*) 9 g, Niuxi (*Radix Achyranthis Bidentatae*) 10 g, and Lulutong (*Fructus Liquidambaris*) 10 g. All are decocted with water, one dose a day for oral drinking. The recipe is applicable to all the syndromes of the disease.

(2) The drink consists of 500 g of fresh Maogen (*Rhizoma Imperatae*) and a proper amount of crystal sugar. The herb Maogen, which is washed and broken with a wooden mallet, is decocted with water for 30 minutes, and the liquid is mixed with the crystal sugar by heating and is taken as a tea-drink for 10 to 15 days continously. The function of the recipe is to cool blood for arresting bleeding and to clear away heat for inducing diure-

【其他治疗】

1. 中成药

（1）三七总甙片　每服 3 片，每日 3 次。适用于临床各证。

（2）复方丹参滴丸　每服 10 粒，每日 3 次。适用于气滞血瘀证。

（3）血府逐瘀口服液 每服 10 ml，每日 3 次。适用于气滞血瘀证。

（4）知柏地黄丸　每服 8 粒，每日 2 次。适用于阴虚火旺证。

2. 单验方

（1）连翘 15 g，蒲黄 20 g，侧柏叶 10 g，藕节 10 g，赤芍药 10 g，牡丹皮 10 g，当归 9 g，牛膝 10 g，路路通 10 g。每日 1 次，水煎服。适用于本病各证。

（2）鲜茅根 500 g，冰糖适量。茅根洗净，用木槌轻砸破裂，加水煎煮 30 分钟，取汁入冰糖烊化，代茶饮，连服 10～15 日。其功能为凉血止血，清热利尿。对阴虚火旺之眼底出血、口渴烦热者较为适宜。

sis. It is applicable to optic fundus bleeding with dry mouth and dysphoria due to yin asthenia and fire hyperactivity.

3. External Therapyes

In the cases of massive hemorrhage of the optic fundus, ionotherapy is applied with the solution obtained from the herbs of Sanqi, Danshen, Honghua, and Chuanxiong. The therapy is performed once every day, and ten times make up one course of treatment. After two to three courses, the blood mass is sure to be removed.

2.5.7 Central Serous Chorioretinopathy

[Introduction]

Central serous chorioretinopathy is one of rather common fundus diseases characterized by the neurepithelial serous detachment in the macula as a result of the barrier dysfunction of the retinal pigmentary epithelium. The clinical manifestations of the disease mainly include sudden blurred vision, metamorphopsia and micropsia. Frequently seen in the male at the ages of 20 to 45, it often occurs unilaterally, or sometimes bilaterally, and has the tendency of repeated attack and good prognosis.

The occurrence of the disease is usually due to the fact that the leaking plasma from the choroidocapillary, because of the disturbance of barrier function of the pigmentary epithelium of the retina, enters the subretina through the damaged pigmentary epithelium, which causes the liquid to accumulate between the retinal neurepi-

3. 外治法

眼底瘀血较多者,局部可用三七、丹参、红花、川芎等药液电离子透入,每日 1 次,10 次为 1 个疗程。一般作 2～3 个疗程,以促进瘀血消散。

第七节　中心性 浆液性视网膜 脉络膜病变

【概述】

中心性浆液性视网膜脉络膜病变是由于视网膜色素上皮屏障功能失常,形成黄斑部神经上皮浆液性脱离为特征的较为常见的眼底病之一。临床上主要表现为突发视物模糊,视物变形、变小。本病多发于健康的 20～45 岁男性,女性少见,常单眼发病,有时也可双眼,有自愈和反复倾向,其预后较为良好。

本病的发生主要由于视网膜色素上皮的屏障功能出现障碍,致使脉络膜毛细血管漏出的血浆通过受损的色素上皮进入视网膜下,液体积聚于视网膜神经上皮与色素上

thelium and pegmentary epithelium, causing the disciform detachment of the retina at the posterier pole.

　　From its clinical manifestations, the case should pertain to "Shizhan Hunmiao"(blurring of vision) in traditional Chinese medicine. Its cause, sometimes, belongs to asthenia (or deficiency) and, sometimes, to sthenia (or excess). In the asthenia cases, deficiency of the liver and kidney or deficiency of the heart and spleen gives rise to nutritional deficiency of eye, causing the attack of the trouble. In the sthenia cases, internal accumulation of damp-heat and turbid phlegm leads to qi stagnation and blood stasis that, consequently, affects the eye and blocks the pores, so that the case occurs.

[Main Diagnostic Points]

1. Clinical Manifestations

There abruptly occurs the symptoms of blurred vision, micropsia and metamorphopsia with the sensation of shadow in the way of the central field of vision occasionally.

2. Fundus Examination

At the beginning, localized edema of the macula is found and then the macula becomes protrudent, forming serous disciform detachment of the retina with light-reflecting circle surrounded and the light reflex of the central fovea disappearing. Later yellowish and whitish petechial exudate occurs. During the recovery stage, the edema gradually disappears and the reflex of the central fovea recovers again.

3. Visual Field Examination

Campimetery finds the relatively central scotoma and the test of Amsler's chart indicates metamorphopsia and central scotoma.

4. Fluorescein Fundus Angiography

At the venous stage, there is one or a few small exu-

皮之间,形成后极部视网膜的盘状脱离。

　　根据本病的临床表现,当属于中医学"视瞻昏渺"范畴。本病的发生有虚有实,虚证多为肝肾不足,或心脾两虚,目失所养所致;实证常由湿热痰浊内蕴,气滞血瘀,浊邪上犯等致玄府不利引起。

【诊断要点】

1. 临床表现

突然发生视物模糊,视物变小,视物变形,有时可感觉有暗影遮挡视野中心。

2. 眼底检查

初起可见黄斑部局限性水肿而隆起形成浆液性视网膜盘状脱离,周围有反光圈,中心凹反射消失,继而出现黄白色点状渗出物。恢复期,水肿逐渐消退,中心凹反光重新出现。

3. 视野检查

平面视野可查出相对性中心暗点。Amsler 表检查可见视物变形及中心暗点。

4. 眼底荧光血管造影

静脉期于后极部或远离

dative spots at the posterior pole or far away, which gradually becomes the spurting or inkblot-like strong fluorescein spots at the late stage.

[Syndrome Differentiation and Treatment]

Since the disease is of either sthenia or asthenia type, or of a mixed type sometimes, it is clinically classified into the syndromes of upward invasion of turbid pathogenic factor, damp stagnation due to spleen deficiency, qi stagnation and blood stasis and deficiency of the liver and kidney. The treadment methods, depending on the different syndromes, should respectively include removing heat and dampness, nourishing the spleen to relieve dampness, removing heat and soothing liver, and benefiting the liver and kidney.

1. Syndrome of Upward Invasion of Turbid Pathogenic Factor

Main Symptoms and Signs   Blurred vision or chromaopsia, micropsia, metamorphopsia; optic fudus findings including edema and exudation in the macular part and the absence of light reflex of central fovea; accompanied by the general symptoms of chest distress, poor appetite, a bitter taste in the mouth and scanty yellowish urine; yellowish greasy tongue coating and slippery rapid pulse.

Therapeutic Methods   Removing heat and promoting diuresis

Recipe   The modified Sanren Decoction: Xingren (*Semen Armeniacae Amarum*) 10 g, Baikouren (*Semen Amomi Rotundus*) 6 g, Yiyiren (*Semen Coicis*) 10 g, Huashi (*Talcum*) 10 g, Houpo (*Cortex Magnoliae Officinalis*) 6 g, Banxia (*Rhizoma Pinelliae*) 9 g, Cheqianzi (*Semen Plantaginis*, bagged) 10 g, Chongweizi (*Semen Leonuri*) 10 g, Zexie (*Rhizoma Alismatis*) 10 g, and Zhike (*Fructus Aurantii*) 6 g.

后极部有一或数个很小的荧光素渗漏点,后期逐渐变成喷射状或墨迹样扩大的强荧光斑。

【辨证论治】

本病有虚有实或虚实夹杂,临床上主要分为浊邪上犯证、脾虚湿滞证、气滞血瘀证、肝肾不足证。治疗视其不同证型,分别采用清热利湿、健脾渗湿、清热疏肝、补益肝肾法。

1. 浊邪上犯证

主要证候   视物模糊,或视瞻有色,视大为小,视直为曲。眼底可见黄斑区水肿、渗出,中心凹反光消失等。全身伴头重胸闷,食少口苦,小便黄少,舌苔黄腻,脉滑数等。

治   法   清热利湿。

方   药   三仁汤加减。杏仁10 g,白蔻仁6 g,薏苡仁10 g,滑石10 g,厚朴6 g,半夏9 g,车前子(包煎)10 g,茺蔚子10 g,泽泻10 g,枳壳6 g。

Modification　In the cases with severe damp-heat, 10 g of Huangqin (*Radix Scutellariae*) and 6 g of Shanzhizi (*Fructus Gardeniae*) are added.

2. Syndrome of Damp Stagnation due to Spleen Deficiency

Main Symptoms and Signs　The same ocular symptoms as the above one, often accompanied by anorexia, loose stool, sallow and dim complexion and lassitude; whitish tongue with whitish coating.

Therapeutic Methods　Nourishing the spleen to benefit qi, excreting dampness to remove stagnation.

Recipe　The modified Shenling Baizhusan Decoction: Dangshen (*Radix Codonopsis Pilosulae*) 10 g, Huangqi (*Radix Astragali seu Hedysari*) 12 g, Shanyao (*Rhizoma Dioscoreae*) 10 g, Baizhu (*Rhizoma Atractylodis Macrocephalae*) 10 g, Chenpi (*Pericarpium Citri Reticulatae*) 6 g, Yiyiren (*Semen Coicis*) 10 g, Jiegeng (*Radix Platycodi*) 6 g, Zexie (*Rhizoma Alismatis*) 10 g, and Zhike (*Fructus Aurantii*) 6 g.

Modification　In the cases of serious edema and exudation in the macular part, 10 g of Zhuling (*Polyporus*) and 10 g of Zelan (*Herba Lycopi*) and 6 g of Niuxi (*Radix Achyranthis Bidentatae*) are added; in the cases of deficiency of spleen yang and glossy tongue coating, 10 g of Guizhi (*Ramulus Cinnamomi*) and 6 g of Ganjiang (*Rhizoma Zingiberis*) are added.

3. Syndrome of Qi Stagnation and Blood Stasis

Main Symptoms and Signs　The same ocular symptoms as the above, accompanied by emotional discomfort, chest distress, stenagma, dizziness, hypochondriac pain, bitter taste in the mouth and dry throat; thready, thin and rapid pulse.

Therapeutic Methods　Removing heat to disperse stagnated liver and promoting flow of qi to activate blood

加　减　湿热较重者,加黄芩10 g,山栀子6 g。

2. 脾虚湿滞证

主要证候　眼症同前。多伴有胃纳不佳,大便溏泻,面黄无华,体倦乏力,舌淡苔白。

治　法　健脾益气,渗湿行滞。

方　药　参苓白术散加减。党参10 g,黄芪12 g,山药10 g,白术10 g,陈皮6 g,薏苡仁10 g,桔梗6 g,泽泻10 g,枳壳6 g。

加　减　黄斑区水肿、渗出较甚者,加猪苓10 g,泽兰10 g,牛膝6 g;脾阳虚衰、舌苔滑者,加桂枝10 g,干姜6 g。

3. 气滞血瘀证

主要证候　眼症同前。常伴有情志不舒,胸闷叹息,头晕胁痛,口苦咽干,脉弦细数。

治　法　清热疏肝,行气活血。

circulation.

Recipe The modified Danzhi Xiaoyaosan Decoction: Chaihu (*Radix Bupleuri*) 6 g, Baishaoyao (*Radix Paeoniae Alba*) 10 g, Danggui (*Radix Angelicae Sinensis*) 10 g, Fuling (*Poria*) 12 g, Baizhu (*Rhizoma Atractylodis Macrocephalae*) 10 g, Mudanpi (*Cortex Moutan Radicis*) 10 g, Shanzhizi (*Fructus Gardeniae*) 10 g, Zexie (*Rhizoma Alismatis*) 10 g, Danshen (*Radix Salviae Miltiorrhizae*) 15 g, Yujin (*Radix Curcumae*) 10 g, and Chongweizi (*Semen Leonuri*) 10 g.

Modification In the cases of distending pain in chest and hypochondrium, 10 g of Chuanlianzi (*Fructus Toosendan*) is added.

4. Syndrome of Deficiency of Liver and Kidney

Main Symptoms and Signs The same ocular symptoms as the above, other accompanying symptoms at the late course including dizziness, tinnitus, lassitude in loin and legs, dreaminess, thin pulse.

Therapeutic Method Nourishing the liver and kidney.

Recipe The modified Qiju Dihuangwan Decoction: Gouqizi (*Fructus Lycii*) 12 g, Juhua (*Flos Chrysanthemi*) 9 g, Shudihuang (*Radix Rehmanniae*) 10 g, Zexie (*Rhizoma Alismatis*) 10 g, Shanyao (*Rhizoma Dioscoreae*) 10 g, Heshouwu (*Radix Polygoni Multiflori*) 10 g, Shanzhuyu (*Fructus Corni*) 10 g, Danshen (*Radix Salviae Miltiorrhizae*) 15 g, and Zhike (*Fructus Aurantii*) 6 g.

Modification In the cases of excessive exudation and pigment in the fundus, 10 g of Danggui (*Radix Angelicae Sinensis*) and 10 g of Niuxi (*Radix Achyranthis Bidentatae*) are added; in the cases of poor vision, 10 g of Tusizi (*Semen Cuscutae*) and 6 g of Shichangpu (*Rhizoma Acori Graminei*) are added; in the cases of hyper-

方 药 丹栀逍遥散加减。柴胡6g,白芍药10g,当归10g,茯苓12g,白术10g,牡丹皮10g,山栀子10g,泽泻10g,丹参15g,郁金10g,茺蔚子10g。

加 减 胸胁胀痛者,加川楝子10g。

4. 肝肾不足证

主要证候 眼症同前。多见于病后期,伴有头晕耳鸣,腰膝酸软,夜寐多梦,脉细。

治 法 补益肝肾。

方 药 杞菊地黄丸加减。枸杞子12g,菊花9g,熟地黄10g,泽泻10g,山药10g,何首乌10g,山茱萸10g,丹参15g,枳壳6g。

加 减 眼底渗出及色素较多者,加当归10g,牛膝10g;视力较差者,加菟丝子10g,石菖蒲6g;阴虚火旺者,加知母10g,黄柏10g。

activity of fire due to yin deficiency, 10 g of Zhimu (*Rhizoma Anemarrhenae*) and 10 g of Huangbai (*Cortex Phellodendri*) are added.

[Other Treatments]

1. Chinese Patent Drugs

(1) **Danzhi Xiaoyao Pill**　5 g each time, twice a day, applicable to the syndrome of qi stagnation and blood stasis.

(2) **Qiju Dihuang Pill**　8 pills each time, twice a day, applicable to the syndrome of deficiency of the liver and kidney.

(3) **Jiajian (modified) Zhujing Pill**　5 g each time, twice a day, applicable to the syndrome of deficiency of the liver and kidney.

(4) **Shenling Baizhu Pill**　5 g each time, twice a day, applicable to the syndrome of damp stagnation due to spleen deficiency.

2. Simple and Proved Recipes

(1) The recipe consists of the following ingredients: Xiakucao (*Spica Prunellae*) 15 g, Yimucao (*Herba leonuri*) 9 g, Fuling (*Poria*) 9 g, Huangqi (*Radix Astragali seu Hedysari*) 12 g, and Cheqianzi (*Semen Plantaginis*, bagged) 9 g, which are decocted with water for oral taking one dose a day, and it is applicable to the disease at the edema stage.

(2) The ingredients in the recipe are: Tusizi (*Semen Cuscutae*) 12 g, Cheqianzi (*Semen Plantaginis*, bagged) 15 g, Shudihuang (*Rhizoma Rehmanniae Praeparata*) 30 g, and Gegen (*Radix Puerariae*) 25 g, which are all decocted with water one dose a day for oral taking and it is applicable to the disease in the recovery stage.

【其他疗法】

1. 中成药

（1）丹栀逍遥丸　每服5 g,每日 2 次。适用于气滞血瘀证。

（2）杞菊地黄丸　每服 8 粒,每日 2 次。适用于肝肾不足证。

（3）加减驻景丸　每服5 g,每日 2 次。适用于肝肾两虚证。

（4）参苓白术丸　每服5 g,每日 2 次。适用于脾虚湿滞证。

2. 单验方

（1）夏枯草15 g,益母草9 g,茯苓9 g,黄芪12 g,车前子（包煎）9 g。水煎服,每日 1 剂,适用于本病水肿期。

（2）菟丝子12 g,车前子（包煎）15 g,熟地黄30 g,葛根25 g。水煎服,每日 1 剂,适用于本病恢复期。

2.5.8 Pigmentary Degeneration of Retina

[Introduction]

Pigmentary degeneration of retina which is hereditary is a kind of chronic progressive disease of fundus. In clinic, it mainly manifests the symptoms of night blindness and gradual contraction of visual field. Monocular attacking occasionally, it is often characterized by the binocular onset, obviously familial heredity, consanguineous marriage of parents and more male patients than the female (a proportion of three to two). The morbidity of the disease, according the survey in some parts of China, is about 1/3 500.

The inheretary modes of the disease include autosomal recessive, autosomal dominant and sex-linked recessive types.

Clinically, the disease pertains to "Gaofeng Neizhang" (pigmentary degeneration of retina) in traditional Chinese medicine. Extreme asthenia of kidney yang due to inherent defect, deficiency of essence and blood due to asthenia of the liver and kidney, and unrisen lucid yang due to asthenia of the spleen and stomach, any deficient factor of these, togethor with other elements, can give rise to the unfilling of vessels, further stagnated blood circulation which leads to nutritional deficiency of eye and visual diminishment, thus causing night blindness. In the course of its pathogenic change, vascular stagnation or obstruction is usually accompanied and, at the late stage, blindness results from the vascular obstruction which leads the eye lack of nutrition of qi and blood.

[Main Diagnostic Points]

1. Clinical Manifestations

There occur the symptoms of night blindness, con-

第八节　视网膜色素变性

【概述】

视网膜色素变性是一种遗传性疾病。临床上主要表现为夜盲和视野日渐缩窄。本病为慢性进行性的眼底疾病，偶见单眼，有明显的家族遗传性，父母常有近亲联姻史，男性患者多于女性，约为3：2。本病的发病率，根据中国部分地区调查资料，群体患病率约为1/3500。

本病的遗传方式有常染色体隐性、显性和性连锁隐性三种。

根据本病的临床表现，当属于中医学"高风内障"范畴。多由先天禀赋不足，命门火衰；或肝肾亏损，精血不足；或脾胃虚弱，清阳不升等诸种不足，导致脉道不充，血流滞涩，目失所养而神光衰弱，夜不见物。病变过程多兼脉道瘀塞，后期常因脉道闭塞，气血失养而失明。

【诊断要点】

1. 临床表现

夜盲、视野缩窄，晚期形

traction of visual field, tubular visual field at the late stage, diminishment of vision and even blindness.

2. Fundus Examination

(1) **Initial stage**　the retina is normal or filthy, and a small amount of osteocyte-like pigmentation is found in the equatorial part.

(2) **Middle stage**　the optic disc becomes wax yellow atrophy, the retinal vessels are contracted, and spider-like or osteocyte-like pigmentation spreads to the surrounding.

(3) **Late stage**　the optic disc turns yellowish white and the retina to bluish gray, with choroid vessels being sclerotic.

3. Visual Field Examination

At the beginning, ring scotoma can be seen and, at the late stage, the visual field is progressively and concentrically contracted until tubular visual field is formed. With the automatic perimeter for static quatitative vision, the contrast sensitivity of retina, at the early pathogenic change, is reduced in the corresponding pathogenic part before the dynamic visual anomalies, and the light threshold value increases.

4. Electrophysiological Examination of Visual Function

ERG is in a low wave form or without wave and the wave of EOG is often missing or severely descending. The dark adaptation test shows that retinal cone cell is normal initially and that the function of rod cell is decreased, which causes the terminal threshold value in the rod curve to arise, the actinic difference to shrink, and finally the dysfunction of rod and the increase of the cone threshold value so as to form a high monophasic curve.

[Syndrome Differentiation and Treatment]

Being asthenia in most cases, the disease is clinically

成管状视野,视力减退,甚至失明。

2. 眼底检查

（1）早期　正常或视网膜污秽,赤道部可见少许骨细胞样色素沉着。

（2）中期　视乳头呈蜡黄色萎缩,视网膜血管普遍狭窄,蜘蛛样或骨细胞样色素沉着向周边部扩散。

（3）晚期　视乳头黄白,视网膜呈青灰色,并可透见硬化的脉络膜血管。

3. 视野检查

早期可见环状暗点,晚期视野进行性向心性缩小,终成管状。应用自动静态定量视野仪可于病变早期发现动态视野异常之前病变对应区域内视网膜对比敏感度降低,光阈值增高。

4. 视觉电生理检查

ERG 呈低波型或无波型,EOG 也常消失或严重下降。暗适应检查早期锥细胞功能正常,杆细胞功能下降使杆体曲线终末阈值升高,造成光色间差缩小,最后杆体功能丧失,锥体阈值亦升高形成高位单项曲线。

【辨证论治】

本病多虚证,临床上主要

classified into the syndromes of deficiency of kidney yang, yin deficiency of the liver and kidney, and deficiency of spleen qi. The common treatment methods, therefore, should include warmly tonifying kidney yang, nourishing the liver and kidney, invigorating the spleen to replenish qi, supported simultaneously with drugs to remove blood stasis by activating blood circulation.

1. Syndrome of Deficiency of Kidney Yang

Main Symptoms and Signs　Blurred vision in twilight or dim light, difficulty in action, gradual contraction of visual field or even tubular visual field, and blindness at last; the fundus findings including wax yellow astrophy of optic disc, contraction of retinal vessels, osteocyte-like or irregular pigmentation of the retina in the equatorial part spreading to the posterior pole and zigzag edge, and filthy colour of the whole retina; accompanied by the symptoms of fever with cold limbs, lassitude in loin and legs, and profuse urine; whitish tongue and thin pulse.

Therapeutic Method　Recuperating kidney yang warmly.

Recipe　The modified Youguiwan Decoction: Shudihuang (*Radix Rehmanniae Praeparata*) 12 g, Shanyurou (*Fructus Corni*) 10 g, Shanyao (*Rhizoma Dioscoreae*) 12 g, Danggui (*Radix Angelicae Sinensis*) 10 g, Gouqizi (*Fructus Lycii*) 12 g, Tusizi (*Semen Cuscutae*) 12 g, Duzhong (*Cortex Eucommiae*) 12 g, Rougui (*Cortex Cinnamoni*) 6 g, Zhifuzi (*Radix Aconiti Praeparata*) 10 g, Yemingsha (*Faeces Vespertilionis*, bagged) 15 g, Danshen (*Radix Salviae Miltiorrhizae*) 15 g, and Jixueteng (*Caulis Spatholobi*) 15 g.

2. Syndrome of Yin Deficiency of Liver and Kidney

Main Symptoms and Signs　The same ocular symp-

分为肾阳不足证、肝肾阴虚证、脾气虚弱证。治疗以温补肾阳，滋补肝肾，补脾益气为常法，同时在上述治疗中，均可配合活血化瘀药物。

1. 肾阳不足证

主要证候　入暮或黑暗处视物不清，行动困难，且视野日渐缩窄，甚至缩窄成管状，最终可失明。眼底可见视乳头呈蜡黄色，视网膜血管变细，赤道部网膜有骨细胞样或不规则形状色素沉着，渐向后极部及锯齿缘方向发展，整个网膜颜色污秽。全身伴有形寒肢冷，腰膝酸软，小便长，舌淡脉细。

治　法　温补肾阳。

方　药　右归丸加减。熟地黄12 g，山萸肉10 g，山药12 g，当归10 g，枸杞子12 g，菟丝子12 g，杜仲12 g，肉桂6 g，制附子10 g，夜明砂（包煎）15 g，丹参15 g，鸡血藤15 g。

2. 肝肾阴虚证

主要证候　眼部症状同

toms as the above one, accompanied by dizziness, tinnitus, dreaminess, seminal emission, vexation, insomnia and lassitude in loin and legs; reddish tongue with a little coating and thin rapid pulse.

Therapeutic Method　Nourishing the liver and kidney.

Recipe　The modified Mingmu Dihuangwan Decoction: Shudihuang (*Radix Rehmanniae Praeparata*) 12 g, Mudanpi (*Cortex Moutan Radicis*) 9 g, Zexie (*Rhizoma Alismatis*) 10 g, Shanyao (*Rhizoma Dioscoreae*) 12 g, Fuling (*Poria*) 12 g, Danggui (*Radix Angelicae Sinensis*) 10 g, Wuweizi (*Fructus Schisandrae*) 9 g, Gouqizi (*Fructus Lycii*) 12 g, Danshen (*Radix Salviae Miltiorrhizae*) 15 g, Shanyurou (*Fructus Corni*) 12 g, Nüzhenzi (*Fructus Ligustri Lucidi*) 12 g, and Zhike (*Fructus Aurantii*) 6 g.

Modification　In the cases of filthy retina and massive pigmentation, 10 g of Niuxi (*Radix Achyranthis Bidentatae*) and 15 g of Yemingsha (*Faeces Vespertilionis*, bagged) are added; in the cases of severe asthenia heat, 10 g of Huangbai (*Cortex Phellodendri*) is added.

3. Syndrome of Asthenia of Spleen Qi

Main Symptoms and Signs　The same ocular symptoms as the above, accompanied by metal fatigue, hypodynamia, dim complexion, poor appetite and loose stool; whitish tongue with whitish coating and thin pulse.

Therapeutic Methods　Nourishing the spleen and benefiting qi.

Recipe　The modified Buzhong Yiqi Decoction: Huangqi (*Radix Astragali seu Hedysari*) 15 g, Dangshen (*Radix Codonopsis Pilosulae*) 10 g, Danggui (*Radix Angelicae Sinensis*) 10 g, Baishaoyao (*Radix Paeoniae Alba*) 10 g, Chenpi (*Pericarpium Citri Reticulatae*) 6 g, Shengma (*Rhizoma Cimicifugae*) 6 g, Gouqizi

上。伴头晕耳鸣，多梦遗精，心烦失眠，腰膝酸软，舌红少苔，脉细数。

治　法　滋养肝肾。

方　药　明目地黄丸加减。熟地黄12 g，牡丹皮9 g，泽泻10 g，山药12 g，茯苓12 g，当归10 g，五味子9 g，枸杞子12 g，丹参15 g，山萸肉12 g，女贞子12 g，枳壳6 g。

加　减　视网膜污秽，色素较多者，加牛膝10 g，夜明砂（包煎）15 g；虚热重者，加黄柏10 g。

3. 脾气虚弱证

主要证候　眼症同前。伴神疲乏力，面色少华，食少便溏，舌淡苔白，脉细。

治　法　补脾益气。

方　药　补中益气汤加减。黄芪15 g，党参10 g，当归10 g，白芍药10 g，陈皮6 g，升麻6 g，枸杞子12 g，白术10 g，灵芝15 g，柴胡6 g，丹参15 g，川芎10 g。

(*Fructus Lycii*) 12 g, Baizhu (*Rhizoma Atractylodis Macrocephalae*) 10 g, Lingzhi (*Ganoderma Lucidum seu Japonicum*) 15 g, Chaihu (*Radix Bupleuri*) 6 g, Danshen (*Radix Salviae Miltiorrhizae*) 15 g, and Chuanxiong (*Rhizoma Ligustici Chuanxiong*) 10 g.

[Other Treatments]

1. Chinese Patent Drugs

(1) Jingui Shenqi Pill　5 g each time, twice a day and applicable to the syndrome of asthenia of kidney yang.

(2) Mingmu Dihuang Pill　5 g each time, twice a day and applicable to the syndrome of deficiency of the liver and kidney.

(3) Buzhong Yiqi Pill　5 g each time, twice a day and applicable to the syndrome of asthenia of spleen qi.

(4) Mingmu Zishen Tablet　5 g each time, twice a day and applicable to the syndrome of yin deficiency of the liver and kidney.

(5) Shihu Yeguang Pill　5 g each time, twice a day and applicable to the syndrome of yin deficiency of the liver and kidney.

2. Simple and Proved Recipes

(1) The ingredients in the recipe are 100 g of Sangshenzi (*Fructus Mori*) and 500 g of Longyanrou (*Arillus Longan*) which are softly decocted with a proper amount of water into a kind of soft extract. Orally taken 10 g each time and twice every day, the extract has the function of nourishing the liver and kidney, benefitting blood to improve vision, and is applicable to the syndrome of deficiency of the liver and kidney and of asthenia of qi and blood.

(2) The recipe consists of 30 g of Shenghuangqi (*Radix Astragali seu Helysari*) and ten Chinese-dates,

【其他疗法】

1. 中成药

（1）金匮肾气丸　每服 5 g,每日 2 次。适用于肾阳不足证。

（2）明目地黄丸　每服 5 g,每日 2 次。适用于肝肾不足证。

（3）补中益气丸　每服 5 g,每日 2 次。适用于脾气虚弱证。

（4）明目滋肾片　每服 5 g,每日 2 次。适用于肝肾阴虚证。

（5）石斛夜光丸　每服 5 g,每日 2 次。适用于肝肾阴虚证。

2. 单验方

（1）桑椹子100 g,龙眼肉 500 g。加水适量,文火熬膏。每次服10 g,每日 2 次。滋补肝肾,养血明目,可用于肝肾阴亏,气血不足证。

（2）生黄芪30 g,大枣 10 个。水煎两次分服,每日 1

which are decocted with water one dose a day and the liquid is taken in the morning and evening. It is applicable to
the syndrome of asthenia of spleen qi.

剂。适用于脾气虚弱证。

2.5.9 Senile Macular Degeneration

第九节 老年性黄斑变性

[Introduction]

Senile macular degeneration, also called the age-con-
cerned degeneration of macula, is one of the most common ocular diseases leading to blindness in the western
world. Clinically, it mainly manifests the symptoms of
visual deterioration and severe disturbance of vision in the
late course. It is common among persons in their fifties
and, the elder people are, the higher incidence is. Little
associated with the sex, the disease attacks both eyes simutaneously or one after the other.

Its cause and pathogenesis, though unclear at present, is believed to be probably connected with the factors
of heredity, nutritional imbalance, chronic light injury,
poisoning, immune diseases and so on, or may be the result of the complicated action of multiple factors.

From the clinical manifestations, the disease should
pertain to "Shizhan Hunmiao" (blurring of vision) in traditional Chinese medicine. Its occurrence is associated
with the irregulation among the organs of the liver,
spleen, stomach and kidney, and it often arises as a result of
deficiency of the liver and kidney, asthenia of primordial essence, or is caused by the incoordination between the liver
and spleen and obstruction or stagnation of meridian and vessels.

[Main Diagnostic Points]

1. Clinical Manifestations

Initially, the vision is diminished, probably with
metamorphopsia and central scotoma of visual field and,

【概述】

老年性黄斑变性,亦称年
龄相关性黄斑变性,是西方国
家老年人最常见的致盲眼病
之一。临床上主要表现为视
力下降,后期发生严重的视力
障碍。本病大多始发于 50 岁
左右,年龄越大,发病率越高。
发病与性别无明显关系。双
眼同时或先后发病。

本病的病因和发病机理
尚未确定,可能与遗传、营养
失调、慢性光损害、中毒、免疫
性疾病等有关,可能是多种因
素复合作用的结果。

根据本病的临床表现,当
属于中医学"视瞻昏渺"范畴。
本病的形成与肝脾胃肾失调
有关,多因肝肾不足,元精亏
虚,不能上注于目;或肝脾失
和,脉络阻滞,精气不能上乘
所致。

【诊断要点】

1. 临床表现

视力下降,早期可能有视
物变形,视野有中心暗点,后

later on, severe disturbance of vision occurs.

2. Fundus Examination

(1) **Atrophic (dry or non-exudative) type** At the beginning, pigmentary disturbance exists in the macular part, the central fovea reflect of light is cloudy or missing, and there scatters the glass membrance wart unclearly bordered. At the late stage, there can be seen golden reflect of light, atrophic area of pigmentary epithelium in geographic form, cystic degeneration or lamellar hiatus.

(2) **Exudative (moist) type** At the initial stage, pigmentary disturbance appears in the macular part, the central fovea reflect of light is missing, and glass membrane wart become confluent. In the middle of the course, there occurs in the macula bleeding, exudation, edema and even preretinal hemorrhage in severe conditions. At the late stage, the bleeding and exudation is absorbed so that a large area of yellowish and whitish scar is formed.

3. Fluorescein Angiography of Fundus

(1) **Atrophic type** There is massive glass membrane wart or transmitting fluorescein in geographic shape, which turns to an area of weak fluorescein as a result of choroidocapillary atrophy in the late course of the disease.

(2) **Exudative type** Neonatal vessels and fluorescein effusion beneath the retina can be seen at the beginning; at the intermediate stage, fluorescein effusion increases in the pathogenic part; and, at the late stage, the fluorescein is covered by cicatricial tissues, with the transmitting fluorescein found in the depigmentation part.

[**Syndrome Differentiation and Treatment**]

In clinic, the disease is classified into the syndromes of deficiency of the liver and kidney, asthenia of spleen qi, accumulation of endogenous phlegm-heat and hemorrhage due to blood heat. The treatment, therefore, should respectively consist of the nourishing, phlegm-re-

期发生严重视力障碍。

2. 眼底检查

(1) 萎缩性(干性或非渗出性) 早期黄斑部色素紊乱,中心凹反光不清或消失,散在边界不清晰的玻璃膜疣。晚期可见金箔样反光,地图状色素上皮萎缩区,囊样变性或板层性裂孔。

(2) 渗出性(湿性) 早期黄斑部色素紊乱,中心凹反光消失,玻璃膜疣常有融合。中期黄斑部出现出血、渗出、水肿,出血严重者可有视网膜前出血。晚期黄斑部出血、渗出吸收,形成一片黄白色瘢痕。

3. 眼底荧光血管造影

(1) 萎缩性 黄斑部有大量玻璃膜疣或地图状的透见荧光;病程晚期因脉络膜毛细血管的萎缩而成一片弱荧光区。

(2) 渗出性 早期可见视网膜下新生血管,荧光素渗漏;中期病变区荧光素渗漏增强;晚期瘢痕性组织遮蔽荧光,色素脱失区有透见荧光。

【辨证论治】

本病临床主要分为肝肾不足证、脾气虚弱证、痰湿内蕴证、血热妄行证。分别采用补益、化痰、凉血法。

moving and blood-cooling methods.

1. Syndrome of Deficiency of the Liver and Kidney

Main Symptoms and Signs　Dim eyesight, metamorphopsia, glass membrane wart and pigmentary disturbance in mucula; neonatal vessels in choroid; accompanied by the general symptoms of dizziness, tinnitus, lassitude in loin and legs; blackish tongue with thin coating and thready thin or thin unsmooth pulse.

Therapeutic Method　Nourishing the liver and kidney to improve vision.

Recipe　The modified Mingmu Dihuangwan Decoction: Shudihuang (*Radix Rehmanniae Praeparata*) 12 g, Gouqizi (*Fructus Lycii*) 15 g, Shanzhuyu (*Fructus Corni*) 10 g, Shanyao (*Rhizoma Dioscoreae*) 10 g, Fuling (*Poria*) 15 g, Tusizi (*Semen Cuscutae*) 10 g, Nüzhenzi (*Fructus Ligustri Lucidi*) 10 g, Gegen (*Radix Puerariae*) 15 g, Roucongrong (*Herba Cistanchis*) 10 g, and Zhike (*Fructus Aurantii*) 6 g.

2. Syndrome of Asthenia of Spleen Qi

Main Symptoms and Signs　The same ocular symptoms as the above one, accompanied by the general symptoms of mental fatigue, lassitude, loss of appetite, short breath and no desire to speak; whitish tongue with thin coating and thready thin pulse.

Therapeutic Method　Nourishing spleen qi.

Recipe　The modified Buzhong Yiqi Decoction: Huangqi (*Radix Astragali seu Hedysari*) 15 g, Dangshen (*Radix Codonopsis Pilosulae*) 12 g, Baizhu (*Rhizoma Atractylodis Macrocephalae*) 10 g, Chenpi (*Pericarpium Citri Reticulatae*) 6 g, Shengma (*Rhizoma Cimicifugae*) 6 g, Fuling (*Poria*) 15 g, Baishaoyao (*Radix Paeoniae Alba*) 10 g, Gegen (*Radix Puerariae*) 15 g, Wuweizi (*Fructus Schisandrae*) 6 g, and Danggui (*Ra-*

1. 肝肾不足证

主要证候　视物模糊,视物变形,黄斑部有玻璃膜疣及色素紊乱,脉络膜新生血管膜形成。全身伴有头晕耳鸣,腰膝酸软,舌暗苔薄,脉细弱或细涩。

治　法　补益肝肾明目。

方　药　明目地黄丸加减。熟地黄12 g,枸杞子15 g,山茱萸10 g,山药10 g,茯苓15 g,菟丝子10 g,女贞子10 g,葛根15 g,肉苁蓉10 g,枳壳6 g。

2. 脾气虚弱证

主要证候　眼部症状同前。全身伴有神疲乏力,胃纳不佳,气短懒言,舌淡苔薄,脉细数。

治　法　健脾益气。

方　药　补中益气汤加减。黄芪15 g,党参12 g,白术10 g,陈皮6 g,升麻6 g,茯苓15 g,白芍药10 g,葛根15 g,五味子6 g,当归10 g。

dix Angelicae Sinensis) 10 g.

Modification In the cases of loose stool, 10 g of Yiyiren (*Semen Coicis*) and 10 g of Biandou (*Semen Dolichoris*) are added.

3. Syndrome of Accumulation of Endogenous Phlegm-dampness

Main Symptoms and Signs Exudative degeneration of macula in fundus examination, accompanied by the general symptoms of dizziness, tinnitus, short breath, palpitation, obesity physique and massive sputum; whitish smooth or yellowish greasy tongue coating and thready slippery pulse.

Therapeutic Method Removing phlegm and dampness.

Recipe The modified Linggui Zhugan Decoction and Erchen Decoction: Fuling (*Poria*) 15 g, Baizhu (*Rhizoma Atractylodis Macrocephalae*) 10 g, Zhibanxia (*Rhizoma Pinelliae Praeparata*) 10 g, Chenpi (*Pericarpium Citri Reticulatae*) 6 g, Guizhi (*Ramulus Cinnamomi*) 6 g, Cheqianzi (*Herba Plantaginis*, bagged) 10 g, Zelan (*Herba Lycopi*) 10 g, and Chushizi (*Fructus Broussonetiae*) 10 g.

Modification In the cases of hemorrhage in the macula, Guizhi is removed and 10 g of Cebaiye (*Cacumen Platycladi*) and 15 g of Baimaogen (*Rhizoma Imperatae*) are added.

4. Syndrome of Hemorrhage due to Blood Heat

Main Symptoms and Signs In addition to the above ocular symptoms, others including hemorrhage of macula and general accompanying symptoms of dizziness, dryness in the mouth and throat, sleeplessness, dreaminess and constipation; reddish tongue and rapid pulse.

Therapeutic Method Removing heat by cooling blood.

加　减　大便溏泻者,加薏苡仁10 g,扁豆10 g。

3. 痰湿内蕴证

主要证候　眼底可见黄斑渗出性变性。全身伴有头晕目眩,气短心悸,体胖痰多,舌苔白滑或黄腻,脉弦滑。

治　法　化痰祛湿。

方　药　苓桂术甘汤合二陈汤加减。茯苓15 g,白术10 g,制半夏10 g,陈皮6 g,桂枝6 g,车前子(包煎)10 g,泽兰10 g,楮实子10 g。

加　减　黄斑部出血者,去桂枝,加侧柏叶10 g,白茅根15 g。

4. 血热妄行证

主要证候　眼症同前,黄斑出血。全身伴有头晕头昏,口干咽燥,失眠多梦,大便干结,舌体红,脉数。

治　法　凉血清热。

Recipe　The modified Shihuisan Decoction: Daji (*Herba seu Radix Cirsii Japonici*) 15 g, Xiaoji (*Herba Cephalanoploris*) 15 g, Cebaiye (*Cacumen Platycladi*) 10 g, Baimaogen (*Rhizoma Imperatae*) 15 g, Mudanpi (*Cortex Moutan Radicis*) 10 g, Hanliancao (*Herba Ecliptae*) 10 g, Nüzhenzi (*Fructus Ligustri Lucidi*) 10 g, Shengdihuang (*Radix Rehmanniae*) 10 g, Chishaoyao (*Radix Paeoniae Rubra*) 10 g, Zhike (*Fructus Aurantii*) 6 g, and Shengpuhuang (*Pollen Typhae*) 10 g.

[Other Treatments]

Chinese Patent Drugs

(1) **Mingmu Dihuang Pill**　9 g each time, twice a day and applicable to the syndrome of deficiency of the liver and kidney.

(2) **Yiqi Congming Pill**　9 g each time, twice a day and applicable to the syndrome of asthenia of spleen qi.

(3) **Sanqi Powder**　1.5 g each time, twice a day and applicable to the cases of macular hemorrhage.

2.5.10　Optic Neuritis

[Introduction]

Optic neuritis is a kind of pathogenic change of the optic nerve which is characterized by diminishment of vision and the corresponding changes of visual field. Because the damaged part of lesion is different, the disease is divided into two types: intraglomerular papillitis of the optic nerve and retrobulbar neuritis. The latter, according to the greater or less emergency of inflammation, is again classified into the acute and chronic cases. The main manifestations of the disease in clinic are abrupt diminishment of vision and even blindness. Common in the young

方　药　十灰散加减。大蓟 15 g，小蓟 15 g，侧柏叶 10 g，白茅根 15 g，牡丹皮 10 g，旱莲草 10 g，女贞子 10 g，生地黄 10 g，赤芍药 10 g，枳壳 6 g，生蒲黄 10 g。

【其他疗法】

中成药

（1）明目地黄丸　每服 9 g，每日 2 次。适用于肝肾不足证。

（2）益气聪明丸　每服 9 g，每日 2 次。适用于脾气虚弱证。

（3）三七粉　每服 1.5 g，每日 2 次。适用于黄斑出血者。

第十节　视神经炎

【概述】

视神经炎是视力下降，视野相应损害的视神经病变。因病变损害的部位不同而分为球内段的视乳头炎及球后段的球后视神经炎两大类。球后视神经炎根据炎症发病的缓急，又分为急性和慢性球后视神经炎两种。本病临床上主要表现为视力急剧下降，甚至失明。本病好发于中青

and middle-aged, it can sometimes be seen in children but less in the aged. It often occurs monocularly and sometimes binocularly and develops rather rapidly with the vision severely damaged.

The causes of the disease which are complicated include, besides some local inflammatory infections, not only demyelinating disease, poisoning, denutrition, heredity, dysbolism but other unidentified factors as well.

The clinical manifestations of the disease show that the case should pertain to "Baomang" (sudden blindness) or "Shizhan Hunmiao" (blurring of vision) in traditional Chinese medicine. Usually, the disease is caused by the fact that exogenous pathogenic heat attacks the viscera and gives rise to hyperactivity of liver fire that affects upwards the eye, or that fire hyperactivity due to yin deficiency disturbs the orifices in head, or that disorder of liver qi by emotional depression leads to qi and blood stagnation. And the deficiency of qi and blood in breast feeding period can also cause the disease.

[Main Diagnostic Points]

1. Clinical Manifestations

The vision of one eye or both is rapidly diminished with serious visual disturbance occurring within a few hours or days. In some severe cases, light perception may disappear, accompanied by the pain of eyeball movement sometimes and the feeling of headache and dizziness in a few cases.

2. Photoreaction

There is disturbance of pupillary reaction in accordance with visual diminishment. The photoreaction is unstable or obtuse, even disappears.

3. Fundus Examination

(1) Papillitis The optic papilla is congested and

年,儿童亦常见,老年人较少。单眼或双眼发病,病情发展较快,视力损害严重。

本病病因复杂,除局部炎症感染外,还包括脱髓鞘疾病、中毒、营养缺乏、遗传性、代谢障碍等,另外还有部分无法确定病因。

根据本病的临床表现,当属于中医学"暴盲"、"视瞻昏渺"范畴。常由外感热邪,内传脏腑,肝火上炎,上攻于目;或阴虚火旺,上扰清窍;或情志抑郁,肝气不舒,气滞血瘀;或产后哺乳,气血虚衰而导致本病。

【诊断要点】

1. 临床表现

双眼或单眼视力迅速减退,可于数小时或数日内发生严重的视力障碍,重者光感消失,有时可伴有眼球转动时疼痛,少数患者有头痛、头晕感觉。

2. 对光反应

有与视力减退相一致的瞳孔反应障碍,对光反应不稳定或迟钝,甚至消失。

3. 眼底检查

(1) 视乳头炎 视乳头

slightly protruded with edema. The retinal vein is ectatic with the artery often unchanged. There is hemorrhage or exudation in the surface of optic papilla or in the surrounding retina.

(2) Retrobulbar neuritis　Normally there is no change in the fundus, but slight congestion occurs in the optic papilla when inflammation approaches.

4. Visual Field Examination

(1) Papillitis　The central scotoma can be found and sometimes the periperal visual field becomes concentrically contracted.

(2) Retrobulbar neuritis　Besides the central scotoma or dumbbell-shaped scotoma, there can also be found fan-shaped defect or periperal visual field contraction.

[Syndrome Differentiation and Treatment]

Clinically, the disease is mainly classified into the syndromes of hyperactivity of liver fire, stagnation of qi and blood, fire hyperactivity due to yin deficiency and asthenia of both qi and blood. The treatment, therefore, should include the respective methods of removing liver heat, soothing stagnated liver, nourishing yin and the therapy for invigoration and restoration.

1. Syndrome of Hyperactivity of Liver Fire

Main Symptoms and Signs　Abrupt visual diminishment or even blindness of the affected eye, tenderness of eyeball and pain in the deep eyeball in movement; findings of the fundus examination including congestion of optic papilla with edema unclearly edged, retinal phlebectasis; edema, exudation and hemorrhage nearby the optic papilla, or no obvious changes of fundus at the start of the disease (retrobulbar neuritis); accompanied by the general symptoms of headache, dizziness, tinnitus and bitter taste in the mouth; reddish tongue with yellowish coating and thready rapid pulse.

Therapeutic Method　Removing liver fire.

充血、水肿,轻度隆起,视网膜静脉扩张,动脉一般无改变,视乳头表面或其周围网膜有时有出血或渗出。

(2)球后视神经炎　通常眼底无改变,但炎症临近视乳头可出现轻度充血。

4. 视野检查

(1)视乳头炎　可查见中心暗点,有时周边视野也可向心性缩小。

(2)球后视神经炎　可查出中心暗点或哑铃状暗点、扇形缺损或周边视野缩窄。

【辨证论治】

本病临床主要分为肝火亢盛证、气滞血郁证、阴虚火旺证、气血两虚证。治疗分别采用清肝、疏肝、滋阴、补益法。

1. 肝火亢盛证

主要证候　患眼视力急降,甚至失明。常伴有眼珠压痛及转动时眼珠深部疼痛。眼底可见视乳头充血、水肿、边界不清,视网膜静脉扩张,视乳头附近网膜有水肿、渗出、出血等,或发病时眼底无明显改变(球后视神经炎),全身可伴有头痛头昏,耳鸣口苦,舌红苔黄,脉弦数。

治　法　清肝泻火。

Recipe The modified Longdan Xiegan Decoction:
Longdancao (*Radix Gentianae*) 10 g, Chaoshanzhizi
(*Fructus Gardeniae*, fried) 10 g, Huangqin (*Radix Scutellariae*) 10 g, Shengdihuang (*Radix Rehmanniae*)
10 g, Cheqianzi (*Semen Plantaginis*, bagged) 10 g,
Danshen (*Radix Salviae Miltiorrhizae*) 15 g, Mutong
(*Caulis Akebiae*) 6 g, Chaihu (*Radix Bupleuri*) 6 g,
Danggui (*Radix Angelicae Sinensis*) 10 g, and Yejuhua
(*Flos Chrysanthemi Indici*) 10 g.

Modification In the cases of severe congestion and
edema of optic papilla, 10 g of Mudanpi (*Cortex Moutan Radicis*) and 10 g of Chishaoyao (*Radix Paeoniae Rubra*) are added; in the cases of massive hemorrhage of
retina, 20 g of Baimaogen (*Rhizoma Imperatae*) is added.

2. Syndrome of Stagnation of Qi and Blood

Main Symptoms and Signs In addition to the same
ocular symptoms as the above one, the other common
symptoms include emotional depression, distending pain in
chest and hypochondrium, loss of appetite; dark reddish
tongue with petechiae and thready unsmooth pulse.

Therapeutic Methods Soothing depressed liver
and activating qi and blood circulation.

Recipe The modified Chaihu Shugansan Decoction:
Chaihu (*Radix Bupleuri*) 10 g, Xiangfu (*Rhizoma Cyperi*) 10 g, Danggui (*Radix Angelicae Sinensis*) 10 g,
Chishaoyao (*Radix Paeoniae Rubra*) 10 g, Danshen
(*Radix Salviae Miltiorrhizae*) 15 g, Fuling (*Poria*)
15 g, Yujin (*Radix Curcumae*) 10 g, Shengdihuang
(*Radix Rehmanniae*) 10 g, Honghua (*Flos Carthomi*)
10 g, Lianqiao (*Fructus Forsythiae*) 12 g, and Gancao
(*Radix Glycyrrhizae*) 3 g.

Modification In the cases of pathogenic fire due to
stagnation of liver qi, 10 g of Shanzhizi (*Fructus Gar-*

方 药 龙胆泻肝汤加
减。龙胆草 10 g,炒山栀子
10 g,黄芩 10 g,生地黄 10 g,车
前子(包煎) 10 g,丹参 15 g,木
通 6 g,柴胡 6 g,当归 10 g,野菊
花 10 g。

加 减 视乳头充血、水
肿较重者,加牡丹皮 10 g,赤芍
药 10 g;视网膜出血较多者,加
白茅根 20 g。

2. 气滞血瘀证

主要证候 眼 症 同 前。
患者常有情志抑郁,胸胁胀
痛,脘闷食少,舌暗红或有瘀
点,脉弦涩。

治 法 疏肝解郁,行气
活血。

方 药 柴胡疏肝散加
减。柴胡 10 g,香附 10 g,当归
10 g,赤芍药 10 g,丹参 15 g,茯
苓 15 g,郁金 10 g,生地黄 10 g,
红花 10 g,连翘 12 g,甘草 3 g。

加 减 肝郁化火者,加
山栀子 10 g,牡丹皮 10 g,黄

deniae）, Mudanpi（*Cortex Moutan Radicis*）and Huang-qi（*Radix Astragali seu Hedysari*）are added.

3. Syndrome of Fire Hyperactivity due to Yin Deficiency

Main Symtoms and Signs　Besides the same ocular symtoms as the above, the general accompanying symptoms include dizziness, tinnitus; feverish sensation in chest, palms and soles; bitter taste in the mouth and dry mouth; reddish tongue with little coating and taut, thin and rapid pulse.

Therapeutic Methods　Nourishing yin and removing pathogenic fire.

Recipe　The modified Zhibai Dihuangwan Decoction: Zhimu（*Rhizoma Anemarrhenae*）10 g, Huangbai（*Cortex Phellodendri*）10 g, Shengdihuang（*Radix Rehmanniae*）12 g, Mudanpi（*Cortex Moutan Radicis*）10 g, Zexie（*Rhizoma Alismatis*）12 g, Fuling（*Poria*）10 g, Shanyao（*Rhizoma Dioscoreae*）12 g, Nüzhenzi（*Fructus Ligustri Lucidi*）12 g, Shanyurou（*Fructus Corni*）10 g, and Danshen（*Radix Salviae Miltiorrhizae*）15 g.

Modification　In the severe cases of fire hyperactivity due to yin deficiency, 12 g of Xuanshen（*Radix Scrophulariae*）, 15 g of Hanliancao（*Herba Ecliptae*）and 10 g of Guiban（*Plastrum Testudinis*）are added.

4. Syndrome of Asthenia of Both Qi and Blood

Main Symptoms and Signs　The same ocular symptoms as the above, frequent occurrence in women in breast feeding period, accompanied by short breath, hypodynamia, and dim complexion; pale tongue and thin weak pulse.

Therapeutic Methods　Invigorating qi and nourishing blood.

Recipe　The modified Bazhen Decoction: Shudi

芩10 g。

3. 阴虚火旺证

主要证候　眼症同前。常伴有头晕耳鸣,五心烦热,口苦口干,舌红少苔,脉弦细数。

治　法　滋阴降火。

方　药　知柏地黄丸加减。知母10 g,黄柏10 g,生地黄12 g,牡丹皮10 g,泽泻12 g,茯苓10 g,山药12 g,女贞子12 g,山萸肉10 g,丹参15 g。

加　减　阴虚火邪盛者,加玄参12 g,旱莲草15 g,龟版10 g。

4. 气血两虚证

主要证候　眼部症状同前。多见于哺乳期妇女,伴有气短乏力,面色少华,舌淡,脉细无力。

治　法　补益气血。

方　药　八珍汤加减。

huang (*Radix Rehmanniae Praeparata*) 10 g, Danggui (*Radix Angelicae Sinensis*) 10 g, Chuanxiong (*Rhizoma Ligustici Chuanxiong*) 10 g, Dangshen (*Radix Codonopsis Pilosulae*) 12 g, Baizhu (*Rhizoma Atractylodis Macrocephalae*) 15 g, Fuling (*Poria*) 12 g, Sangshenzi (*Fructus Mori*) 12 g, Danshen (*Radix Salviae Miltiorrhizae*) 12 g, and Zhigancao (*Radix Glycyrrhizae Praeparata*) 3 g.

[Other Treatments]

1. Chinese Patent Drugs

(1) Longdan Xiegan Pill　6 g each time, twice a day and applicable to the syndrome of hyperactivity of liver fire.

(2) Shugan Liqi Pill　6 g each time, twice a day and applicable to the syndrome of stagnation of qi and blood.

(3) Zhibai Dihuang Pill　9 g each time, twice a day and applicable to the syndrome of fire hyperactivity due to yin deficiency.

(4) Shiquan Dabu Pill　9 g each time, twice a day and applicable to the syndrome of asthenia of both qi and blood.

2. Simple and Proved Recipes

(1) Qingying Decoction　The ingredients in the decoction are: Shuiniujiao (*Cornu Bubali*) 30 g, Xuanshen (*Radix Scrophulariae*) 12 g, Maimendong (*Radix Ophiopogonis*) 10 g, Lianqiao (*Fructus Forsythiae*) 15 g, Shengdihuang (*Radix Rehmanniae*) 10 g, Huanglian (*Rhizoma Coptidis*) 6 g, Jinyinhua (*Flos Lonicerae*) 12 g, and Zhuyejuanxin (*Folium Phyllostachydis Henonis et Bambusae Juvenile*) 6 g. All the herbs are decocted with water one dose a day for oral taking. The recipe is applicable to acute optic neuritis.

(2) Jueming Tea　A proper amount of Juemingzi

熟地黄10 g,当归10 g,川芎10 g,党参12 g,白术15 g,茯苓12 g,桑椹子12 g,丹参12 g,炙甘草3 g。

【其他疗法】

1. 中成药

（1）龙胆泻肝丸　每服6 g,每日2次。适用于肝火亢盛证。

（2）疏肝理气丸　每服6 g,每日2次。适用于气滞血郁证。

（3）知柏地黄丸　每服9 g,每日2次。适用于阴虚火旺证。

（4）十全大补丸　每服9 g,每日2次。适用于气血两虚证。

2. 单验方

（1）清营汤　水牛角30 g,玄参12 g,麦门冬10 g,连翘15 g,生地黄10 g,黄连6 g,金银花12 g,竹叶卷心6 g。水煎服,每日1剂。适用于急性视神经炎。

（2）决明茶　取决明子

(*Semen Cassiae*), which is cleanly washed with the impurity removed, is fried with mild fire to a light yellowish colour after dried in the sunlight. The prepared ingredient is then boiled to a kind of strong tea which is orally taken by adding a small amount of sugar. In summer, 30 g of Shijuemingzi is boiled to a sort of strong tea which, with the dregs being relieved, is mixed with a small amount of sugar and taken as a tea drink. The tea can remove hepatical heat to improve vision and nourish the kidney to replenish vital essence. It is applicable to patients with distending pain of eye and constipation because of excession of liver yang.

(3) Proved Recipe　The herbs in the recipe are: Shengdihuang (*Radix Rehmanniae*) 10 g, Xiakucao (*Spica Prunellae*) 12 g, Lianqiao (*Fructus Forsythiae*) 15 g, Mudanpi (*Cortex Moutan Radicis*) 10 g, Shanzhizi (*Fructus Gardeniae*) 10 g, Huangqin (*Radix Scutellariae*) 10 g, Chishaoyao (*Radix Paeoniae Rubra*) 10 g, Shijueming (*Concha Haliotidis*, to be decocted first) 20 g, Juhua (*Flos Chrysanthemi*) 10 g, and Gancao (*Radix Glycyrrhizae*) 3 g. Decocted with water one dose a day, the recipe is applicable to the syndrome of hyperactivity of liver fire.

Western medicine can be applied as a supporting treatment method if the case of optic neuritis shows severe congestion and edema of optic papilla.

2.5.11 Optic Atrophy

[Introduction]
Optic atrophy is a kind of ophthalmopathy in which the retrograde degeneration of the optic nerve causes the blanching of the optic papilla accompanying the functional

适量,将决明子洗净,除去杂质,晒干后微火炒嫩黄色。夏季时可取决明子30 g煮成浓茶,弃渣,放入适量白糖,加盖待冷却后即可服用,有清肝明目,补肾益精的作用,可用于肝阳偏亢,眼胀痛,大便干结者。

（3）经验方　生地黄10 g,夏枯草12 g,连翘15 g,牡丹皮10 g,山栀子10 g,黄芩10 g,赤芍药10 g,石决明(先煎)20 g,菊花10 g,甘草3 g。水煎服,每日1剂。适用于肝火亢盛证。

视神经炎乳头充血、水肿严重者,可配合应用西药。

第十一节　视神经萎缩

【概述】
视神经萎缩是指视神经发生退行性改变,使视神经乳头变白,并有视功能损害的一

injury of vision. It is the final results of various diseases of the retina and optic nerve in serious conditions and can cause severe visual disturbance because of the extensive injury of the photoreceptor, ganliocyte and neuraxon and because of the loss of nerve fiber and gliosis. Clinically, the disease mainly manifests the symptoms of diminishment of vision, contraction of visual field and total blindness of the sick eye in severe cases. In ophthalmology, it is an obstate and severe disease which has a very high incidence and can easily give rise to blindness.

Optic atrophy can be caused by different pathogenic changes of the retina and optic nerve such as inflammation, degeneration, ischemia, trauma, compression, poisoning and tumor. The specific examples are retinal pigment degeneration, chorioretinitis, demyelinating disease, optic neuritis, papilloedema, disease of the retinal vessels, drug or heavy metal poisoning, compression from the intracranial space-occupying lesions, hereditary disease, Leber's optic neuropathy, syphilis, trauma of the optic nerve, glaucoma and so on.

Although optic atrophy is the final results of retinal and optic troubles, different eyeground diseases and some hereditary changes may also cause the disease, which is classified into primary, secondary and ascending types according to the different indications of the part of lesion and the affection to the optic disc under the ophthalmoscope.

The disease should pertain to "Qingmang" (optic atrophy) in traditional Chinese medicine. Although knowledge on optic atrophy in TCM can be traced back to the ancient times, its cause and pathogensis, in a word, is nothing more than the various factors which finally lead to

种眼病。它是多种严重的视网膜和视神经疾病的最终结局。因视网膜的光感受器、神经节细胞及其轴突广泛损害，以及神经纤维丧失、神经胶质增生，而引起严重的视功能障碍。临床主要表现为视力减退、视野缩小，严重者患眼全盲。是一种有很高发病率的易致盲的眼科疑难重症。

视网膜、视神经的炎症、退变、缺血、外伤、压迫、中毒、肿瘤等多种病变均可引起视神经萎缩。如视网膜色素变性、脉络膜视网膜炎症、脱髓鞘疾病、视神经炎、视乳头水肿、视网膜血管疾病、药物或重金属的中毒、颅内占位病变的压迫、遗传性疾病、Leber 视神经病变、梅毒、视神经外伤、青光眼等。

由于视神经萎缩是视网膜、视神经疾病发展的终末结果，多种眼底疾病及某些遗传病变均可导致视神经萎缩。由病变发生的部位及对视乳头的影响，根据眼底镜下的不同表现，将本病分为原发性、继发性及上行性萎缩三种。

本病当属于中医学"青盲"范畴。中医对青盲的认识源远流长，其病因病机总括而言，不外是各种原因最终导致了目中玄府的闭阻而神光不

the obstruction of ocular pores (tissues) so that visual diminishment or loss occurs. Its specific causes, however, are of quite variety. When asthenia of essence and blood, because of congenital defect or deficiency of the liver and kidney, can not have the eye nutritioned, for instance, the optic disc may become atrophic and the eyesight falls down. When the depression of seven emotions and stagnation of liver qi results in stagnancy of qi and blood circulation and blockage of pores, the vision may be blinded. If the trauma of eye and head involves the ocular connectors to cause obstruction of collaterals, the essence and blood cannot move up to the eye, giving rise to blindness or blurred vision. Or when the obstruction of meridian by wind-phlegm blocks the ocular pores (tissues), the vision can also be blurred or darkened.

[**Main Diagnostic Points**]

1. Clinical Manifestations

(1) The vision is obviously diminished and the light perception disappears.

(2) The pupillary light reaction is slow or even disappears in terms of the pathogenic changes.

(3) The fundus examination finds that the optic disc becomes pale or whitish pale or wax yellow with clear or unclear boundaries, that the retinal vessels turn thin, and that there exist a large number of atrophic foci or spots of pigmentation in the retina.

(4) The visual field is of concentric diminution which is obviously characterized by red and green diminution. Sometimes, there may appear obvious central scotoma, fan-like defect and biocular temporal hemianopia or homonymous hemianopia. The changes of visual field and diminishment of vision synchronize.

能外达所致。但具体病因可有所不同,如先天禀赋不足,或肝肾亏损,精血虚衰,不能上荣于目,则目窍萎闭,神光衰微;或七情郁结,肝失条达,气血不行,玄府郁闭,神光不得外达;或头目外伤,目系受损,脉络瘀滞,精血不能上运于目而至目暗不明;或风痰阻络,闭塞目中玄府,致神光内闭而不能视物。

【诊断要点】

1. 临床表现

(1) 视力明显下降,甚至无光感。

(2) 瞳孔对光反应可根据病变的程度,由迟缓甚至消失。

(3) 眼底检查可见视乳头颜色变淡,或苍白,或蜡黄,边界清楚或模糊不清,或有视网膜血管变细,或可见视网膜上大面积萎缩病灶或色素斑块沉着。

(4) 视野多呈向心性缩小,以红、绿色视野缩小尤为明显。也可出现明显的中心暗点、扇形缺损、双眼颞侧偏盲或同侧偏盲等。视野的改变常同视力的减退同步发展。

2. Laboratory Examinations

(1) Electrophysiological examination of the visual function The wave form of the evoked potential of figure vision or flashing vision is clearly low. The potential peak time is prolonged and the wave is even absent. The wave of the figure electroretinogram is reduced or totally disappears while that of the flasing electroretinogram may appear normal.

(2) Fluorescein fundus angiography At the beginning, there is no abnormal finding in the examination but, in the course of the disease, the fluorescein of optic disc, when examined, usually becomes weak till the strong fluorescein of optic disc is found because of the effusion of papillary vessels at the late stage.

[Syndrome Differentiation and Treatment]

In clinic, the disease is mainly classified into the syndromes of asthenia of the liver and kidney, deficiency of spleen and kidney yang, stagnation of liver qi, stagnancy of qi and blood stasis, and obstruction of excessive wind and phlegm. In the syndrome differentiation, asthenia and sthenia or deficiency and excess should be discriminated, and the treatment, in accordance with the causes of the disease, should be put on the reinforcing and reducing methods, supported with the drugs of dredging meridians and inducing resuscitation.

1. Syndrome of Asthenia of the Liver and Kidney

Main Symptoms and Signs Gradual diminishment of vision or even blindness, pale or wax yellow optic disc and filthy retina with pigmentation under the ophthalmoscope, accompanied by the general symptoms of dizziness, tinnitus, sleeplessness, dreaminess, lassitude in loin and legs, spermatorrhea and night sweat; pale reddish tongue with whitish thin coating and deep thin pulse.

Therapeutic Methods Nourishing the liver and

2. 实验室检查

（1）视觉电生理检查 图形视诱发电位或闪光视诱发电位波形明显低下，峰潜时延长甚至波形完全熄灭。图形视网膜电图波形降低或完全消失，而闪光视网膜电图有可能正常。

（2）眼底荧光血管造影 病变早期，荧光造影无异常发现，但随病情的发展，造影时视乳头荧光普遍减弱，直至造影后期因视乳头血管渗漏而见到视乳头强荧光。

【辨证论治】

本病临床主要分为肝肾不足证、脾肾阳虚证、肝气郁结证、气滞血瘀证、风痰闭阻证。辨证应分清虚实，治疗应针对病因，补虚泻实，并配用通络开窍药物。

1. 肝肾不足证

主要证候 视力渐降，甚至失明，眼底检查见视乳头色白或蜡黄，网膜污秽有色素沉着。全身兼见头昏耳鸣，失眠多梦，腰膝酸软，遗精盗汗，舌质淡红，苔薄白，脉沉细。

治 法 滋养肝肾，开窍

kidney and improving eyesight by resuscitation.

Recipe　The modified decoction of Mingmu Dihuan-gwan Decoction plus the modified Zhujingwan Decoction: Shudihuang (*Radix Rehmanniae Praeparata*) 10 g, Shengdihuang (*Radix Rehmanniae*) 10 g, Shanzhuyu (*Fructus Corni*) 10 g, Huaishanyao (*Rhizoma Di-oscoreae*) 10 g, Zexie (*Rhizoma Alismatis*) 10 g, Fu-shen (*Poriacum Ligno Hospite*) 10 g, Mudanpi (*Cortex Moutan Radicis*) 10 g, Chaihu (*Radix Bupleuri*) 8 g, Danggui (*Radix Angelicae Sinensis*) 10 g, Wuweizi (*Fructus Schisandrae*) 6 g, Cheqianzi (*Semen Plan-taginis*, bagged) 10 g, Gouqizi (*Fructus Lycii*) 10 g, Chushizi (*Fructus Broussonetiae*) 10 g, Tusizi (*Semen Cuscutae*) 10 g, Chuanjiao (*Pericarpium Zanthoxyli*) 3 g, Shichangpu (*Rhizoma Acori Graminei*) 10 g, Niuxi (*Radix Achyranthis Bidentatae*) 10 g, Gandilong (*Lum-bricus*) 10 g, and Lulutong (*Fructus Liquidambaris*) 10 g.

Modification　In the cases of severe dizziness, 10 g of Tianma (*Rhizoma Gastrodiae*) is added; in the cases of severe lassitude in loin and legs, Xuduan (*Radix Dip-saci*), Sangjisheng (*Ramulus Loranthi*) and Buguzhi (*Fructus Psoraleae*), each 10 g, are added; in the cases of serious night sweat, 15 g of Longgu (*Os Draconis Fos-silia Ossis Mastodi*, to be decocted first) and 15 g of Muli (*Concha Ostreae*, to be decocted first) are added; in the cases of serious sleeplessness and dreaminess, 10 g of Suanzaoren (*Semen Ziziphi Spinosae*) and 10 g of Ye-jiaoteng (*Caulis Polygoni Multiflori*) are added.

2. Syndrome of Deficiency of Spleen and Kidney Yang

Main Symptoms and Signs　Gradual diminishment of vision or even blindness, pale optic disc under the oph-thalmoscope; accompanied by the general symptoms of pale complexion, cold body, lassitude in loin and legs,

明目。

方　药　明目地黄丸合加减驻景丸加减。熟地黄10 g,生地黄10 g,山茱萸10 g,怀山药10 g,泽泻10 g,茯神10 g,牡丹皮10 g,柴胡8 g,当归10 g,五味子6 g,车前子(包煎)10 g,枸杞子10 g,楮实子10 g,菟丝子10 g,川椒3 g,石菖蒲10 g,牛膝10 g,干地龙10 g,路路通10 g。

加　减　头晕甚者,加天麻10 g;腰腿酸软甚者,加续断10 g,桑寄生10 g,补骨脂10 g;盗汗甚者,加龙骨(先煎)15 g,牡蛎(先煎)15 g;失寐多梦甚者,加酸枣仁10 g,夜交藤10 g。

2. 脾肾阳虚证

主要证候　视力渐降,甚至失明,眼底检查见视乳头色苍白。全身兼见面白形寒,腰膝酸冷,少气乏力,食少便溏,

short breath, fatigue, poor appetite and loose stool; a pale tongue with whitish coating and a deep thin pulse.

Therapeutic Methods Nourishing the spleen and kidney and warming yang for resuscitation.

Recipe The modified Fuzi Lizhong Decoction: Fuzi (*Radix Aconiti Praeparata*) 5 g, Baizhu (*Rhizoma Atractylodis Macrocephalae*) 10 g, Ganjiang (*Rhizoma Zingiberis*) 3 g, Dangshen (*Radix Codonopsis Pilosulae*) 10 g, Rougui (*Cortex Cinnamomi*) 2 g, Buguzhi (*Fructus Psoraleae*) 10 g, Huangqi (*Radix Astragali seu Hedysari*) 10 g, and Zhigancao (*Radix Glycyrrhizae Praeparata*) 3 g.

Modification In the cases of deficiency of essence and blood, Shudihuang (*Radix Rehmanniae Praeparata*), Shengdihuang (*Radix Rehmanniae*), Danggui (*Radix Angelicae Sinensis*) and Shanyurou (*Fructus Corni*), each 10 g, are added.

3. Syndrome of Stagnancy of Liver Qi

Main Symptoms and Signs Dim eyesight, pale optic disc with clear or unclear boundaries under the ophthalmoscope, often accompanied by the general symptoms of dizziness with a distending sensation in the eye, irritability, fullness in the chest and hypochondrium, bitter taste in the mouth and dry throat; pale or thin yellowish tongue coating and thready or rapid pulse.

Therapeutic Method Relieving stagnated liver qi.

Recipe The modified Danzhi Xiaoyaosan Decoction: Mudanpi (*Cortex Moutan Radicis*) 10 g, Shanzhizi (*Fructus Gardeniae*) 10 g, Chaihu (*Radix Bupleuri*) 8 g, Fuling (*Poria*) 10 g, Baizhu (*Rhizoma Atractylodis Macrocephalae*) 10 g, Danggui (*Radix Angelicae Sinensis*) 10 g, Baishaoyao (*Radix Paeoniae Alba*) 10 g, Gancao (*Radix Glycyrrhizae*) 3 g, Bohe (*Herba*

舌质淡,苔白,脉沉细。

治　法　补脾益肾,温阳通窍。

方　药　附子理中汤加减。附子5 g,白术10 g,干姜3 g,党参10 g,肉桂2 g,补骨脂10 g,黄芪10 g,炙甘草3 g。

加　减　若兼有精血不足者,加熟地黄10 g,生地黄10 g,当归10 g,山萸肉10 g。

3. 肝气郁结证

主要证候　目视不明,眼底检查见视乳头色白,边界清楚或模糊不清。全身多伴有头昏目胀,急躁易怒,胸胁胀满,口苦咽干,舌苔白或薄黄,脉弦或数。

治　法　疏肝解郁。

方　药　丹栀逍遥散加减。牡丹皮10 g,山栀子10 g,柴胡8 g,茯苓10 g,白术10 g,当归10 g,白芍药10 g,甘草3 g,薄荷(后下)5 g,生姜2 片。

Menthae, to be decocted later) 5 g, and 2 slices of Shengjiang (*Rhizoma Zingiberis Recens*).

Modification　In the cases of severe fullness in the chest and hypochondrium, Zhike (*Fructus Aurantii*), Chuanlianzi (*Fructus Toosendan*), Xiangfu (*Rhizoma Cyperi*) and Guangyujin (*Radix Curcumae*), each 10 g, are added; in the cases of the sign of blood stasis, the Taohong Siwu Decoction is added to the recipe.

4. Syndrome of Qi Stagnation and Blood Stasis

Main Symptoms and Signs　Blurred vision or visual injury even with the loss of light perception due to the trauma in head and eye, fundus findings including pale optic disc and obviously thinned vessels of retina, often accompanied by a general sign of blood stasis after trauma; dim-pale tongue with ecchymosis and thin whitish coating and thready unsmooth pulse.

Therapeutic Method　Removing blood stasis and meridian obstruction by activating qi and blood circulation.

Recipe　The modified Xuefu Zhuyu Decoction: Danggui (*Radix Angelicae Sinensis*) 10 g, Shengdihuang (*Radix Rehmanniae*) 10 g, Taoren (*Semen Persicae*) 10 g, Honghua (*Flos Carthomi*) 10 g, Zhike (*Fructus Aurantii*) 10 g, Chishaoyao (*Radix Paeoniae Rubra*) 10 g, Chaihu (*Radix Bupleuri*) 8 g, Gancao (*Radix Glycyrrhizae*) 3 g, Jiegeng (*Radix Platycodi*) 6 g, Chuanxiong (*Rhizoma Ligustici Chuanxiong*) 10 g, and Niuxi (*Radix Achyranthis Bidentatae*) 10 g.

Modification　In the chronic cases of asthenia of healthy qi, 15 g of Huangqi (*Radix Astragali seu Hedysari*) and respective 10 g of Dangshen (*Radix Codonopsis Pilosulae*) and Baizhu (*Rhizoma Atractylodis Macrocephalae*) and Chenpi (*Pericarpium Citri Reticulatae*) are added.

加　减　胸胁胀满甚者，加枳壳10 g，川楝子10 g，香附10 g，广郁金10 g；有血瘀现象者，加桃红四物汤。

4. 气滞血瘀证

主要证候　视物昏朦，或头目外伤后，视力严重受损，甚至不辨三光，眼底见视乳头色苍白，甚则视网膜血管明显变细。全身常有伤后生瘀之象，舌质暗，有瘀斑，苔薄白，脉弦涩。

治　法　行气活血，祛瘀通络。

方　药　血府逐瘀汤加减。当归10 g，生地黄10 g，桃仁10 g，红花10 g，枳壳10 g，赤芍药10 g，柴胡8 g，甘草3 g，桔梗6 g，川芎10 g，牛膝10 g。

加　减　病久正虚，加黄芪15 g，党参10 g，白术10 g，陈皮10 g。

5. Syndrome of Obstruction of Excessive Wind and Phlegm

Main Symptoms and Signs   Abrupt attacking with sudden diminishment of vision, the ophthalmoscope findings including pale optic disc with clear or unclear boundaries and thinned retinal vessels, accompanied by the general symptoms of obesity physique, dizziness, headache, vertigo, chest distress, facial hemiparalysis or hemiplegia; whitish greasy or pale yellowish tongue coating and thready rapid pulse.

Therapeutic Methods   Removing wind and phlegm and dredging meridians to improve visual acuity.

Recipe   The modified Zhengrong Decoction: Baifuzi (*Rhizoma Typhonii*) 6 g, Dannanxing (*Arisaema cum Bile*) 6 g, Baijiangcan (*Bombyx Batryticatus*) 10 g, Fangfeng (*Radix Ledebouriellae*) 10 g, Qianghuo (*Rhizoma seu Radix Notopterygii*) 10 g, Qinjiao (*Radix Gentianae Macrophyllae*) 10 g, Banxia (*Rhizoma Pinelliae*) 10 g, Mugua (*Fructus Chaenomelis*) 10 g, Songjie (*Lignum Pini Nodi*) 10 g, and two slices of Shengjiang (*Rhizoma Zingiberis Recens*).

Modification   In the cases of obvious dizziness, 10 g of Caojueming (*Herba Cassiae*) and 10 g of Xiakucao (*Spica Prunellae*) are added; in the cases of severe obstruction of the fundus vessels, 15 g of Danshen (*Radix Salviae Miltiorrhizae*) and 10 g of Yujin (*Radix Curcumae*) and of Chuanxiong (*Rhizoma Ligustici Chuanxiong*) are added; in the cases of excessive pathogenic wind, 10 g of Gouteng (*Ramulus Uncariae cum Uncis*) and 10 g of Dilong (*Lumbricus*) and 5 g of Quanxie (*Scorpio*) are added.

［Other Treatments］

1. Chinese Patent Drugs

(1) Qiju Dihuang Pill   6 g each time, twice a day

5. 风痰闭阻证

主要证候　起病急骤,视力剧降,眼底见视乳头色白,边界清楚或模糊不清,视网膜血管变细。全身伴素体肥胖,头晕头痛,眩晕胸闷,或口眼歪斜,半身不遂,苔白腻或淡黄,脉弦数。

治　法　祛风化痰,通络明目。

方　药　正容汤加减。白附子6 g,胆南星6 g,白僵蚕10 g,防风10 g,羌活10 g,秦艽10 g,半夏10 g,木瓜10 g,松节10 g,生姜2 片。

加　减　头昏明显者,加草决明10 g,夏枯草10 g;眼底血脉闭阻严重者,加丹参15 g,郁金10 g,川芎10 g;风邪盛者,加钩藤10 g,地龙10 g,全蝎5 g。

【其他疗法】

1. 中成药

（1）杞菊地黄丸　每服

and applicable to the syndrome of asthenia of the liver and kidney.

(2) Mingmu Dihuang Pill　6 g each time, twice a day and applicable to the syndrome of asthenia of the liver and kidney.

(3) Liuwei Dihuang Pill　6 g each time, twice a day and applicable to the syndrome of asthenia of the liver and kidney.

(4) Shihu Yeguang Pill　6 g each time, twice a day and applicable to the syndrome of asthenia of the liver and kidney.

(5) Zhibai Dihuang Pill　6 g each time, twice a day and applicable to the syndrome of deficiency of the spleen and kidney plus deficient fire.

(6) Fuzi Lizhong Pill　6 g each time, twice a day and applicable to the syndrome of deficiency of spleen and kidney yang.

(7) Yougui Pill　6 g each time, twice a day and applicable to the syndrome of deficiency of spleen and kidney yang.

(8) Xiaoyao Pill　6 g each time, twice a day and applicable to the syndrome of stagnancy of liver qi.

(9) Danzhi Xiaoyao Pill　6 g each time, twice a day and applicable to the syndrome of stagnancy of liver qi causing pathogenic fire.

(10) Compound Danshen Tablet　3 tablets each time, twice a day and applicable to the syndrome of qi stagnation and blood stasis.

2. Simple and Proved Recipes

(1) Chuanxiong Tea　Chuanxiong (*Rhizoma Ligustici Chuanxiong*) and green tea, each 6 g, are decocted with water, and the liquid, mixed with proper amount of brown sugar, is taken as tea for 10 to 15 days. The tea can invigorate qi and activate blood circulation to relieve

6 g,每日 2 次,适用于肝肾不足者。

（2）明目地黄丸　每服 6 g,每日 2 次,适用于肝肾不足者。

（3）六味地黄丸　每服 6 g,每日 2 次,适用于肝肾不足者。

（4）石斛夜光丸　每服 6 g,每日 2 次,适用于肝肾不足者。

（5）知柏地黄丸　每服 6 g,每日 2 次,适用于肝肾不足,兼有虚火者。

（6）附子理中丸　每服 6 g,每日 2 次,适用于脾肾阳虚者。

（7）右归丸　每服6 g,每日 2 次,适用于脾肾阳虚者。

（8）逍遥丸　每服6 g,每日 2 次,适用于肝气郁结者。

（9）丹栀逍遥丸　每服 6 g,每日 2 次,适用于肝气郁结,日久化热者。

（10）复方丹参片　每服 3 片,每日 2 次,适用于气滞血瘀者。

2. 单验方

（1）川芎茶　川芎、绿茶各6 g,水煎,加红糖适量当茶饮,可饮 10～15 日。能益气活血止痛,适用于本病视乳头苍白,视网膜动脉变细,头痛

pain and is applicable to the cases of the symptoms and signs of pale optic disc, thinned arteries of the retina, headache with distending sensation in the eye, dim tongue with ecchymosis and thin unsmooth pulse.

(2) Yinqi Mingmu Soup　15 g of tremella (soaked first), 100 g of chicken liver (sliced) and 5 g of Gouqizi (*Fructus Lycii*), all the ingredients are boiled in water with some condiments. As it starts boiling, the floating foams are removed and, when the chicken liver is just well done, the soap is put in a bowel and 20 jasmine flowers are mixed into it. The soap is taken one dose a day for 10 to 15 days and it can nourish the liver and kidney to improve eyesight and mental ability and is applicable to the syndrome of yin deficiency of the liver and kidney.

(3) Longyanrou Porridge　15 g of Longyanrou (*Arillus Longan*), 5 to 10 Chinese dates and 100 g of rice fruit, all are cooked with water to a kind of porridge which is taken in the morning and evening for several weeks. The porridge can nourish the heart and stomach to invigorate blood and is applicable to the syndrome of deficiency of heart blood.

(4) Turtle Meat Soup　One turtle with its head and viscera removed, 50 g of Gouqizi (*Fructus Lycii*) and of Shanyao (*Rhizoma Dioscoreae*), 15 g of Shudihuang (*Radix Rehmanniae Praeparata*) and 9 g of Chenpi (*Pericarpium Citri Reticulatae*), all the ingredients are boiled together with water. When the soup is done, the dregs are removed and the soup and turtle meat is taken once a proper amount every day for 10 to 15 days. The soup can nourish the kidney and liver to benefit blood and increase the blood circulation in the eye and the nutrition of optic nerve to improve the visual acuity. It is applicable to the syndrome of yin deficiency of the liver and kidney.

(5) Huanghua Foshou Beverage　30 g of day lily

目胀,舌质瘀暗,脉细涩者。

（2）银杞明目汤　选用银耳15 g(先发泡开),鸡肝100 g(切片),枸杞子5 g。加水和佐料烧沸后去浮沫,待鸡肝刚熟,装入碗内撒入茉莉花20朵即食,每日1剂,连服10～15日。可补肝益肾,明目养神,适用于肝肾阴虚证。

（3）龙眼肉粥　龙眼肉15 g,大枣 5～10 枚,粳米100 g,加水适量共煮粥,早晚服用,连服数周。能养心补血益胃,适用于心血不足证。

（4）鳖肉汤　用鳖1只,去头及内脏,枸杞子50 g,山药50 g,熟地黄15 g,陈皮9 g。以上共煮熟后去药渣,喝汤吃肉,酌量摄食,每日1次,连服10～15日。能益肾补肝养血,有增进眼部血液循环,改善视神经营养,增加视力之作用,适用于肝肾阴虚证。

（5）黄花佛手饮　黄花

and of Foshou (*Fructus Citri Sarcodactylis*) are made into soup which, by adding sugar or salt, is taken once or twice a day for 10 to 15 days. It can soothe the liver and regulate qi circulation and is applicable to the syndrome of stagnancy of liver qi.

(6) Qingjuhua Porridge　100 g of rice is boiled with proper amount of water into a kind of porridge which, when nearly done, is mixed with 15 g of Baijuhua (*Flos Chrysanthemi*) and 2 g powder of Qingpi (*Pericarpium Citri Reticulatae Viride*) and boiled again in two to three minutes. The porridge is taken every morning and evening for 10 to 15 days. It can soothe the liver to regulate qi circulation, remove obstruction and stagnation, and relieve heat to brighten the eye. The porridge is applicable to the syndrome of stagnated heat in liver meridian.

(7) Taoren Porridge　100 g of rice fruit and 15 g of Taoren (*Semen Persicae*) powder, both are cooked with a proper amount of water to a kind of porridge which is orally taken once a day for a few days. The porridge can activate blood circulation and remove collateral obstruction and blood stasis to stop pain. It is applicable to the optic atrophy with headache caused by collateral obstruction or trauma of head and eye.

3. External Therapy

The disease can be treated with the massage of optic nerve accompanied by the thread burial therapy.

菜30 g,佛手30 g,做汤加糖或盐后食用,每日 1～2 次,连服10～15 日。可舒肝理气,适用于肝气郁结证。

（6）青菊花粥　用白米100 g加水适量煮粥,粥熟时加入白菊花15 g,青皮末2 g,再煮2～3 分钟,早晚服用,连服10～15 日。能疏肝理气,散结解郁,清热明目。适用于肝经郁热证。

（7）桃仁粥　粳米100 g,桃仁15 g研粉,加水适量同煮粥。每日服 1 次,连服数日。能活血通络,散瘀止痛。适用于脉络阻滞或头眼部外伤引起之视神经萎缩、头痛等。

3. 外治法

应用视神经按摩兼埋线术治疗。

Postscript

The Compilation of *A Newly Compiled Practical English-Chinese Library of TCM* was started in 2000 and published in 2002. In order to demonstrate the academic theory and clinical practice of TCM and to meet the requirements of compilation, the compilers and translators have made great efforts to revise and polish the Chinese manuscript and English translation so as to make it systematic, accurate, scientific, standard and easy to understand. Shanghai University of TCM is in charge of the translation. Many scholars and universities have participated in the compilation and translation of the Library, i.e. Professor Shao Xundao from Xi'an Medical University (former Dean of English Department and Training Center of the Health Ministry), Professor Ou Ming from Guangzhou University of TCM (celebrated translator and chief professor), Henan College of TCM, Guangzhou University of TCM, Nanjing University of TCM, Shaanxi College of TCM, Liaoning College of TCM and Shandong University of TCM.

The compilation of this Library is also supported by the State Administrative Bureau and experts from other universities and colleges of TCM. The experts on the Compilation Committee and Approval Committee have directed the compilation and translation. Professor She

后　记

《(英汉对照)新编实用中医文库》(以下简称《文库》)从2000年中文稿的动笔,到2002年全书的付梓,完成了世纪的跨越。为了使本套《文库》尽可能展示传统中医学术理论和临床实践的精华,达到全面、系统、准确、科学、规范、通俗的编写要求,全体编译人员耗费了大量的心血,付出了艰辛的劳动。特别是上海中医药大学承担了英语翻译的主持工作,得到了著名医学英语翻译家、原西安医科大学英语系主任和卫生部外语培训中心主任邵循道教授,著名中医英语翻译家、广州中医药大学欧明首席教授的热心指导,河南中医学院、广州中医药大学、南京中医药大学、陕西中医学院、辽宁中医学院、山东中医药大学等中医院校英语专家的全力参与,确保了本套《文库》具有较高的英译水平。

在《文库》的编撰过程中,我们始终得到国家主管部门领导和各中医院校专家们的关心和帮助。编纂委员会的国内外学者及审定委员会的

Jing, Head of the State Administrative Bureau and Vice-Minister of the Health Ministry, has showed much concern for the Library. Professor Zhu Bangxian, head of the Publishing House of Shanghai University of TCM, Zhou Dunhua, former head of the Publishing House of Shanghai University of TCM, and Pan Zhaoxi, former editor-in-chief of the Publishing House of Shanghai University of TCM, have given full support to the compilation and translation of the Library.

With the coming of the new century, we have presented this Library to the readers all over the world, sincerely hoping to receive suggestions and criticism from the readers so as to make it perfect in the following revision.

Zuo Yanfu

Pingju Village, Nanjing

Spring 2002

专家对编写工作提出了指导性的意见和建议。尤其是卫生部副部长、国家中医药管理局局长佘靖教授对本书的编写给予了极大的关注,多次垂询编撰过程,并及时进行指导。上海中医药大学出版社社长兼总编辑朱邦贤教授,以及原社长周敦华先生、原总编辑潘朝曦先生及全体编辑对本书的编辑出版工作给予了全面的支持,使《文库》得以顺利面世。在此,一并致以诚挚的谢意。

在新世纪之初,我们将这套《文库》奉献给国内外中医界及广大中医爱好者,恳切希望有识之士对《文库》存在的不足之处给予批评、指教,以便在修订时更臻完善。

左言富

于金陵萍聚村

2002 年初春

A Newly Compiled Practical English-Chinese Library of Traditional Chinese Medicine

（英汉对照）新编实用中医文库

Basic Theory of Traditional Chinese Medicine	中医基础理论
Diagnostics of Traditional Chinese Medicine	中医诊断学
Science of Chinese Materia Medica	中药学
Science of Prescriptions	方剂学
Internal Medicine of Traditional Chinese Medicine	中医内科学
Surgery of Traditional Chinese Medicine	中医外科学
Gynecology of Traditional Chinese Medicine	中医妇科学
Pediatrics of Traditional Chinese Medicine	中医儿科学
Traumatology and Orthopedics of Traditional Chinese Medicine	中医骨伤科学
Ophthalmology of Traditional Chinese Medicine	中医眼科学
Otorhinolaryngology of Traditional Chinese Medicine	中医耳鼻喉科学
Chinese Acupuncture and Moxibustion	中国针灸
Chinese Tuina (Massage)	中国推拿
Life Cultivation and Rehabilitation of Traditional Chinese Medicine	中医养生康复学